THE KID-FRIENDLY
ADHD&
AUTISM
C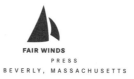OKBOOK

THE ULTIMATE GUIDE TO THE
GLUTEN-FREE, MILK-FREE DIET

Pamela J. Compart, M.D. and Dana Laake, R.D.H., M.S., L.D.N.

Foreword by Jon B. Pangborn, Ph.D., F.A.I.C. and Sidney MacDonald Baker, M.D.

FAIR WINDS
PRESS
BEVERLY, MASSACHUSETTS

First published in the USA in 2009 by
Fair Winds Press, a member of
Quayside Publishing Group
100 Cummings Center
Suite 406-L
Beverly, MA 01915-6101
www.fairwindspress.com

First edition published in 2006
Second edition published in 2009

16   15   14   13   3   4   5

ISBN: 978-1-59233-472-8

Library of Congress Cataloging-in-Publication Data available

Cover design by Danny Yee, Yee Design
Book design by Sue Yee, Yee Design

Printed and bound in USA

*The information in this book is for educational purposes only. It is not intended to
replace the advice of a physician or medical practitioner. Please see your health care
provider before beginning any new health program.*

This book is dedicated to all the courageous

children and to all who love and serve them.

We are humbled in your presence.

Preface

When I went to medical school over twenty years ago, nutrition was given very little attention. While I attended a very open-minded, cutting-edge school, my nutrition training consisted of one week of lectures. This left my colleagues and me with the impression that, at the time, nutrition was not felt to be very relevant to the practice of medicine. As I proceeded through my traditional training, not much happened to dispel that notion. It was only after I completed my formal training and began practicing in the "real world" of developmental pediatrics that I realized how critically important nutrition is to overall health and, in particular, to brain functioning.

Early on in my training, when parents would ask me if they should try special diets or nutritional supplements for their special-needs children, I distinctly remember advising them not to waste their time, as there was no evidence to show that they helped. I wish now that I could find all those parents and tell them they were right to be thinking outside the box. Parents have always been motivated to look at all options to help their children, especially those with special needs. It is only now that science is catching up with what those parents asked many years ago. Part of the role of this book is to explain the science behind the diets and why these diets may be worth trying with your child.

I am grateful that I came to an understanding of nutrition via a traditional medical route. I was not at all predisposed to believing that diets would help change behavior, development, and brain function. So when I saw diets working, I knew it was not a placebo effect. Still, I wanted to know *why* they worked and have now devoted my medical practice to understanding these nontraditional approaches. My traditional training also reminds me that there is no one way to treat children with special needs. Many people in both camps (traditional and nontraditional) assume that the type of intervention they favor is the right one. I believe strongly in using all the tools I have at my disposal to help children reach their potential, whether those tools are traditional (therapy, school placement, medications, etc.) or nontraditional (diet change, nutritional supplements, digestive support, etc.). This book addresses some of these less traditional tools, specifically diet and nutrition.

Dr. Sidney Baker, in his book *Detoxification and Healing*, outlines a helpful context for thinking about the role of diet in brain function. In essence, he asks two basic questions that, for me, form the basic foundation of my approach to caring for children with special needs. Paraphrased here, these two questions are:

1. Is this child's body and brain getting all that is needed to perform optimally?

2. Is there something getting to this child's brain that interferes with its ability to perform optimally?

Diet and nutrition are clearly involved in answering both of these questions. An optimized diet, along with nutritional supplements, provides nutrients that are essential for body and brain functioning. In addition, breakdown products from certain foods (particularly dairy and glutens) can interfere with brain functioning. These concepts will be explained further in the chapters that follow. The recipes in this book are designed to give the body and brain what is needed, and to eliminate those substances that are most likely to interfere with function.

In medicine, there is a saying that you don't have to remember everything, you just have to remember where you filed the article. In the same way, I don't have to know everything about nutrition; I have to know who my good resources are to complement my medical knowledge of health and nutrition; Dana Laake, my coauthor, is such a resource.

Pamela J. Compart, M.D.

My introduction to nutrition began through a career in dentistry. I learned the powerful effects of food on the body and mind from Emanuel Cheraskin, a physician and dentist, who was an internationally renowned researcher and expert in the field of nutritional medicine, dental health, and the role of vitamins and minerals in health and disease. While attending a course led by this pioneer, who would influence my career for the next 25 years, I fell in love with the fields of nutrition and preventive medicine. Cheraskin opened the first of many doors in this challenging and rapidly evolving field. His legacy was great, but I remember him most for the simplicity of his favorite statement, "Man is a food-dependent creature; if you don't feed him he will die. If you feed him improperly, a part of him will die."

In 1979, George Mitchell, our family physician, invited me to join him in opening a preventive medicine practice in Washington, D.C. Dr. Mitchell provided me the opportunity of traveling throughout the country to learn from the innovators and visionaries in nutrition and alternative medicine.

My first special child presented early on in the practice, when a distraught mother brought her seven-year-old son for evaluation and treatment. He was a conundrum to his family, teachers, and physicians. Beginning at two years of age, problem behaviors had developed. He eventually became physically violent toward others, including routinely striking his father. He was unable to function in school because of poor attention span, impulsivity, acting out, and aggression. He had chronic bowel problems, wet his bed nightly, and was in a constant state of agitation and unhappiness. Showing the reports from his teachers, his mother cried as she confessed, "Each teacher tells me that he is the worst child they have ever encountered."

A review of his diet revealed that milk products and glutens (wheat) were his most common and favorite foods. This occurred in the era when there was little acceptance of the connection between food and behavior. In fact, to suggest this relationship was considered medical quackery. I had only read about the results of removing milk products and gluten from diets to achieve improvement in behavior and function—I had not yet experienced it with a patient. We did not have the quality and accuracy of testing so prevalent today, but the anecdotal evidence was abundant. Since a trial of food avoidance fits the medical dictum, "Do no harm," I recommended a trial of strict avoidance of milk products and gluten.

The results elated me as much as the parents. After the first few days withouth milk products and gluten, the boy became worse. But within a week of avoidance, he began to improve, and at the end of one month they had their good son back. He cooperated at school, began to progress in achievements, received outstanding behavior reports, and stopped aggressive and impulsive behaviors. His bowels improved, and he no longer wet the bed at night. Most important, he stopped hitting his father and began hugging again. Thinking he was "cured," his parents allowed him to have cake and ice cream at a birthday party, only to have him relapse into the full spectrum of symptoms. They returned to the diet, and his symptoms resolved once again. I am eternally grateful for what this child taught me; he sparked the beginning of my quest to help other children.

Dana Laake, M.S., L.D.N

Foreword

When it comes to autism and attention deficit hyperactivity disorder (ADHD), diet does matter! Children with these disorders suffer from maldigestion, the inability to completely digest food down to the simple molecules that our bodies need. Many of those with autism and ADHD produce partially digested and unabsorbed substances that serve as food for unfriendly and possibly pathogenic flora in their intestinal tracts. In addition, some of what is absorbed into the bloodstream acts as false neurotransmitters and as allergens that provoke inflammatory responses. Of course, the nature of these partially digested substances depends upon the foods that are eaten. That's what this book is about—identifying offending foods and safe foods, and making those safe foods palatable.

For many years the Autism Research Institute (ARI) in San Diego has kept track of parent-recorded responses of their autistic children to special diets. Twice a year, ARI updates these responses on a one-page tabulation called, "ARI Publication 34." According to the February 2006 edition, 50 percent of autistics improved by avoiding milk products (based on 5,847 responses); 49 percent improved with avoidance of wheat (3,367 responses); and 65 percent improved on a gluten- and casein-free diet (1,818 responses). Thousands of parents are *not* wrong! You can join their successes. Read this book and learn how to determine if a special diet will benefit your autistic or ADHD child.

One of the most difficult activities that parents can undertake is implementing a diet that their children may resist. Often, these children become addicted to some of the foods that actually are troublemakers for them. Also, their peers don't have to avoid these dietary goodies, so why should they? The authors help you with these issues. In this book, Pamela Compart, M.D. and Dana Laake, R.D.H., M.S., L.D.N. remove the how-to-do-it stumbling blocks that confront so many parents.

Jon B. Pangborn, Ph.D., F.A.I.C.
Cofounder, Defeat Autism Now!

The *Kid-Friendly ADHD & Autism Cookbook* is appropriately described by it's subtitle *The Ultimate Guide to the Gluten-Free, Casein-Free Diet.* This is an "all-in-one" book that is a combination resource guide and multilevel cookbook. Other cookbooks that provide gluten and casein-free recipes alone are insufficient, providing parents with only a fraction of the help that they need.

In addition to being concerned about preparing good, healthy food for their children, parents are more concerned about the difficulty of feeding their children who have unusually limited appetites, crave foods that cause them problems, and have strong food aversions—especially to vegetables.

By offering solutions, the authors present ways to increase the acceptability of the substitute foods.

Through the "Trojan Horse Technique," they teach parents how to "hide" nutritionally healthy foods so they are readily accepted. There are also many suggestions for overcoming sensory problems with texture, color, and taste. For busy parents who are also trying to cook special meals, the authors provide two kinds of solutions: "Quick N Easy" versions of recipes and ways to use commercially prepared foods" successfully.

Remember, your child is the real expert. Changing his or her diet is only a way of asking the question, "Will this help?" It is a diagnostic step that cannot be replaced by any lab test and it simply depends on your child's response. It doesn't become a treatment until you get a "thumbs-up" from changes you accomplish and the results you observe—followed by surprise and infinite relief.

Sidney MacDonald Baker, M.D.
Fellow, American Academy of Pediatrics
Former Director of Gesell Institute of
  Human Development
Cofounder, Defeat Autism Now!

Contents

Part I Get Ready! Get Set!

Part II Go! The Kid-Friendly Recipes

Introduction

There is one thing stronger than all the armies in the world,
and that is an idea whose time has come.
                  —Victor Hugo

Why Buy This Book?

Although written for children with Attention Deficit Hyperactivity Disorder (ADHD) or autism spectrum disorders (ASD), it can be helpful for any child with a variety of behavioral or developmental challenges. Because it may be easier to change the entire household's diet at the same time, this book is also written for the families. Other family members are often surprised by improvements in their own health and behavior.

You may wonder how this book is different from other gluten- or milk-free recipe books. We believe this book is different in several ways:

- When implementing a special diet, it is hard to take "on faith" that it may help. This book explains the reasons why diet changes may help your child's brain and body function better.

- We recognize that it is much easier to recommend a specialized diet than to actually implement it. This book includes helpful suggestions on how to begin and how to maintain a specialized diet.

- We are aware that changing diets in children, especially children who are picky, can be a challenging undertaking. This book includes many helpful hints for dealing with the picky eater.

- Not everyone likes or has time to cook. We have included "Quick N Easy" versions of recipes for parents on the go. For those who prefer more complex recipes, we have included those as well.

- Children with ASD often have additional challenges, both in behavior and biochemistry, which can make feeding an even more difficult task. This book includes ways to hide or disguise nutritious and healthy foods in ways children will accept.

- Many books about specialized diets focus only on the elimination of gluten and casein. There are subsets of children who may also react to other common offending foods such as soy, egg, corn, and nuts; yeast-promoting foods; and food components such as phenols (including salicylates), double sugars (disaccharides), and oxalates. This book includes recipes that are free of multiple offending foods.

- This book focuses not only on what is being taken out of a diet, but also on what is put back in. The goal of elimination diets is not just removing unhealthy or potentially harmful foods, but also providing nutritious, appealing foods in their place.

- The second edition includes 100 new recipes, including those from a variety of cultures, and updated diet information and guidelines.

What Is Attention Deficit Hyperactivity Disorder?

ADHD is a collection of symptoms including inattention, hyperactivity, and impulsivity. There is no blood test that can diagnose ADHD. It is diagnosed by presenting a certain number of symptoms in a particular combination. A paraphrasing of these symptoms from the manual that provides the current definition of ADHD, the *Diagnostic and Statistical Manual of Mental Disorders, 4th edition,* or *DSM–IV,* follows:

- **INATTENTION SYMPTOMS:** Failure to pay close attention to details or making careless mistakes in schoolwork or other activities, difficulty sustaining attention, often not seeming to listen when spoken to directly, often not following through on instructions or failure to complete tasks, difficulty organizing tasks and activities, avoiding tasks that require sustained mental effort (such as homework), losing things necessary for tasks and activities, easy distractibility, and frequent forgetfulness in daily activities (tying shoes, zipping up pants, etc.).

- **HYPERACTIVITY SYMPTOMS:** Fidgeting or squirming, difficulty staying seated when expected to, running or climbing in situations in which it is inappropriate, difficulty playing quietly, often acting as if driven by a motor, and talking excessively.

- **IMPULSIVITY SYMPTOMS:** Blurting out answers before questions finished, difficulty awaiting turn, and often interrupting conversations or intruding.

Children who have at least six symptoms of inattention are described as having ADHD, Predominantly Inattentive Type. Children who have at least six symptoms in some combination of hyperactivity and impulsivity are described as having ADHD, Predominantly Hyperactive-Impulsive Type. Children who meet both of these requirements are described as ADHD, Combined Type.

There are some important things to keep in mind regarding the diagnosis of ADHD:

- Everyone can experience periods of difficulty with attention or hyperactivity. An ADHD diagnosis requires that symptoms be present for at least six months.

- By definition, ADHD symptoms begin before age seven. This does not mean symptoms were significantly impairing before seven, because prior to this age, children are not often in settings where they must sit still for long periods. Symptoms often do not become apparent or problematic until children reach school age and are required to sit still for hours.

- To have ADHD, symptoms must be impairing to social or academic functioning. ADHD symptoms are not always a problem; it is a matter of degree. They must also occur in more than one setting, such as at home and at school.

- Symptoms must be inappropriate for the child's developmental age, not chronologic age. If a four-year-old child has developmental delays and is functioning at a two-year-old level, his ADHD symptoms must be out of the norm for a two-year-old, not a four-year-old.

- Most important, not every child who presents with ADHD symptoms has ADHD. Part of the definition is that these symptoms must not be better explained by some other diagnosis. Children who are anxious or depressed or who have learning disabilities or allergies and food intolerances will also not pay attention well.

There are many approaches to treating ADHD. This book is not meant to diagnose ADHD or take the place of advice from your child's medical professional. Rather, it provides ideas for how to optimize your child's nutrition so that his or her brain can work at its best. For some children, diet changes alone may be sufficient to treat symptoms. For others, some combination of diet, nutritional supplements, school accommodations, therapies, tutoring, and/or medication results in the best outcome. When the brain is working at its best, a child can be more responsive to these other treatments.

What Is Autism? Why Are They Called Autism Spectrum Disorders?

Autism is a developmental disorder that is also defined according to the *DSM–IV*. It is a much more complex disorder than ADHD, but like ADHD, it has no specific blood test or brain scan that can make the diagnosis. It is also a collection of symptoms. It requires a total of six symptoms from the following three major areas, with at least two symptoms in the first area and at least one each from the second and third areas.

- **QUALITATIVE IMPAIRMENT IN SOCIAL INTERACTION:** Marked difficulty in the use of nonverbal behaviors such as eye contact, facial expressions, body postures, and gestures to regulate social interaction; failure to develop age-appropriate relationships with peers; lack of a spontaneous seeking to share enjoyment or interests with others; and lack of social or emotional reciprocity (the "give and take" that occurs in relationships)

- **QUALITATIVE IMPAIRMENTS IN COMMUNICATION:** Delay or lack of development of spoken language; lack of gesture communication (such as pointing); marked difficulty in initiating or sustaining conversation with others; stereotyped or repetitive use of language or unusual language (such as quoting memorized dialogue from TV or videos or using phrases totally out of context); and lack of spontaneous make-believe play or social play appropriate to the child's developmental level

- **RESTRICTED, REPETITIVE, AND STEREOTYPED PATTERNS OF BEHAVIOR, INTERESTS, AND ACTIVITIES:** Unusual preoccupation with a particular area of interest that is abnormal in either intensity or focus; apparently inflexible adherence to specific, nonfunctional routines or rituals; stereotyped and repetitive motor behaviors (e.g. hand flapping, whole-body rocking); and persistent preoccupation with parts of objects (e.g. spinning the wheels on a car rather than using it in play)

There must also be delays or abnormal functioning occurring before age three years in at least one of the following: (1) social interaction, (2) language as used in social communication, or (3) symbolic or imaginative play.

An important feature of ASD is that the diagnosis is not just about delayed development or lack of certain skills. Much of it is about the quality of a skill or interaction. A child can amass a great deal of language, but if it is not used to communicate, that is unusual. For example, a child may be able to recite an entire book from memory but not be able to have a conversation. His language may seem advanced, but his ability to communicate is not typical.

The term "autism spectrum disorders" is used to indicate that there is a wide variety of possible combinations and severity of symptoms. Not every child will meet the exact number or combination of symptoms comprising autism. However, children with autism are different from children who have only speech-language delays or overall developmental delays because of the unusual quality or lack of development of social and interaction skills. The term "pervasive developmental disorder" is often used to indicate children who have many of the symptoms of autism, but not in the right number or combination to be given a diagnosis of autism. There is debate whether children with Asperger's syndrome are also on the autism spectrum or have a separate disorder. They share many of the same characteristics of children with autism, with some differences. The main diagnostic difference is that children with autism must have delays in their early language development. By definition, children with Asperger's syndrome have normal early language development. Children with Asperger's syndrome also often have an encompassing preoccupation with particular areas of interest that interferes with their social interactions. For the purposes of this book, we will use the term "autism" to refer to all of these ASDs.

Regardless of the label given to a particular child's symptoms, many children with ADHD or ASD respond very well to changes in diet and nutrition. The purpose of optimizing nutrition is to also optimize brain and body function, so that children can respond to all the other treatments provided and have the best possible outcome. Other chapters in this book will describe some of the unique biochemical problems children with ASD have that are different from those seen in children with ADHD.

What If I'm Not Sure If My Child Has ADHD or Autism? Can This Book Still Help?

Your child does not need to have a specific diagnosis in order to benefit from this book. Again, this book provides help in giving the brain and body what is needed, and taking away what is not needed in order to achieve optimum results.

Will Diet Alone Be Enough to Treat My Child's Symptoms?

Children with ADHD or ASD often require a comprehensive set of treatments. There is no one cause of ADHD or autism and, therefore, no single treatment. Particularly for the child with autism, he or she may come into the world with genetic predispositions, inborn errors of metabolism, immune dysfunction, maldigestion, malabsorption syndromes, and food reactions. That predisposition is then modified by a wide range of environmental factors which can potentially increase susceptibility to autism: birth trauma, pathogen exposure, toxins, heavy metal exposures, unusual vaccination reactions, allergens, pesticides, poor diet, nutritional deficiencies, and other stressors. Typically, it is not any single factor that is the cause, but the cumulative effect known as the "total load" that tilts the balance in these children. The current research focus is aimed toward identifying the many potential risk factors, establishing more preventive measures, improving early diagnosis, establishing early interventions, and expanding the effectiveness of therapies and treatments.

We visualize our approach as three "legs" on the treatment "table," all of which are important for keeping the table steady and balanced.

- **THERAPIES.** These can include behavioral therapies or organizational strategies and educational interventions (special education, speech or occupational therapy, etc.).

- **MEDICATIONS.** Depending on the need, medications are used as appropriate to each child.

■ **BIOMEDICAL COMPONENT.** Diet and nutrition are critical components of the overall treatment plan because they address underlying core problems. We are much more than what we eat—we are what we eat, digest, absorb, and utilize. Unfortunately, diet and nutrition are often overlooked or dismissed, when, in fact, many of the symptom presentations in ADHD or autism are directly related to nutritional deficiencies, disturbances in nutrient metabolism, poor diet, and the negative effects of specific foods.

For optimum results, all three legs need to be considered. This book focuses on one part of the biomedical leg of that table—the diet.

What Exactly Is "The Diet"?

The elimination diet for autism and ADHD, commonly called "the diet," is a regimen of eating and drinking that focuses on the elimination of gluten and casein. Although other foods may also be bothersome, these two proteins are by far the most common offenders. Casein is the main protein found in milk products, but don't confuse "milk-free" with "casein-free," as casein is found in products other than milk. It is found in other dairy products such as yogurt and ice cream, and also in many baked goods and other unexpected places such as certain canned tuna.

Gluten is a protein found in wheat and other grains. Again, "wheat-free" is not the same as "gluten-free." A more in-depth discussion of these proteins, their sources, and substitutes can be found in chapter 2.

For most children, the elimination of casein and gluten is enough. However, some may also be sensitive to other foods such as soy or corn. All of the recipes in this book are gluten- and casein-free; some are also free of soy, corn, and other potentially bothersome foods. We hope that these recipes provide guidance for the broadest group of children on specialized diets.

Are There Tests to Help Determine If My Child Needs a Specialized Diet?

This question will be discussed in detail in later chapters. In general, nutritional and dietary treatment approaches should be based on determining the underlying biochemical, metabolic, and nutritional imbalances present for each child. Fortunately, the science of nutrition has caught up with the decades of clinical and anecdotal observations. Now there is an abundance of sophisticated testing that has improved our diagnostic abilities. Tests include analysis for maldigestion and malabsorption syndromes; food allergies, sensitivities, and intolerances; bowel pathogens, inflammation and disorders; exposure to toxic metals and other harmful substances; immune status; nutrient levels; and defects in the metabolism of amino acids, fatty acids, carbohydrates, vitamins, and minerals. In particular, many of the children have problems in digestion and absorption, in addition to accumulation of toxic metals. Almost all of the children with ADHD or autism have nutritional deficits, and those with the most severe presentations have multiple significant nutrient deficits and metabolic disturbances.

Most of these specialized tests are not always part of the routine work-up for people with ADHD and autism. Without these tests, significant problems can be missed, rendering treatment plans incomplete.

How Will This Book Help?

This book includes chapters that address the following issues:

- Identifying sources and substitutes for the main culprits—gluten and casein—as well as soy, corn, eggs, salicylates, phenols, and disacchardies.
- What makes a food "good" or "bad" for you
- How to determine if your child is sensitive to particular foods
- How to change your child's diet
- How to get your picky eater to accept new foods
- Suggestions for dealing with common problems encountered when changing diets

In Their Own Words

No one tells the story better than the parents who have tenaciously sought and found the right treatment path for their children—and the children who have courageously walked it! The stories we've included throughout the book may differ because each child's response is unique. While some respond dramatically to a single intervention, others respond best when a combination of treatments is utilized. It is important for parents not to give up when the results are not immediate and dramatic. Remember to be persistent and patient. We start with Anne Evans's poignant dedication in her book, *Autism Treated and Cured,* a detailed description of her daughter's path from autism to dramatic recovery.

Increasing Prevalence in Autism: 500,000 and growing

May 2006: The Centers for Disease Control and Prevention (CDC) presented data on surveys from 2003 to 2004 on the prevalence of autism.

These are the first national estimates.

- 1 out of 175 school-age children (age 4 to 17) currently has autism. The real prevalence likely exceeds the current numbers because so many of the children under 4 years of age are not diagnosed until they are older.
- Current CDC estimate: 500,000 from birth to age 21
- Fastest growing developmental disability (2003 comparison)
  806% growth in autism
  31% growth in all other disabilities
- 24,000 new cases per year

Prior to 1985	3 to 5 per 10,000
1998 to 2000	30 to 35 per 10,000
2006	67 per 10,000

The number of children "born autistic" has not changed significantly over time. What has escalated exponentially is regressive autism, which occurs between twelve and twenty-four months, after a period of normal development and behavior.

Since autistic behaviors are usually present prior to the age of 3 years, early diagnosis is critical. The best success results from early-intervention treatments.

CHAPTER 1

Food Reactions:
What They Are and How to Test for Them

*The important thing in science is not so much to obtain new facts
as to discover new ways of thinking about them.*

—William Bragg

Food Allergies versus Food Sensitivities and Intolerances

MANY PEOPLE USE THE TERM "FOOD ALLERGIES" TO describe all reactions to food, but this is not accurate. Allergy is one type of reaction to food. There are also numerous sensitivities and intolerances to foods that are not classified as allergic reactions. Many children with ADHD or ASD have multiple types of reactions to foods, ranging from allergies to a variety of types of sensitivities and intolerances. The type of reaction least likely to cause behavioral symptoms is the traditional type of food allergy with obvious symptoms such as sneezing, hives, and wheezing. Children with ADHD or ASD tend to have food reactions best labeled as "sensitivities" or "intolerances." Some of the most common foods that cause food intolerances and sensitivities are similar to those that cause allergies—milk, wheat, and soy. Corn is also a frequent offending food, but almost any food can trigger reactions due to sensitivity and intolerance.

*"The real voyage of discovery consists not
in seeking new landscapes but in having new eyes."*
—Marcel Proust

There are many types of food sensitivities and intolerances that result from poor digestion and/or poor absorption of specific food substances. For the purposes of this chapter, when we refer to food sensitivities, we are referring to the delayed (immunoglobulin G, or IgG) type of food reactions. Food intolerances can include a wider range of reactions, such as intolerances to lactose, fructose, other carbohydrate sugars, phenols, salicylates, and gluten (in celiac disease), and intolerance to byproducts of abnormal digestion, such as opiate peptides from milk/casein, gluten, and soy.

Food Allergies

The antibodies (immune cells) in the body that result in traditional allergies are called immunoglobulin E (IgE) antibodies, which trigger the release of histamine. The antibodies that result in one type of food sensitivity are immunoglobulinG (IgG) antibodies. The reactions are different and the testing is different. This distinction will be important when we discuss types of blood tests commonly available to test for food reactions later in this chapter. The most confusion comes from testing for traditional (IgE) allergy reactions versus delayed (IgG) reactions.

IgE reactions are obvious and fast. We are all familiar with traditional allergic reactions in some fashion. A person eats a food and develops hives or wheezing. A person with a severe peanut allergy can develop a life-threatening allergic reaction after eating peanuts. The immune pathway in the body that results in these reactions is very fast-acting. Cause and effect is usually easy to figure out because the reaction happens so quickly. These reactions do not have a direct negative effect on the brain. While people may become irritable from the discomfort of the allergy symptom, such as itching or wheezing, they are not irritable due to a specific effect of the food on the brain. The most common foods that provoke allergic reactions are milk, eggs, peanuts, tree nuts (almonds, cashews, pecans, and walnuts), fish, shellfish, soy, and wheat.

Food Sensitivities

Most types of food reactions, however, are not IgE reactions; most fall into the other categories. IgG food sensitivities can result in physical symptoms similar to allergies. However, they may also result in a much broader array of symptoms, including behavioral or developmental symptoms. A striking difference between food allergies and food sensitivities is the time it takes for the reaction to occur. While food allergy symptoms occur quickly, symptoms of food sensitivities can occur at any time within three days of eating the food. Most commonly, these reactions occur within one to two days. This often makes it very difficult to figure out which food caused which behavioral reaction. With food allergies, keeping a food diary can be very helpful. Because of the delayed nature of food sensitivities, food diaries are less helpful.

For those with compromised systems, the number of IgG sensitivities may be high and include most of what the person eats. For that reason, rotation diets are frequently recommended to limit the damaging effect on the immune system. The concept behind a rotation diet is to limit the exposure to the same food, and more specifically the same family of foods. By not repeating the suspect or reactive foods daily, the body's reactions to the foods will be more limited. The most common food rotation programs suggest not eating the same foods more often than once per day in four or more days. Resources for food rotation programs are included in the appendix.

Food Intolerances

These reactions are not immunoglobulin (IgE or IgG) reactions. Intolerances include problems with digestion of foods due to the lack of specific enzymes including maldigestion of lactose, carbohydrate double sugars (disaccharides), and proteins from gluten and milk (casein). Celiac gluten intolerance is not due to maldigestion but to an autoimmune response that damages the intestinal villi in response to gluten exposure.

Intolerances also include inability to metabolize a component of a food such as fructose, phenylalanine, phenols and salicylates. Food intolerances may result in immediate and also delayed reactions, depending on the situation. With lactose intolerance, the effects (diarrhea, cramps) may be notable within hours. Gluten celiac type reactions may also be immediate (stomach pain, cramps, diarrhea) and long–term (growth delay, skin conditions, fatigue, and neurological or behavioral/development symptoms). For intolerance to phenols and salicylates (a type of phenol), some reactions may be more immediate (stomach ache, red face or ears, hyperactivity, hives, and headaches) while others are more delayed (dark circles under the eyes, short attention span, sleep disorders, speech difficulties, tics, behavioral problems, and head banging).

Symptoms of Food Sensitivities and Intolerances

Symptoms of food sensitivities and food intolerances can be broad:

- **GENERAL SYMPTOMS:** Fatigue, food cravings

- **SKIN:** Eczema, unexplained rashes, allergic shiners (dark circles under the eyes), red face/ears

- **DIGESTION:** Stomach aches, loose stools or diarrhea, constipation, alternating diarrhea and constipation

- **RESPIRATORY:** Mucus production, congestion

- **IMMUNE, INFLAMMATORY, AND AUTOIMMUNE REACTIONS**

- **CARDIOVASCULAR:** Abnormal pulse, elevated blood pressure

- **NEUROLOGIC:** Headaches (e.g., migraines), ringing in the ears, tingling, dizziness, tics

- **PSYCHOLOGICAL:** Depression, mood disorders, anxiety, panic attacks, aggression, sleep disorder

- **BEHAVIOR/DEVELOPMENT:** ADHD symptoms (decreased attention, hyperactivity, impulsivity), mood swings, irritability, anxiety, autism symptoms (poor eye contact, social withdrawal, decreased language, obsessions, repetitive behaviors)

Causes of Food Reactions: The Digestive Connection

Normally, when foods are digested in the small intestine (the upper part of the intestine), they break down into their smallest components: proteins to amino acids, fats to fatty acids, and carbohydrates to simple sugars. Along with nutrients, these are allowed to cross the intestinal lining into the bloodstream, where they travel to other parts of the body, including the brain.

A critical part of this healthy system is the lining of the intestine. This lining needs to be a good barrier so that foods cannot enter the blood until they have been fully digested. It functions like a window screen, letting in good air but not larger items like pesky flies or harmful bugs. When the intestinal lining is damaged, potentially harmful large food molecules can enter the bloodstream—like holes in the window screen letting in bugs. This condition is commonly referred to as a "leaky gut," since food molecules leak through the microscopic holes in the intestinal lining.

Many children with ADHD or autism have problems with their intestinal lining. Children with autism also may not have enough digestive enzymes or the body may not release them at the right times or in sufficient amounts. The type of food that causes the most problems for children with ADHD or autism is protein, specifically proteins from milk, wheat, and soy. Dietary proteins (fish, fowl, meat, eggs, dairy, beans, nuts, seeds, and grains) consist of many chains of amino acids and are not useful until they are broken down into individual amino acids by digestive enzymes. The foods themselves are like dollar bills that will not work in a coin machine. They must be broken down first into individual coins (amino acids). Visualize these proteins as long metal chains, with each link being an amino acid; digestive enzymes break the connection between links and free the amino acids (links) for further use. The amino acids are very small and are absorbed through the intestinal lining into the body. The amino acids can then be put back together in different combinations to make peptides and proteins again. These can be used to build important structures in the body, such as muscle, or to send messages in the body, for example, as hormones or transmitters in the brain.

During digestion, not all of the amino-acid chains are completely digested. What results are residues of short chains of amino acids called peptides. The peptides, however, are large and should not be absorbed unless the gut is damaged and, therefore, too permeable or leaky. Think of amino acids like Scrabble letters. Peptides are the "words" made from those letters. Depending on how the letters (amino acids) are arranged, different "words" (peptides) are formed. The body recognizes these "words". If, however, the letter arrangement does not spell a "word", the body considers it to be foreign. Likewise, if the intestinal lining is damaged, the body may consider the peptides that leak into the bloodstream to be foreign. If they are not recognized because they are foreign, the body sends specialized cells to get rid of them. When the peptides are "words" the body recognizes, the body allows them to remain. If the "words" have receptors in the brain, they may cross the brain and send a signal. If the signal is not one that should normally occur in the brain, there can be a short circuit in brain functioning. This can contribute to many of the symptoms seen in children with ADHD or autism.

"I used to lie down and cry and hold my stomach. I had continuous stomachaches. No one knew how bad it hurt. No one believed me. They thought that I was telling stories. I did not pay attention in school. I was in the bathroom all of the time. The teachers used to complain. I wasn't good at reading. I had bad grades. I think I was failing. I didn't really like school. Learning wasn't fun. I used to be in a daze."

—Ashley Stilson,
age fourteen, originally diagnosed with pervasive developmental disorder

The Dope on Opiates

While short-circuiting of the brain from "misspelled words" can occur in a variety of conditions, a feature that is more common in autism but occasionally found in ADHD is the creation of "words" or peptides that have an opiate-like effect on the brain. If the amino acid "letters" in the peptide "word" are arranged in a specific order, the peptide looks like an opiate and acts like an opiate—similar to morphine. "Opiates" refers to the narcotic alkaloids found in opium such as morphine and heroin. An "opioid" has an opiate-like reaction. Casein and gluten are the most common foods that result in these opiate-like substances. Soy is also a likely a source of these opiates. Casein and gluten contain a similar sequence of amino acids. They have, embedded within their long chains of amino acids, sequences of these short opiate-like peptides. These peptides are not available or active unless the proteins are incompletely broken down due to digestive enzyme deficiencies such as lack of dipeptidyl peptidase IV

(DPP-IV). The resulting opiate-like endorphins have very specific amino acid sequences. For gluten the result is gliadorphin (tyr-pro-gln-pro-gly-pro-phe) and milk casein, the result is casomorphin (tyr-pro-gln-pro-gly-pro-ile). These opiate-like peptides are generally large and unable to pass through the intestinal lining. When the lining is leaky, these peptides can enter the bloodstream and travel to the brain, having an opiate-like effect there. These opiate peptides have been found in the spinal fluid and the urine of children with autism. The effect of opiates on the brain can certainly explain some of the symptoms seen in autism.

Many children crave dairy and wheat products. There are some children whose parents describe them as "milk-aholics" because of the intensity of their craving for milk. These cravings may be similar to drug-seeking types of behaviors. A child may not want other foods because they don't give the brain the same "high" as the opiate-producing foods. Food "hunger strikes" and refusal to eat can occur. This may also account for the behaviors—from irritability to rage—seen in many children when dairy and wheat are initially removed from the diet. They are, in effect, having drug-withdrawal symptoms.

These opiate-like peptides mimic the effects of drugs like morphine and have been shown to react with areas of the brain that are involved in speech and auditory processing. Opiate-like effects on the brain could also result in social withdrawal. A child may "zone out" or "be in his/her own world." He/she may laugh or giggle for no apparent reason. In addition, a child may have a high pain tolerance since opiates, like morphine, are excellent painkillers.

We are aware that there are likely other psychoactive and neruoative peptide possibilities. It is not unusual for the casomorphin and gliadorphin tests to be negative, yet the child shows a significant improvement in behavior and focus when either milk casein and/or glutens are removed from the diet. It is certainly likely that there are other types of reactions occurring. Recent studies indicate that gluten and casein can be a source for increased propionic acid, another compound that can elicit the symptoms of autism when exposure is elevated. For these reasons, when a child presents with an extremely limited diet and/or an addictive focus to the classical problem foods (e.g., milk products, glutens, and possibly soy), these are signs that an avoidance trial is important.

Support for the Opioid Theory

According to the research of Kalle Reichelt, M.D.:

- Food-source opioids have been reported in the cerebrospinal fluid, breast milk, blood, and urine, particularly in patients with autism, depression, and schizophrenia.

- Addictive behaviors are present when on glutens and casein, and withdrawal symptoms can occur with removal.

- Opioids decrease in the urine of those on a GFCF diet.

- For those with autism, as with morphine users, their pupils are small while "under the influence" and large when going through a period of abstinence.

- Constipation, self-absorption, and insensitivity to pain are markers for opiate use and autism.

http://www.gluten-free.org/reichelt.html

Lab Tests: What They Tell Us and What They Don't

In medical practice, where possible, we like to have information about whether certain treatments are indicated. Sometimes we can tell this simply based on examining a child. Other times, lab tests are ordered. So it seems logical that testing for food reactions (allergies, sensitivities/intolerances) would be a reasonable thing to do. However, this is actually a source of some debate among practitioners. Some believe food testing should always be done before starting an elimination diet; others believe it is not necessary or can be deferred to a later date. Regardless of when food testing is done, it is important to understand what the tests tell us and, equally important, what they do not reveal.

Like the misunderstanding of the difference between food allergies and food sensitivities, many people use the words "allergy testing" to describe testing for all types of food sensitivities or intolerances. Testing for food allergies is different from testing for food sensitivities. If you take your child to a traditional allergist, testing will be done for food allergies, the immediate, fast-acting immune response (IgE). This is either done by skin testing or blood testing. The blood testing, or radioallergosorbent testing (RAST), can be ordered through a traditional laboratory. This type of testing provides reliable information about the immediate types of allergy reactions, the types that can cause hives, wheezing, and a host of other physical symptoms. Neither the skin nor the IgE blood testing gives any information about food IgG sensitivities, which is the type of reaction related to ADHD, autism, and other behavioral symptoms. Therefore, if you want to have your child tested for food sensitivities, a referral to a traditional allergist may not provide the answers you are looking for.

There is another type of testing, for those delayed food reactions, called IgG testing. This type of blood testing is offered only through specialized laboratories and is often not covered by insurance plans. While some traditional laboratories may offer it for casein and/or gluten, traditional laboratories typically do not offer a full panel that includes a variety of foods and food groups. These tests are expensive, and cost needs to be considered as one factor in determining whether or when to test your child.

Reactions that indicate a problem with foods are called positive reactions. They are reported in various degrees, based on the strength of the reaction. There are a number of points to keep in mind when interpreting food IgG test results:

- Finding a positive reaction in blood testing does not guarantee that removal of the food will result in improvement. It is revealing that molecules from that food "leaked" into the bloodstream, triggering a response from the body's immune system, resulting in an increase in these IgG antibodies. Removal of the offending foods and/or rotation does reduce the total load and hence can potentially reduce symptoms. The IgG reaction is common in many with autism. IgG reactions contribute to overall body burden.

- The absence of a food reaction does not guarantee your child is not reactive to that food in another category of reactions, sensitivities, or intolerances.

- Reactions may be positive to foods your child has never eaten. This is because certain food groups can cross-react, causing false positive reactions.

- Some children have positive reactions, of varying degrees, to a large number of foods. If fifteen or more reactions are present, this is thought to be more of an indicator that the intestinal lining is leaky (too permeable to large molecules) rather than each individual food being a problem. In other words, this shows that the intestinal barrier is unable to keep out a variety of food molecules and the immune system has responded by making antibodies against all of those foods. It does not necessarily mean that all fifteen foods need to be eliminated from the diet. Also, when the number is large, the foods are usually those most commonly consumed.

So what to make of these tests? How best to use them to help guide treatment? It is our opinion that food testing generally does not need to be done initially. Again, removing foods based solely on food IgG results does not guarantee improvement in symptoms.

Given these caveats, why and when should you consider food IgG testing? Food testing may be more helpful if conducted after other treatments have already been completed, such as those that help heal the "leakiness" of the intestinal lining. When the intestinal lining is a better barrier, it will be harder for food molecules to enter the bloodstream. The food molecules that do enter and still trigger immune reactions might then have more significance. Food testing may also be helpful in a situation in which the most common offending foods have been removed from the diet and other treatments (such as nutritional supplements) have been started and the child is still not showing adequate improvement. In that case, food testing may then provide guidance on which of all the foods in a child's diet might still be causing problems. This would help guide further dietary elimination trials.

"Be not astonished at new ideas; for it is well known to you that a thing does not therefore cease to be true because it is not accepted by many."

—**Spinoza** *(1632-1677)*

Are There Any Helpful Tests to Do Before Starting the Diet?

It is our opinion that there are two types of tests that are often helpful to have at the beginning of this process:

- For children with ADHD or autism: Blood testing for a disorder known as celiac disease.
- For children with autism: Urine testing for opiate peptide residues caused by gluten, casein, and soy.

CELIAC DISEASE

Celiac disease is a medical disorder in which gluten is not tolerated. In this disease, intake of gluten results in what is called an autoimmune reaction; the result is that the body recognizes the cells in the lining of the small intestine as foreign and reacts against them. This changes the anatomy of the intestinal lining and makes it "leaky."

The traditional view of celiac disease was that it had to cause diarrhea or affect a child's growth. However, recent studies reveal that bowel movements and growth may be normal, and a child may instead exhibit behavioral, developmental, or neurological effects from this disease. Celiac disease may also be present in a small percentage of children with ADHD or ASD. Celiac disease also occurs in 10–15% of children with Down Syndrome. The reason for testing for celiac disease before starting a gluten-free diet is that the only current treatment for celiac disease is 100 percent strict, lifelong elimination of gluten. Even 99 percent elimination of gluten will not cure the disease. In children, with 100 percent strict elimination of gluten, this disease is virtually completely reversible, and the intestinal lining will return to normal. This often results in improvement in behavioral and developmental symptoms. In addition, if celiac disease is present and not treated for years, the risk of other autoimmune disorders (such as rheumatoid arthritis or lupus) is increased. It is felt that treating celiac disease lowers the future risk of these disorders.

While some children with ADHD or autism require 100 percent strict elimination of gluten in order to see benefit, there is not a medical con sequence to only partial elimination. With celiac disease, partial treatment may result in medical problems in the future. Testing for celiac disease includes two kinds of tests, one that identifies specific antibodies to gluten (anti-endomysial, anti-gliadin, tissue transgluaminase, reticulin) and one that identifies genetic markers (HLA DR by PCR, specifically HLA DQ2 and/or HLA DQ8). The antibody tests must be accomplished while gluten is still in the diet. For the genetic test, exposure to gluten is not required. Genetic testing is generally done if there is a family history or if the screening antibody tests are abnormal. Therefore, it may be worth asking your child's physician to order blood testing for celiac disease before you start eliminating gluten.

According to the experts in celiac disease, there can also be gluten intolerance that is not celiac disease (i.e., specific celiac testing will be negative). As with gluten, individuals can also react in more than one way to milk products and to soy. Testing for food sensitivities or intolerances can produce a false negative result. It is our experience that avoiding suspect foods is the most reliable means of determining the culprits and their effects.

URINE OPIATE PEPTIDES

Urine testing is available to measure the opiate-like peptides made from casein, gluten, and soy. This testing is available only in specialized laboratories and is often not covered by insurance. It must be ordered by a physician or other practitioner such as a nutritionist. Testing directly measures opiate-like peptides from casein and gluten. Soy peptides cannot yet be directly measured and may be included in the measurements of casein and gluten peptides.

"Travis underwent the stool, urine, and blood tests this summer. The doctors found abnormal yeast overgrowth, inefficient production of digestive enzymes, deficiency in vitamin A, and food sensitivities to many more foods, the foods he ate the most—including eggs, soy, tomatoes, yeast, canola, cantaloupe, and coconut. He has been off these foods for four weeks now. There was a regression for the first two weeks, but now Travis is much better and more energetic."

—Letter from
Michele Pacifico in 2000, regarding son Travis

The degree of elevation of peptides can provide helpful information regarding the amount of withdrawal symptoms to expect. When a child has high levels of opiates, it may be more difficult to remove the foods due to the intensity of the "addiction" and subsequent withdrawal symptoms. Finding opiates in the urine also provides good motivation for following the diet, as it provides evidence that the foods are creating substances that can have a negative effect on brain functioning.

The Body Doesn't Lie: The Wisdom of Trial and Response

The best test is the child's own body. We know the most common offending foods are casein, gluten, and soy. Removing these foods gives "the biggest bang for the buck" for the largest number of children.

The gold standard for food reactions is the child's response to elimination of a food. It is better than any blood test. The goal of treatments is not to make the blood tests better; the goal is to make the child better. Some children will show obvious improvement when offending foods are removed from their diet. For other children, the response is less clear. The standard way of doing a food test is to do what is called an "elimination and challenge." An offending food is removed for a period of time. If improvement is not obvious, the body is then challenged by reintroduction of that food. Often, after an offending food is removed, there will be a more obvious and stronger reaction when the food is reintroduced. This method

John is in first grade—on time and independent. He is above grade level in language arts, including comprehension. His teacher states that his writing skills are excellent for content (less so for handwriting). There are no "behaviors"; however, he still jumps and flaps a little when excited, and his attention is not typical. Since his performance is fine, no medications have been recommended. He has an individualized education program (IEP) for next year, with one hour a week of special-education teacher oversight for executive functioning skills. There is no need for speech or occupational therapy. John still has issues that require more work; however, they are subtle and involve only social and executive functioning skills. We are told that, eventually, he will not require an IEP for autism spectrum disorder.

—Kathy Rivers, M.D.,
mother of a child recovering from autism

identifies offending foods and the symptoms they cause. A complicating issue is that children may be reactive to more than one food. Even if they react to a food that is removed, other stronger food reactions may mask any improvement from removal of that single food. Sometimes improvements are not seen until more than one food is removed from the diet. Paraphrasing Dr. Sidney Baker, if you are sitting on four pins, removing only one will not make much of a difference in your comfort level.

Chapter Summary

- Food reactions include food allergies, food sensitivities, and food intolerances, and they are not the same. The reactions that can cause ADHD or autism symptoms are food sensitivities and intolerances.

- Food IgG sensitivities are delayed reactions and can be difficult to determine.

- Food sensitivity and food intolerance reactions are much more varied than food allergy reactions and can affect skin, digestion, brain, behavior, and development.

- Children with ADHD or autism can have problems with their digestion, such as not enough digestive enzymes and/or leakiness of the intestinal lining.

These problems allow partly digested food substances (peptides) to enter the blood, cause problems in the body, and potentially short-circuit brain functioning. This can contribute to behavioral symptoms such as those seen in ADHD or autism.

- Opiate-like effects from problem foods can result in symptoms of autism, such as social withdrawal, inappropriate laughing, zoning out, high pain tolerance, and cravings for the foods that cause the problems.

- Lab tests provide important information regarding food reactions; however, the gold standard is still an elimination trial called "trial and response."

CHAPTER 2

The Culprits:
Glutens, Casein, Soy, and Others

"No gluten, no milk, no problem!"
— Will, brother of a child with autism on the gluten-free, casein-free diet

"I was blessed to have a child who was an immediate and
dramatically positive responder to dietary intervention.
Within thirty-six hours after we stopped casein, his inces-
sant screaming and head banging were almost gone, and we
had some eye contact back. Within five days after we stopped
gluten, his life-long rash was gone, and his stools improved.
Dietary infractions have produced equally dramatic results,
so we have been very motivated to continue the diet.
Maintaining his special diet is very difficult, but not nearly as
hard as living with a severely autistic child. For us, diet has
been one of the top three interventions that have aided in his
recovery from autism."

—MOTHER OF JOHN, *a five-year-old recovering from autism*

*It's not the food you avoid that makes you sick.
It's the food you crave and eat every day!*

What Are They, Where Are They, and What Are the Substitutes?

Glutens, animal milk, and soy are extremely complex foods, which may explain why so many people have problems with one or more of them. They are listed among the most common food allergens—but the reactions (intolerances) we are discussing are not classical allergic responses like hives, rashes, and itching.

As explained in chapter 1, glutens, casein, and also soy can digest poorly in the intestinal tract to groups of undigested amino acid chains called peptides, some of which can have opiate-like activity. When these peptides are absorbed into the bloodstream, they can cross the blood-brain barrier and negatively affect mood, mental and neurologic function, and behavior. When these peptides are opiate-like, they can cause addiction to the food source. Hence, the child craves the foods causing the problem and begins to limit the diet to primarily opiate-forming foods. This is why it is common for children to experience significant withdrawal symptoms when the foods are eliminated.

Knowledge is power, and we will try and simplify what can be complex.

Don't Be a Gluten for Punishment

WHAT AND WHERE ARE THEY?

Glutens are plant proteins in the subclass Monocotyledonae, found in wheat, semolina, bulgur, couscous, wheat berries, graham flour, whole meal flour, groats, malt, oats, barley, rye, triticale, and possibly spelt and kamut. Gluten is elastic and provides the stretchiness necessary in making yeast and non-yeast breads.

Gluten-containing grains are the most common ingredient in breads, pastas, crackers, cookies, cakes, cereals, pretzels, matzah, Passover flour, farfel, cream sauces, thickening agents, and breading. Gluten derivatives are also found in malt, modified food starches, hydrolyzed vegetable protein (HVP), hydrolyzed plant protein (HPP), textured vegetable proteins (TVPs), and dextrin, and they are used in the following unless labeled gluten-free: soy sauce, flavorings, instant coffee, some ketchups, mustards, commercial mixes, cake decorations, marshmallow crème, canned soups, deli meats, sausage, and hot dogs. Products labeled as corn bread or rice pasta may contain glutens. Breaded items contain glutens unless otherwise labeled. Gluten is also found in some of the binders and fillers found in vitamins and medications, and even pastes and glues on envelope flaps.

Gluten problems are not new in medicine. A portion of gluten called gliadin is known to exacerbate a genetic condition known as celiac disease by damaging the small intestine villi and to cause dermatitis herpetiformis, a celiac-associated serious skin condition. Celiac and nonceliac gluten intolerances have increased. These conditions are not the same as the ADHD- or autism-related gluten intolerances that result in absorption of peptides from incomplete digestion of these foods. However, the information about gluten avoidance found in the celiac literature is still very helpful.

A wheat-free food is not gluten-free unless all of the gluten sources are avoided. If the label does not state "gluten-free," then it is likely not gluten-free. It is not necessary to label foods that would not be expected to have gluten in them—such as unprocessed meats, eggs, vegetables, fruits, beans, nuts, and seeds.

WHAT IS LEFT TO EAT?

Grains that can be eaten on a gluten-free diet include rice of all varieties (white, brown, basmati, wild, sweet, poha), millet, corn, quinoa, amaranth, tapioca, buckwheat (not related to wheat at all), sorghum (jowar), ragi, teff, corn (if tolerated), and Montina (Indian ricegrass).

Nongrain substitutes for flours include potato starch and flours made from potato, taro, yam, arrowroot, almond, hazelnut, cassava, malanga, lotus, water chestnut, artichoke, chestnut, and beans, including chickpeas, peas, mung bean, and soy (if tolerated).

Since glutens provide the elastic quality needed in making baked goods, the substitutes must include safe ingredients that give the same result as gluten: xanthan gum, methylcellulose (indigestible polysaccharide of beta-glucose), or guar gum (soluble fiber from the Indian cluster bean). Substitutes for thickeners include the following: agar, arrowroot, bean flour, cornstarch, gelatin powder, guar gum, kudzu powder, sweet rice flour, tapioca flour, tapioca, and xanthan gum.

Remember to keep in your kitchen gluten-free baking powder and baking soda along with vanilla without alcohol (Frontier Vanilla). Successful gluten-free baked goods are possible; they just require a combination of flours, thickeners, and baking supplements to achieve an acceptable texture and flavor.

The Communion Conundrum

In most Christian churches, the communion wafer is traditionally made of wheat flour, and there is controversy over whether there can be a gluten-free substitute. Most churches have become liberal on the subject, allowing members to provide their own gluten-free host, which is wrapped separately (to avoid cross-contamination). These can be made or purchased and must be provided in time to be consecrated prior to the service. Make these arrangements individually with your priest or minister. See recipes and suggestions on page 131.

CATEGORY	SOURCES OF GLUTEN	GLUTEN-FREE (GF) SUBSTITUTES
Grains	**Wheat:** wheat berry, couscous, flour, graham, semolina, durum, bran, bulgur, cracked wheat, rusk **Oat:** oat bran, oat germ, oatmeal, oat flour, rolled oats **Barley:** flour, malt, starch, barley pearl **Rye:** rye starch **Triticale:** hybrid of wheat and rye **Spelt:** species of wheat **Kamut:** ancient wheatlike grain **Groats:** mixture of oat, wheat, buckwheat **Products of gluten grains:** bagels, biscuits, cakes, cereals, cookies, crackers, croutons, doughnuts, pasta, pretzels, stuffing, thickeners, tortillas, wafers, matzah, Passover flour, Communion wafers	**GF grains:** amaranth, buckwheat, corn, millet, Montina (Indian rice grass), quinoa, rice (basmati, black, brown, sweet, white, wild), sorghum (jowar), teff, tapioca. Exception: certified GF Lara's oats **Nongrain substitutes:** arrowroot, artichoke, cassava, lotus, malanga, sago, sweet potato, taro, water chestnut, yam **Nuts:** almonds, chestnuts, hazelnuts **Legumes:** beans, chickpeas, flava, mung bean, peas, soy **Thickeners:** agar, arrowroot, bean flour, gelatin, guar gum, kudzu powder, starch, sweet rice flour **Gluten-like elastic items:** guar gum, maltodextrin from corn or rice, methylcellulose, xanthan gum **Pasta/Noodles:** GF flours, rice noodles, spaghetti squash
Beverages	Malted drinks or malt in drinks	Water, including plain seltzer
	Ovaltine, Postum, flavored tea or coffee	Herbal teas, tea, coffee (unflavored)
	Beer and ale (fermented)	Wines
	Some grain alcohols, especially if flavored	Distilled liquors
	Flavored water, seltzer	Fresh or frozen juices
	Juice punch or drinks (additives, flavorings)	Fresh or frozen juices
Sweets Sweeteners Flavoring Spices Baking aids	Artificial flavors	Pure flavors, distilled or labeled GF
	Artificial colors	Pure colors or labeled GF
	Candy	GF candy
	Caramel coloring—foreign brands	Caramel (U.S. brands made from corn)
	Confectioners' sugar (flour, cornstarch)	GF confectioners' sugar
	Commercial cake decorations	GF cake decorations
	Syrup (unless GF)	GF rice syrup
	Seasonings may have wheat	Pure seasoning or labeled GF
	Spice mixes (may have wheat)	Single spices usually are pure
	Nutritional yeast (may contain gluten), Brewer's yeast	Yeast (Baker's, Autolyzed)

CATEGORY	SOURCES OF GLUTEN	GLUTEN-FREE (GF) SUBSTITUTES
Condiments Sauces	Soy sauce	Wheat-free tamari soy sauce
	Worcestershire sauce	Lea & Perrin
	Ketchup, mustard, mayonnaise	GFCF ketchup, mustard, mayo
	Flavored vinegar, malt vinegar	Distilled vinegar
	Yogurts and yogurt drinks with thickeners	Organic/natural yogurts/drinks w/o thickeners
	Processed cheeses	Natural and organic cheeses
Additives	Dextrin (foreign brands)	Dextrin (U.S. brands made from corn)
	Monosodium glutamate (MSG)	No MSG of any kind
	Citric acid	Citric acid if GF (corn)
	Hydrolyzed plant protein (if wheat)	HVP if nongluten TVP (soy)
	Modified food starch can be wheat	Starch on food labels (means corn)
	Malt (barley)—assume "malt" means barley	Corn malt (must be labeled as such)
Foods	Canned soups, bouillon cubes, or powdered broth	Homemade GF soups, broths
	Deli meats, sausages, hot dogs	Fresh meat, poultry, fish, eggs
	Flavored yogurts, malted milk	Pure milk products (if not intolerant)
	Imitation seafood and bacon	Fresh or frozen seafood and GF, casein-free (CF) bacon
	Processed cheese spreads	Natural cheeses (if not reactive)
	Pudding, marshmallow cream	100% natural oils, fats
	Stuffing mixes, breading	GF breading, stuffing
Other	Chewing gum	
	Glues—stamps, envelopes, stickers	
	Nutritional supplements (binders, fillers)	
	Play-Doh	GF Play Dough Recipe (page 112)
	School glue	
	Nutritional supplements with alcohol if from a grain alcohol. (Note: even if alcohol is "burnt" off, grain residues will remain.)	

Milk Products and Casein: Little Miss Muffet Was Wrong!

WHAT AND WHERE ARE THEY?

Mammal milk (human, cow, goat) has many components, including water, fats, protein, lactose, minerals, acids, enzymes, gases, and vitamins. Milk products include milk (from nonfat to whole), buttermilk, evaporated milk, yogurt, kefir, cream cheese, sour cream, cream sauces, cream dressings, ice cream, sherbet, cheese, curds, cottage cheese, whey, butter, and any food that contains any one of these products.

Milk products are hidden in many unexpected places, including canned tuna, nondairy creamers, whipped toppings, salad dressing, bakery glazes, breath mints, fortified cereals, high-protein beverage powders, infant formulas, nutrition bars, processed meats, and nutritional supplements. Remember the mantra "Read the label." Avoid products with the following ingredients: milk solids, lactose, galactose, lactalbumin, lactoglobulin, casein, and caseinate.

The Case Against Casein

Casein, which accounts for 75 percent of the proteins in milk, is a major culprit in ADHD- or autism-related food sensitivities. It is found in all milk products, with the exception of properly clarified butter, also known as ghee, in which the milk solids have been removed. Dairy-free or milk-free does not mean casein-free. Even nondairy cheese substitutes from soy, almonds, or rice may have casein to improve the texture. Casein is commonly used in meat products such as deli meats, salami, sausage, hot dogs, and pepperoni, and caseinate is a common component in nutritional supplements.

What about Casein in Breast Milk?

Human casein proteins are different from the casein proteins in cow's or goat's milk. The alignment of the amino acids is different. Therefore, the negative effects from casein do not occur with breast-feeding. Breast-feeding is considered a protective factor in autism.

Weighing in on Whey

Whey is the serum, or watery, part of milk that is separated when milk protein/casein coagulates to become curd in the making of cheese. Whey is primarily lactose and soluble proteins. (There are pure forms of lactose-free whey.) Little Miss Muffet's curds and whey are known as cottage cheese. The lumps are the curds (cheese, casein) and the whey is the lactose-containing liquid. Unless the whey is pure and clearly stated as casein-free on the label, it is still to be avoided on the casein-free diet.

WHAT IS LEFT TO EAT?

Substitutes for milk products include rice milk; soy milk; soy yogurt; potato milk; quinoa milk; and nut milks made from almonds, brazil nuts, cashews, coconut, hazelnuts, macadamias, pecans, pine nuts, pumpkin seeds, sesame seeds, sunflower seeds, and walnuts.

MILK PRODUCTS

Animal milk	Cream	Powdered milk
Butter	Curds	Rennet
Buttermilk	Evaporated milk	Sherbet
Cheese—all	Half-and-half	Sour cream
Condensed milk	Ice cream, ice milk	Whey
Cottage cheese	Kefir	Yogurt
Cream cheese	Nougat	

Read Labels & Avoid

Lactobacillus if not dairy-free (DF)	Hydrolyzed milk protein	Lactoglobulin
Casein	Hydrolyzed vegetable protein	Lactose
Calcium caseinate	Lactalbumins	Magnesium caseinate
Caseinate	Lactate	Potassium caseinate
Galactose	Lactic acid	

Non-Food Sources

Cosmetics

Pharmaceuticals (lactose)

Nutritional supplements

Ingredients which sound like they contain milk products but do not contain them:

- Calcium lactate
- Calciums stearoyl lactylate
- Cocoa butter
- Cream of tartar
- Lactic acid
- Oleoresin
- Sodium lactate
- Sodium stearoyl lactylate

BUYER BEWARE – READ THE LABEL – CONTACT THE MANUFACTURER

For products manufactured on or after January 2006, manufacturers are required to declare in the ingredient list the name of any major food allergen that is contained in the product or product spices, flavorings, additives, and colorings.:

- Milk
- Wheat
- Eggs
- Fish (must list specific kind)
- Crustacean shellfish (specific kind crab, lobster, shrimp
- Tree nuts (specific kind almond, pecan, walnut)
- Peanuts
- Soy

If in doubt – find out. Contact the manufacturer.

FOOD SOURCES OF MILK PRODUCTS

Not all listed items will contain milk products—read labels!

Baked Goods

Biscuits, breads, cakes, cookies

Caramel coloring

Doughnuts, pastries

Mixes for baked goods

Pancakes, waffles

Pie crust

Soda crackers, Zwieback

Beverages

Chocolate milk

Cocoa

Malt, malted milk

Ovaltine, chocolate sodas

Sweets

Creams in anything

Custards, puddings

Ice cream, sherbet, gelato

Milk chocolate

Sorbet (not all)

Spumoni

Sauces, Fats, Oils

Butter-fried foods

Cream sauce

Gravies

Margarine

Mayonnaise (some brands)

Salad dressing (some)

Meat/Fish Proteins

Bisques, chowders

Cheese—dairy-free (some have casein)

Creamed foods

Cream soup bases

Deli turkey

Egg dishes—omelets, scrambled eggs, soufflés, casseroles

Processed meats, sausage, hot dogs

Tuna fish (canned)

MILK-PRODUCT SUBSTITUTES

Beware: "dairy-free" does not necessarily mean "casein-free."

Milks/Yogurts

Coconut milk

Coconut Keifer and Yogurt

Hemp milk

Nut milks (almond)

Potato milk

Rice milk

Soy milk

Soy yogurt

Tofu products

Chocolate

GFCF chocolate chips

GFCF semisweet chocolate chips

Ice Cream

Vance's DariFree milk Fruit Popsicles

Sorbets by Haagen-Dazs and Ben & Jerry's

Italian ice

Soy ice and soy ice cream

Tofutti

Buttermilk Substitute

In recipes

1 cup (235 ml) buttermilk equivalent:

2 tablespoons (28 ml) lemon juice in

1 cup (235 ml) milk substitute

Butter

Coconut oil/butter

Earth Balance Whipped Spread (GFCF, no trans-fats)

Ghee (clarified butter— has no casein)

Lard—excellent in baked goods

Kosher items— only pareve

Applesauce can substitute for both milk and butter in mashed potatoes

For a complete listing of all combined GFCF foods, see www.gfcfdiet.com/unacceptable.htm http://freelivingfoods.com/download/list_of_ unacceptable_ingredients.pdf

Fermented Beverages

Julie Matthews (NourishingHope.com) in her *Cooking to Heal* workbook and recipes, emphasizes the importance of fermented foods in achieving excellent digestive and systemic health. Homemade fermented foods, such as yogurt (dairy and non-dairy), kefir, raw sauerkraut, and kombucha (sweetened tea) are abundant with probiotics, a.k.a., the "good" bacteria. Whereas typical probiotic supplements may have 3 to 75 billion as a count, one cup of homemade yogurt has 700 billion per cup. It is important to note that for those who are casein-free/milk-free—animal milk fermented products are to be avoided.

For these purposes, only consume fermented products that are not from animal milk origins.

Anyone with maldigestion, malabsorption, bowel inflammation, and/or impaired digestive flora (dysbiosis) will benefit from high-quality probiotics. They work in the GI tract to regulate bowel function, improve digestion, improve digestive immunity, maintain a stable acid/alkaline balance, break down bile acids, recolonize after antibiotics are given, and produce necessary fatty acids and vitamins, especially biotin. In infants, they prevent colic, diaper rash, and gas. With probiotic use, there is a reduction in allergies, asthma, and eczema in children.

Coconut: The Wonder Food

- Though considered a nut, the coconut is actually a seed.
- Coconut water, the liquid inside the coconut, is a healthy electrolyte drink that is rich in nutrients.
- Coconut milk is made from the coconut "flesh." When chilled, the "cream" and "milk" separate and are useful substitutes for animal source milk products.
- Coconut milk can be fermented into coconut kefir and yogurt, which are abundant in the good probiotics for the digestive tract.
- Coconuts, and the cream, milk, kefir, and yogurt made from the coconut, are health foods. They are helpful in promoting good immunity and alleviating digestive disorders such as gas, indigestion, diarrhea, vomiting, colitis, and ulcers.
- Coconut oil fatty acids do not raise cholesterol or contribute to heart disease. Fifty percent of the coconut oil fatty acids are lauric acid, which has antibacterial, antiviral, and antiprotozoal qualities.

Soy Sorry!

Soy has not been a common food in the American diet until recently. Soy foods include edamame (the immature soy bean harvested while still green and sweet) and fermented products such as miso, natto, tamari/soy sauce, tempeh, tofu, and yuba.

Soy is found in hydrolysed vegetable protein (HVP), lecithin, mono and diglycerides, monosodium glutamate (MSG), and vitamin E products (most all of which are soy-based). It may also be used in baked goods, canned tuna, cereals, infant formulas, margarine, mayonnaise, sauces, soups, vegetable broth, vegetable protein substitutes and vegetable oils.

There is much controversy over soy and its suitability in the human diet. While other beans can be eaten if cooked properly, soybeans require fermentation due to the presence of natural toxins that can deplete or interfere with specific nutrients.

The processing of soy to render it acceptable as a food requires exposure to high heat and chemicals. Today, some soy is also genetically modified. Nongenetically modified sources are preferred and available. Soy remains a common allergen and is also not easily tolerated by many individuals. Like gluten and casein, it can also partially digest to form opiate-like peptides. The testing for this isn't reliable, therefore the best testing is trial and response.

For those who are not allergic to soy and are able to tolerate it easily, the best soy sources are organic and include edamame and the naturally fermented soy products such as tempeh, natto, miso, soy sauce, tofu and yuba.

SOY PRODUCTS

Read labels for soy and soy by-products

Soy bean oil, flour, milk	Tamari
Edamame	Tempeh
Miso	Tempura
Natto	Tofu
Sprouts (soy)	Yuba

Other

Lecithin	MSG
HVP	Vitamin E
Mono- and diglycerides	

FOOD SOURCES OF SOY

Baked Goods

Baking mixes, flours	Crackers
Bread, cakes, cereals	Pasta, pastries, rolls

Meats/Others

Baby foods	Luncheon/deli meats
Cheese substitutes	Sausage (not all)

Oils/Fats

Butter substitutes	Shortening
Oil, margarine	

Beverages

Coffee substitutes	Infant formulas
Soy milk	

Condiments

Butter substitutes	Nut mixes
Salad dressing, sauces, soy sauce	Vegetable broth
	Worcestershire sauce

Sweets

Candy and candy bars	Ice cream—Tofutti
Caramel, custard	

Soy substitutes are the same as those listed earlier as gluten and milk substitutes (with the exception of those containing soy).

Eggs, Corn, and Nuts

Allergies or intolerances to these foods can occur. When casein, gluten, and soy are eliminated, consumption of foods containing eggs, corn, or nuts often increases in order to replace those foods that were eliminated. In some children, reactions to the increase in these foods may then appear.

EGGS

It is not always obvious that a product contains egg. Be aware that the following words on a label mean the product contains egg or egg by-products: albumen, globulin, vitellin, livetin, ovoglobulin, ovamucin, ovamucoid, ovovitellin, ovovitelia, and lysozyme. See the chart below for a thorough listing.

EGG PRODUCTS

Read labels for eggs and egg by-products

Egg whites, yolks	Ovamucin
Egg powder	Ovamucoid
Albumen, globulin	Ovovitellin
Vitellin, livetin	Ovovitelia
Ovoglobulin	Lysozyme

Nonfood Sources

Vaccines—those cultured in chicken eggs

FOOD SOURCES OF EGG

Not all of these products contain eggs. The egg source may not be obvious.

Baked Goods

Baking powder	French toast
Breading	Pastries
Breads, rolls, biscuits	Pancake/waffle mixes
Cake flour	Pastas
Cookies, doughnuts	Pie crusts and fillings

Beverages

Eggnog	Ovaltine

Sweets/Sweeteners/Flavoring

Protein powders	Marshmallows
Gelatin desserts	Meringues, macaroons
Frosting, icing, glazes	Puddings, pie fillings, soufflés
Ice cream, ices, sherbets	

Condiments/Sauces/Oils

Mayonnaise	Salad dressing
Hollandaise	Tartar sauce

Other Foods

Bouillon	Sausage, pâté
Meatballs, loafs, patties	Soup

SUBSTITUTES FOR 1 EGG

2 tablespoons (16 g) cornstarch

2 tablespoons (16 g) arrowroot flour

2 tablespoons (20 g) potato starch

1 tablespoon (8 g) soy milk powder

1 banana (good in cakes)

$1/4$ cup (62 g) tofu

Unflavored Gelatin:
Mix 1 envelope (1 tablespoon, or 7 g) in
1 cup (235 ml) boiling water.
3 tablespoons (45 ml) = 1 egg

Baby food (pureed apples or pears):
3 tablespoons (45 g) = 1 egg

CORN

Corn is one of the most common food allergens for children and adults in the United States, and it is also one of the most difficult to avoid. It is inexpensive and versatile and therefore abundant in processed foods.

CORN PRODUCTS

Read labels for corn and corn by-products

Cornstarch, cornmeal, flour	Fructose
Corn chips, popcorn	High-fructose corn syrup
Maize	Lecithin
Corn syrup	Maltodextrin
Corn oil	MSG
Dextrin	Salt (commercial)
Dextrose	Succotash
Glucose	Thickeners
Fruit pectin	Vegetable starch

Nonfood Sources

Aspirin	Laundry starch	Paper plates
Capsules	Livestock feed	Suppositories tablet (most)
Chalk	Medicines	
Cosmetics	Nutritional supplements (some)	Talcum powder
Glues: stamps, envelopes, stickers		Toothpaste
	Paper cups	

FOOD SOURCES OF CORN

Not all these products contain corn. However, most processed and prepared foods contain corn unless labeled "corn-free."

Beverages

Alcohol: distilled, ale, beer, bourbon, cordials, liqueurs, wine coolers

Coffee: instant, "designer"

Infant/toddler formulas

Fruit-juice "cocktails" (not 100% juice)

Soy milk

Ice cream, sherbets, sorbets

Milk in paper cartons

Sodas, soft drinks

Sweetened condensed milk

Sweetened/flavored drinks

Sweets/Sweeteners/Flavoring

Artificial sweeteners

Candy (almost all)

Caramel

Chewing gum

Custards, puddings

Flavoring extracts

Frosting, icings

Gelatin desserts

High-fructose corn syrup

Ice creams, sherbets, sorbets

Jams, jellies

Marshmallows

Powdered sugar

Sorbitol

Syrups/corn syrup

Gelatin desserts

Vanilla extract

Vinegar (distilled)

Yogurts (sweetened)

Baked Goods

Baking powder (most)

Breads, rolls, biscuits

Cakes

Cereals (prepared)

Doughnuts

Graham crackers

Grits, hominy

Pancake/ waffle mixes

Pastries, pies

Tortillas

Vegetable starch

Xanthan gum

Condiments/Sauces/Oils

Gravies, sauces

Ketchup, chili sauce

Margarine

Mayonnaise

Mustards

Salad dressings

Steak sauce, tartar sauce

Other Foods

Bacon (most)

Bean sprouts

Canned foods (almost all)

Cheese spreads, cheese foods

Coffee "creamer"

Dehydrated soups

Eggs: frozen, dried

Fried foods (in corn oil)

Meats—cured, processed

Oriental foods

Peanut butter (sweetened)

Pickles (sweetened)

NUTS

Of the nuts, the peanut, which is technically a legume, is the most common allergen. Allergic reactions to peanuts are considered the most common cause of anaphylaxis-related deaths in the United States. Identifying obvious sources of nuts is not difficult. It is more difficult to identify nut additives. It is even more challenging to determine which products have trace amounts, especially when not on the label. Cross-contamination occurs when nut parts or dust contaminate other foods during the manufacturing process. Nut oils should not contain nut protein, in theory, but this depends on the manufacturing process. The degree of allergy or sensitivity is the determining factor. Careful label reading is a must. See the following charts for help.

KINDS OF NUTS

Almonds	Macadamia nuts
Brazil nuts	Peanuts (legume)
Cashews	Pecans
Coconuts	Pine nuts
Filberts	Pistachios
Hazelnuts	Walnuts
Hickory nuts	Black walnuts

PRODUCTS CONTAINING NUTS

These are nut products and foods commonly made with nuts.

Amaretto	Mixed nuts
Artificially flavored nuts	Nu-Nuts
Beer nuts	Nut butters, meal, pastes
Bitter almond	
Gianduja	Nut oils, flavorings, syrups
Gingko	Peanutamide
Ground nuts	Pesto
Loramine wax	Pignolia
Mandelonas	Pralines
Marzipan	

NUT-CONTAMINATED PRODUCTS

These are foods that may contain nuts or be cross-contaminated with nuts.

Baked goods	Frozen desserts
Baking mixes	Graham-cracker crusts
Barbeque sauce	HPP, HVP
Batter-dipped foods	Ice cream
Bulk bin foods	Margarine
Candy	Milk formula
Cereals	Nougat
Chili	Oriental sauce
Cookies	Pastry
Dessert toppings	Pie crusts
Egg rolls	Sauces
Emulsifier	Vegetable fat
Flavoring	Vegetable oil

"Don't be afraid to take a big step if one is indicated.
You can't cross a chasm in two small jumps."
—David Lloyd George

CHAPTER 3

More Culprits

Maintaining his special diet is very difficult,
but not nearly as hard as living with a severely autistic child.

—Mother of a recovering autistic son

"MY SON HAD BEEN ON THE SPECIFIC CARBOHYDRATE DIET (SCD) for about a year, which means he couldn't (and still can't) have any starch, sucrose or lactose. After exploring the Air and Space Museum, we went into the food court and I unpacked the turkey burgers and almond cookies I'd made and brought along. Unfortunately, eating with hundreds of other people who didn't bring their own picnic means my son had to watch while all the other kids ate one of his favorite forbidden foods: French fries. Instead of going through the whole explanation of why he couldn't have them, when he asked, I let him have some. In my defense, after a year on the SCD, you're allowed to start slowly adding previously restricted foods back in to see how they're tolerated. But impulsively giving him both potatoes and probably gluten (I doubt they fry battered food in separate oil from the oil in which they fry French fries in the food court) at the same time didn't make sense. After thinking it through, I realized the reason for my lapse: I was mad that my son was deprived of something that most kids can eat. And as a parent, I felt deprived of having a kid who could not have something that most kids get to have. Apparently, this is normal."

—KATHRYN SCOTT *in "Flirting with Disaster," published in* Living Without, *Spring 2006*

Disaccharidase Deficiency and the Specific Carbohydrate Diet (SCD)

As previously discussed, many children with ADHD and autism have damage in their intestinal tracts. When the cells that produce digestive enzymes are damaged, fewer enzymes will be available for digestion. This occurs in the small intestine, where over 90 percent of digestion and absorption occurs. We have discussed the digestive problems resulting from gluten and milk products, but they are not the only culprits.

The SCD diet was developed by Sydney Haas and is described in the book by Elaine Gotschall, *Breaking the Vicious Cycle—Intestinal Health Through Diet*. It distinguishes between the two basic kinds of carbohydrates:

- Simple, monosaccharide sugars, including fructose, glucose, and galactose
- Double-sugar disaccharides, including lactose, sucrose, maltose, and isomaltose

Most people are familiar with lactose intolerance due to poor or no production of the enzyme lactase, which digests lactose from milk. When other disaccharide-digesting enzymes are missing, the symptoms and damage become more severe.

SCD is based on the principle that simple carbohydrates (monosaccharides) require minimal digestion, are well absorbed, and leave no undigested residues. The complex double-sugar carbohydrates (disaccharides) are hard to digest, especially for those who have damaged intestines and inadequate digestive enzymes. The residues of the undigested double sugars become food for intestinal "bad bugs" and yeast, resulting in a "cesspool" within the gut. This leads to digestive distress, including gas, bloating, cramps, abnormal stools, constipation, and diarrhea. The result is poor absorption of nutrients. Disaccharide intolerance is common in many bowel conditions, including Crohn's disease, colitis, inflammatory bowel conditions, and irritable bowel syndrome.

By avoiding the disaccharide carbohydrates, the bad bugs and their harmful by-products starve and decrease while the good bugs thrive and increase. The intestinal lining heals, digestion and nutrient absorption improve, and overall health benefits.

The only carbohydrates allowed in the SCD are the simple sugars. Acceptable foods include honey, most vegetables, most fruits, and noncarbohydrates such as fats, oils, meats, eggs, fish, poultry, some hard cheeses, some legumes, and well-fermented yogurt. The foods to avoid include sugars; canned vegetables and fruits; all grains; breads; pastas and other starchy foods; processed, canned meats; and milk and most milk products, especially those with lactose. See the chart on the pages that follow for a more thorough listing.

The diet is kept as natural as possible, since sugars and starches are added to most processed foods. Just as with the GFCF diet, the more strict the diet, the better the results. However, there are differences between the GFCF diet and SCD diet.

Foods approved for GFCF diet, but not for the SCD:

- Grains: corn, rice, buckwheat, millet, quinoa, tapioca
- Starchy vegetables and some beans
- Double sugars (disacccharides): lactose, sucrose, maltose, isomaltose

Foods approved for the SCD, but not on the GFCF diet:

- Lactose-free cheeses
- Well-fermented yogurt

In addition to the diet, specific carbohydrate-digesting enzymes are prescribed in order to reduce the symptoms from minor infractions. The enzymes, however, cannot make up for not following the diet.

SCD is a difficult diet to do in combination with a GFCF diet. We generally reserve this diet for children who have intestinal yeast overgrowth that has been difficult to eradicate or who have chronic intestinal issues unresponsive to other treatments. This diet is also worth considering in children with autism who continue to have behavioral and developmental symptoms in spite of having pursued other treatments. Parents are often best at deciding if or when it is feasible to consider this diet, given the additional restrictions beyond the GFCF diet.

There is also an expansion of the SCD called Gut and Psychology Syndrome (GAPS). Although the SCD is diet only, GAPS includes an expanded SCD (removal of milk casein) in addition to detoxification and supplementation. GAPS also emphasizes the importance of including homemade broths and fermented vegetables.

For further information:

- *Breaking the Vicious Cycle* by Elaine Gottschall
  Web site: www.breakingtheviciouscycle.info
- *Breaking the Vicious Cycle List, Modified*
  Web site: www.scdiet.org
- Gut and Psychology Syndrome (GAPS)
  Web site: www.gapsdiet.org

"My son, Robb, is on a gluten-free casein-free diet as well as the Specific Carbohydrate Diet. Although I saw nice improvements after several months on the GFCF diet, there was a remarkable change for him THE NEXT DAY after he started the SCD diet. He practically bounced out of bed and ran into our room—MUCH more energy."

—Mother of Robb,
a six-year-old with autism and Down syndrome

THE SPECIFIC CARBOHYDRATE DIET

DOUBLE SUGAR	SOURCES	BREAKS DOWN TO	MISSING ENZYMES =DISACCHARIDASES
Lactose	Milk products	Glucose and galactose	Lactase
Sucrose	Sugars	Glucose and fructose	Sucrase
Maltose	Starch	Glucose and glucose	Maltase
Isomaltose	Starch	Glucose and glucose	Isomaltase

CATEGORY	AVOID	INCLUDE
Protein Animal		Poultry, meat, seafood
	Preserved meats	Gelatin: unflavored
	Processed meats	Eggs
	Canned meats & seafood	Yogurt: well-fermented, homemade
	Flavored gelatin	Dry curd cottage cheese
	Milk products (most)	Hard cheeses
Protein Vegetable	Bean sprouts, pinto, cannellini	String beans, lima beans
	Chick peas, fava, soy, mung	Almonds, –brazil, chestnuts, coconut, filbertshazelnuts, pecans, pistachios, walnuts
	Processed nuts	Nut butters (w/o sugar added)
	Flours from beans, nuts, seeds	

THE SPECIFIC CARBOHYDRATE DIET

CATEGORY	AVOID	INCLUDE
Vegetables Fresh or frozen May need to cook or steam these	Canned vegetables Artichoke (Jerusalem) Butter beans Garlic and onion powder Potato, sweet potato, yams Parsnips Water chestnuts	Artichoke, asparagus, beets, carrots, Celery, cucumbers, garlic, eggplant, Kale, lettuce, mushroom, olive, parsley, Pumpkin, rhubarb, spinach, squash, string beans Tomato, turnips, watercress, zucchini.
Fruits	Canned in syrup Dried fruits! Plantains	May need to use fruit sauces or steamed, baked fruits. Apples, apple cider, applesauce w/o sugar Avocado, apricot, banana, berries, cherries, citrus Dates, grapes, peaches, pears, tropical fruits, Fruit sauces w/o sugar (apple, pear)
Grains	All grains to be avoided	Nut flours Spaghetti squash

> "I feel alive. I am no longer tired. Being sick made me tired. I can walk more. I no longer stare inappropriately at other people. I now make eye contact with other people. I like looking at other people."
>
> —Ashley Stilson

CATEGORY	AVOID	INCLUDE
Sugar	All artificial sweeteners	Some honey
	Candy, carob, chocolate	Stevia
	Corn syrup, HFCS, dates	.
	Maple syrup, molasses, Succanat,	
	Sugar alcohols, sucralose	
Other	Gums: guar, xanthum	Cellulose
	Fried foods	Homemade mayo
	Mayonnaise, margarine	Oils: avocado, canola, coconut, olive, safflower
	Oils: corn, soy	Ketchup homemade
	Commercial ketchup	Balsamic homemade, vinegar
	Soy sauce, Tamari	Pickles, Olives
	Balsalmic vinegar (commercial)	
Beverages	Sodas, fruit punch,	Water, weak coffee, herb teas
	V8 juice, V8 fusion	Weak tea. Weak coffee
	Frozen fruit juice, apple juice	Dilute pure juice (1/3 juice)
	Soy milk,	Nut milks
	Alcohol (most)	Splash of 100% juice to flavor items, apple cider

Yeast/Candida

Intestinal yeast overgrowth is a potential problem in children with ADHD or autism. The digestive tract normally contains multi-trillions of bacteria and a small amount of yeast. This balance is important, as these bacteria are beneficial to the intestine—they produce nutrient factors that keep the intestine healthy. They also, by their sheer numbers, prevent yeast from multiplying and occupying more of the intestine. Yeast overgrowth most commonly occurs after antibiotic use.

Antibiotics, as they pass through the intestine, kill off these good bacteria. This allows an increase in yeast. Yeast overgrowth can also occur when children or adults eat diets low in fiber, since fiber is an important food source for the intestinal bacteria. Yeast releases toxic chemicals. These toxins irritate the intestinal lining and can contribute to a leaky gut (as explained in chapter 1). When there is a leaky gut, these yeast toxins can enter the bloodstream. These toxins can then affect brain functioning.

In our experience, many children respond well to treatment of yeast overgrowth. Treatment includes restocking the intestine with these helpful bacteria (called probiotics) and killing yeast with either natural supplements or medications. There is debate about whether yeast-free diets are also needed when children have yeast overgrowth. We do focus on limiting/avoiding sugars, and we promote healthy foods—both of which are antiyeast. It is important to note that yeast overgrowth occurs because yeast organisms are opportunistic and thrive in an unhealthy environment. Therefore, it is our preference to get the intestine back into a good state of balance so that the yeast has no place to "set up housekeeping" rather than eliminating yet another group of foods. One diet that addresses this issue is the Body Ecology Diet (BED) which utilizes easily digested foods, fermented foods, and the concept of food combining. BED also emphasizes low-acid forming foods and the restriction of sugars and starches. There is a subset of children whose yeast overgrowth seems resistant to treatment; in these cases, a trial of a yeast-free diet or the SCD may be indicated.

Gut Flora and Probiotics

Some important facts about probiotics and the health of your child's gut flora.

- The human body contains about 10 trillion cells, yet the digestive tract has ten times that number of microorganisms, known as gut flora or intestinal microbiotia.

- There are over 500 different bacterial species which make up 60 percent of the dry mass of feces.

- Ninety percent of the bacteria come from 40 to 60 species.

- Because of all the metabolic activity performed by these bacterial, the gut bacteria are known as the "forgotten organ."

- The gut flora have a continuous and profound effect on gut and systemic immunity and inflammation.

- Gut flora protect against overgrowth of pathogenic yeasts and bacteria, metabolize harmful oxalates, and are depleted by antibiotics.

- Dietary sources of good flora come from fermented foods such as homemade yogurt, kefir, kombucha (sweetened mushroom tea) and raw sauerkraut, which have a much higher count than supplements.

- Probiotic supplements may contain millions to 100 billion "good" bacteria, which is not nearly as much as the 500 billion or more possible in naturally fermented foods.

- Children who have a history of a lack of breast milk and repeated antibiotic use are at high risk for intestinal flora destruction and a resulting increase in bowel problems, including inflammatory bowel disorders.

Salicylate Intolerance and The Feingold Diet

The Feingold Diet was established by Benjamin Feingold, MD, a pediatrician and allergist who had observed the effects of salicylate foods and medications on child behavior. Salicylates appear in high levels in aspirin and many over-the-counter and prescription medications. Salicylates also appear naturally in foods and plants and at low levels in some flavoring agents and food preservatives.

Studies indicate that from 10 to 25 percent of all children may be sensitive to salicylates. There are also other conditions linked to salicylate exposures, including asthma and allergic urticaria (hives).

The biochemical explanation behind what Dr. Feingold observed is now better understood. Not all individuals are negatively affected by salicylates. It affects those who are predisposed and have intolerances based on inefficient enzyme functions. Please see the explanation of phenol intolerances and phenol sulfotransferase (PST) deficiency that follows.

The "avoids" list for PST deficiency is very close to the "avoids" list for salicylates.

Stage I of the Feingold program involves eliminating synthetic dyes, artificial flavors, and specific preservatives entirely. It also involves removing naturally occurring salicylates from the diet until a favorable response is seen. In Stage II, some of the fruits and vegetables are reintroduced, according to the level of tolerance. The synthetic and medicinal sources continue to be avoided. The success of the diet will depend on the degree of a person's sensitivity to salicylates and the amount of exposure.

For further information, visit www.feingold.org.

Phenol Intolerance— Phenol Sulfotransferase (PST) Deficiency

To understand the problems with phenols and PST, it is important to have a basic understanding of enzyme functions and metabolism.

Body enzymes are necessary for our body systems to work well. When enzymes function, metabolites or by-products occur. Metabolites are normal, but too many or too few metabolites occur when there are problems in enzyme functions. Children with ADHD and, even more so, children with autism have many inefficiencies in metabolic enzyme functions and deficiencies in nutrients (vitamins, minerals, amino acids, Coenzyme Q10, and glutathione). Children with autism have more profound and more complex inefficiencies and deficiencies.

Enzymes depend on one or more nutrients to function properly. When the enzymes are "lazy" or there is a deficiency in the nutrients the enzymes require, logjams occur. Metabolites that result from normal metabolic pathways back up when enzymes are inefficient, just as traffic in a city backs up when a four-lane bridge becomes a two-lane bridge. The "traffic" metabolites start causing problems on other "roads," or enzyme pathways. When the inefficiency of the enzymes gets worse, the backup gets worse and gridlock can occur. In the city, the solution includes reducing the traffic and repairing the bridge. In the body, the solution includes reducing the substances that must use certain enzymes and providing the nutrients to make the enzymes work better.

Phenols, meanwhile, are widely available, naturally occurring compounds found mostly in fruits, vegetables, some grains and nuts, flavorings, and spices. Phenols have antioxidant qualities and protective functions, so some are beneficial and good to consume for most individuals.

The enzyme PST is an important part of detoxification pathways, which remove from the body toxins resulting from internal sources (metabolism) and from external sources (environmental chemicals, certain additives in foods). When the enzyme is deficient, foods, toxins, and chemicals that are higher in phenols are not well tolerated by these lazy, deficient enzymes, and the metabolite traffic backs up, causing symptoms of agitation and hyperactivity. Remember, the phenols are *beneficial* to the system; it is the PST deficiency that is the problem. Artificial coloring and flavoring are the most significant load on the PST system, but high-salicylate foods are significant too. Salicylates are a type of phenol (however, not all phenols are salicylates). High-phenol foods include apples, tomatoes, oranges, cocoa, red grapes, colored fruits, and cow's milk. Bananas may also be a problem. While it is not clear if they contain phenols, they contain tyramine which can cause headaches and fatigue. Pears are low in phenols, which may be the reason why they are so well tolerated by most people. Environmental chemicals and toxins, especially petroleum by-products, also weigh heavily on the PST system.

The following symptoms may suggest that your child has a phenol sensitivity:

- Known food/chemical intolerance or unusual sensitivity to medications
- Disrupted sleep; unusual laughter when waking in the night
- Regressive behavior after eating food/juice containing artificial colors
- Self-injurious actions perhaps related to headaches
- High consumption of apple juice (or other high-salicylate juices) and high-phenol foods (apples, red grapes, etc.)
- Large variations in functioning ability
- Anger and/or aggression
- Hyperactivity
- Unexplained periodic red ears or red cheeks
- Night sweating
- Wetting the bed

There are laboratory tests, but consider giving a challenge test. This challenge is best done when your child is home all day with you and not in school or involved in other activities. Kelly Dorfman, cofounder of Developmental Delay Resources, suggests giving your child a few chewy fruit snacks or a glass of sugary fruit punch and then observing the reaction.

The solution to curbing phenol sensitivity is to "open up the flow of traffic" by improving PST function and decreasing the load from the environment, additives, and food sources. Add to the diet nutrients that help improve PST function: magnesium, vitamin B6 (but not B6 alone), vitamin C, vitamin E, glutathione, and N-acetyl cysteine. Provide a source of sulfate to help the PST enzyme, thereby improving the handling of phenols in food. One such source is Epsom salts, which consist of magnesium and sulfate and can be added to bathwater. Reduce the burden by avoiding artificial additives, dyes, and coloring, as well as environmental toxins. However, be aware that restricting phenol foods is difficult because they are so widely distributed in the diet. The most common high-phenol foods kids eat are apples and red grapes. See the chart in this chapter for a short list of phenol sources.

PHENOL COMPOUNDS

The medications and synthetic dyes, colorings, flavorings, and additives are a significant problem.

ADDITIVES IN FOODS, CLEANING SUPPLIES, TOILETRIES, ART SUPPLIES	MEDICATIONS	FOODS WITH HIGH PHENOLS/SALICYLATES	
Synthetic/artificial colors: FD&C colors	Aspirin	Almonds	Oranges
Synthetic/artificial flavors: Vanillin	Salicylic acid	Apples	Paprika
Petroleum derivatives: BHA, BHT, TBHQ	Products that contain aspirin or salicylic acid	Apricots	Peaches
Natural flavorings (may contain phenol)		Berries	Peppers (bell, chili)
Salicylate		Cherries	Pickles
MSG		Chili powder	Plums
Hydrolyzed Vegetable Protein		Cider	Prunes
Sulfites		Cider vinegar	Raisins
Benzoates		Cloves	Tangerines
Perfumes		Coffee	Tea
Nitrites, nitrates		Cucumbers	Tomatoes
Corn syrup (made from hydrogen sulfide and cornstarch)		Currants	Wine
		Red grapes	Wine vinegar
		Nectarines	
		Oil of wintergreen	

"Ethan continues to improve. In the past week he has started to ask questions, which is the next step to being able to hold a conversation. I never thought I would be happy to hear 'why?' and 'why not?'"

—**Bea Wolman,** *mother of four-year-old Ethan*

Oxalates and the Low Oxalate Diet (LOD)

Oxalates are abundant in seeds and nuts and many plants and fruits. In a healthy digestive tract, oxalates are not absorbed and are either metabolized by the flora or eliminated via the stool. In damaged digestive tracts that have increased permeability (leaky gut), however, oxalates can be absorbed abundantly.

Eating high oxalate foods is one way to increase oxalates in the body, especially if there is depletion of good flora in the gut; however the body also makes oxalates when enzymes are imbalanced. The oxalate molecules link up with calcium and then crystallize, especially in damaged tissues. The crystals are painful to the tissues where they form and they increase inflammation in the digestive tract.

The authors do not recommend the low oxalate diet as a first-line diet. By focusing on clearing up the digestive issues, the oxalate problem should be resolved. However, it may be worth considering if other diets have been tried—such as the GFCF diet and/or the SCD—and there are still symptoms. Situations in which a trial of this diet may be considered include: GI or other pain soon after eating, persistent gastrointestinal symptoms (constipation, diarrhea or gas), or urinary symptoms. For more about the diet, refer to the Resources section.

HIGH OXALATE FOODS TO BE AVOIDED

LEGUMES, NUTS, AND SEEDS	GRAINS	VEGETABLES	FRUITS	OTHERS
Beans, green, waxed, dried	Bread, whole wheat	Beets	Blackberries	Chocolate, plain
Baked beans in tomato sauce	Cheerios	Celery	Blueberries	Cocoa, dry powder
Nuts	Graham crackers	Eggplant	Grapes, Concord	Ovaltine, powder
Peanuts	Graham flour	Escarole	Currants, red	Fig Newtons
Pecans	Grits, white corn	Green leafies	Dewberries	Fruitcake (1 slice)
Garbanzo beans, canned	Kamut	Leeks	Figs, dried	Marmalade
Peanut butter	Oatmeal	Okra	Gooseberries	Beer
Sesame seeds	Popcorn	Peppers, green	Kiwi	Chocolate milk
Soybean curd (tofu)	Spelt	Potatoes	Lemon peel	Cocoa
Soy products	Stone ground flour	Potatoes, sweet	Lime peel	Oxalate fruit juices
Sunflower seeds	Wheat bran	Rhubarb	Orange peel	Ovaltine
	Wheat germ	Rutabagas	Raspberries	Tea, black, Indian
	Whole wheat flour	Sorrel	Rhubarb	Bigelow herbal teas
	Yellow Dock	Squash	Strawberries	Cinnamon, ground
		Tomato sauce	Tangerines	Pepper
		Watercress		Ginger
		Yams		Soy sauce

CHAPTER 4

Eater Beware!
Improving Your Nutritional I.Q. and Shooting Down Myths

The doctor of the future will give no medicine,
but will interest . . . patients in the care of the human frame,
in diet, and in the cause and prevention of disease.

—Thomas Edison

"OUR DAUGHTER, A PREMATURE INFANT, HAD SIGNIFICANT HEALTH issues when she met Dr. Compart at age five and a half. These issues have included failure to thrive as an infant, looking dazed and overwhelmed much of the time in classroom settings, and constant vomiting of meals. Dr. Compart suggested we try her on a gluten-free and casein-free diet. This diet change has made a significant impact on her health and life, as well as ours. She has been on the diet for nearly four years now, has gained enough weight to move from the fifth percentile mark to the twenty-fifth percentile, rarely vomits her meals, and although she still struggles with attention issues, she no longer looks dazed. This diet feels like a lifesaver to us!"

—MOTHER OF NICOLE,

a nine-year-old with multiple health and developmental issues

Garbage In, Garbage Out: Good Nutrition Is Not Optional

Beyond the challenges of developmental delays and disorders of sensory, language, processing, and motor functions, many children with autism have additional burdens to their systems: food allergies and intolerances, toxic metal accumulation, extremely restricted appetites, poor nutritional status, inhalant allergies (grass, trees, pollens, molds), and frequent infections. Added to this are environmental toxins and pesticides. All of these straws are on the backs of these precious children, who are biochemically less strong and resilient. Any one of these issues may be tolerated, but their sum total and complexity become overwhelming.

Any effort to reduce the burden on children's systems will help them improve more steadily. Any positive change is helpful. Therefore, a healthy diet and good nutritional status are cornerstones—not options. This holds true for the child with ADHD as well as the child with autism.

Diet is what is eaten. Nutrition is what the cells derive. When poor-quality food is put in the body, the nutritional status cannot be anything but poor. However, a healthy diet may still result in poor nutrition if there are problems in one or more of the following bodily processes: digestion, absorption, transportation to the tissues, uptake and utilization of nutrients by the tissues, and higher nutritional demands created by the presence of interfering substances, including toxic metals.

Public Food Enemy #1: Hydrogenated Oils/Trans-Fatty Acids

When healthy oils become unhealthy mutant saturated fats, it is analogous to good Dr. Jekyll becoming evil Mr. Hyde. Hydrogenation is the industrial processing of unsaturated refined vegetable oils (corn, sunflower, safflower, canola, peanut, cottonseed, or soy) to form an unhealthy, chemically hardened, saturated mutant plastic fat. The process involves bubbling hydrogen through the oil at high temperatures using toxic metal catalysts such as nickel and cadmium. The natural fatty acids are mutated or rearranged to unnatural "trans" fatty acids, which are far worse than any naturally occurring saturated fatty acid. In fact, trans-fatty acids from commercial hydrogenation do not occur in nature at all and do not belong in the human body.

Partial hydrogenation is still hydrogenation—and all of it is bad. Trans-fatty acids from commercial hydrogenation are found in margarines, shortening, junk foods, baked goods, crackers, cookies, doughnuts, pastries, fries, peanut butter, processed cheese, chicken nuggets, and movie popcorn. The trans-fatty acids from commercial hydrogenation are nutritionally inferior due to high heat processing, have absolutely no health benefit, and are detrimental to health in ways that affect all people.

So how bad can trans-fatty acids be and why are they important when it comes to children with ADHD or autism? In the body, trans-fatty acids look like and take the place of the natural and essential fatty acids. They are similar to a key that looks like your door key, fits in the lock, but does not turn and won't come out. Trans fats become part of the cell membranes, hardening them. This interferes with the ability to transport nutrients into the cell and remove metabolic waste (garbage) from the cells. Children with ADHD or autism already have problems with cell function and toxic accumulation without adding hydrogenated oils to the diet.

Trans-fatty acids from commercial hydrogenation do the following to the human body:

- Cause problems in energy metabolism
- Decrease good HDL and increase total cholesterol and other problem fats
- Increase risk for arterial plaque and cardiovascular disease
- Interfere with essential fatty acid metabolism—critical to brain development
- Increase risk for diabetes
- Increase inflammation
- Have a negative effect on immunity—also a core problem in autism
- Interfere with enzymes that metabolize medications, toxins, and cancer-promoting chemicals
- Contribute to neurological problems
- Negatively affect fat-cell size and number and fat composition
- Interfere with reproduction (female fertility and male sperm quality)
- Alter the quality of breast milk
- Correlate to low birth weight in human infants

So when it comes to spreads, butter is better, but not for those with casein/milk problems. The alternative is ghee, which is clarified butter—also called drawn butter.

In an effort to identify and reduce trans-fatty acids in the diet, the Food and Drug Administration (FDA) has recently established labeling regulations. Unfortunately, the FDA has not banned trans-fatty acids (from commercial hydrogenation), and the regulations have a loophole. According to the FDA, "if the serving contains less than 0.5 gram [of trans fat], the content, when declared, shall be expressed as zero." If the word "hydrogenated" is on the label, then trans-fatty acids are in the food. Depending on how much is consumed, the trans-fatty acid intake could increase significantly. So although the regulations are a step in the right direction, a full ban is what is needed. It's time to return to the "good ol' days" when people ate real food.

Jack Sprat Was Wrong: Good Fats to the Rescue

A common diet myth is that animal fats are all saturated and vegetable fats are all unsaturated. Dietary fats and oils are combinations of saturated and unsaturated fatty acids, both of which occur naturally in animal and plant sources.

Saturated fatty acids are not all the same and include short-, medium-, and long-chain fatty acids. The short-chain fatty acids are found in butter, coconut oil, and palm kernel oil and have lower melting points than longer-chain saturated fatty acids. Medium-chain saturated fatty acids are found in foods as medium-chain triglycerides and are used in special medical formulas for those who cannot absorb the longer-chain fatty acids. These are especially important in infant formulas where they duplicate the medium-chain saturated fatty acids found in human milk. The longer-chain saturated fatty acids are the most common found in foods. The long-chain fatty acids are important in membranes, especially in the brain.

Unsaturated fatty acids include monounsaturates and polyunsaturates. The most common monounsaturated fatty acid is oleic acid which is found in avocados, nuts, and many oils, including olive, canola, and in high-oleic safflower and sunflower oils. Oleic acid is also abundant in animal fats such as lard and tallow. The best known polyunsatured fatty acids are omega-6 and omega-3. Omega-6 is found in vegetables, nuts, seeds and their oils. Omega-3 includes alpha-linolenic acid (ALA), which is important for vision, skin health, and in neurological and brain development. It is less abundant in the diet and found in beans, green leafy vegetables, nuts and seeds and their oils. The best concentrated sources are unhydrogenated flax oil, canola oil and soybean oils (and also hemp and perilla oils). The importance of omega-3 ALA is its conversion to eicosapentaenoic acid (EPA) and docosahexaenoic acid (DHA) which are found naturally in fish. EPA and DHA are especially important for brain function and it is noted that some children with ADHD or autism have higher needs for these omega-3 fatty acids.

Coconut oil and other tropical oils are not the enemies. These healthy natural fats and oils were abandoned with the saturated-fat scare and replaced with hydrogenated oils and their trans-fatty acids, which are mutant, plastic fatty acids more harmful to human health than any naturally occurring fatty acid. The lauric acid found in coconut oil and mother's milk has antifungal, antimicrobial properties and is especially beneficial to infants and children. Tropical oils have been demonstrated to raise good cholesterol (HDL) levels.

> "We started in the summer of 2000, when Sarah was four, with just nutritional changes. Other treatments began in spring 2001. By the first of the year 2003, she was reviewed by a Ph.D. from Kennedy Krieger [Institute] who stated that she no longer had any symptoms of autism. She continued with symptoms of a visual memory problem for a little over another year, until spring 2005. Now she is typical in development and behavior."
>
> —Anne Evans,
> *mother of Sarah*

Fishy Facts

Seafood is abundant in healthy nutrients, especially protein, zinc, omega-3 fatty acids, and iodine. Seafood is generally much easier to digest than animal protein (meats, poultry). The concerns lie in environmental issues, which include inadequate conservation efforts to avoid depletion of certain species of fish and the increasing contamination from industrial pollutants. The species of sea life that are most likely to have higher levels of toxins and pesticides include the large steak fish that feed on smaller fish and the bottom feeders. Farming techniques also have an impact on the toxic content of the farm-raised fish, depending on what they are fed. The location of the seafood determines the level of toxins present. Currently in the United States, there is no USDA organic certification in seafood, so the consumer must be educated.

Problems:

- Chemicals and contaminants: mercury, polychlorinated biphenyls (PCBs), chlordane, dioxins, DDT, cadmium.
- Toxins work their way up the food chain (big fish eat small fish).
- Toxins are higher in the organs and fatty tissues (shellfish "mustard" or "tamale").
- Government monitoring is poor. There is no USDA organic certification.
- The more contaminated seafood consumed, the higher the risk.
- Fetuses, young children, and those with immune problems are at highest risk.

Suggestions:

- Eat seafood caught away from major cities.
- Buy the whole fish and ask to have it filleted. Flesh should look moist and shiny.
- Gills should be red; eyes should be bright, not dull.
- Less healthy fish are used in processed fish products such as fish sticks.

Preparing:

- Store in the refrigerator, cook and eat or freeze immediately.
- Keep mussels, clams, oysters, and shellfish alive. If dead, do not cook or eat.
- Remove the skin. Trim off the dark meat and fat. Cook fish so the fat drips away.
- Broil, bake, or grill and avoid the drippings. Poaching removes some contaminants.

SAFER CHOICES (farm-raised only if organic)

Bass (freshwater, giant sea)	Monkfish, mullet
Blue Crab (Atlantic)	Perch, pike, pollack, porgie
Burbot	Rockfish, sablefish
Butterfish	Salmon
Cobia	*(Wild or farm-raised with organic methods Atlantic or Pacific [sockeye, coho])*
Cod	
Croaker	Sardines
Cusk	Sculpin, smelt, snapper
Drum	Spotted sea trout
Haddock	Trout (rainbow, brook)
Herring	Whitefish, whiting

AVOID (highest risk for pregnancy, fetus, infants, children, and immune disorders)

Mercury (found in big, old fish)	High in PCBS (Polychlorinated biphenyls)
Blue fish	Catfish
Halibut	Carp
Kingfish	Lake trout
Mackerel	Muskellunge
Mahi Mahi	Northern pike
Marlin	Striped bass
Shark	Shark
Swordfish	Walleyes
Tilefish	
Tuna	

Higher in other contaminants	Higher in contaminants
Carp	Farm raised fish—*raised in crowded pens with processed feed. Farm raised with organic methods is better.*
Catfish	
Farm raised fish (unless organic)	
Flounder	The mustard in blue crabs or tamale in lobsters
Grouper	
Shellfish	Oysters
Trout	
Raw fish—sushi, sashimi *Risk of parasite exposure*	

Good News about Cholesterol!

Some people have the idea that if high cholesterol is bad, the lower the cholesterol, the better. This is not true. Without cholesterol, the body can not function. Cholesterol is so important to human health that the liver makes approximately 1,000 milligrams per day. Scientific studies have documented that dietary cholesterol has little effect on blood cholesterol levels. The body regulates the amount of cholesterol so that when more is consumed, the body makes less, and when less is consumed, the body makes more.

Why would the body make a substance purported to be so dangerous? Why would mother's milk be so rich in cholesterol? Cholesterol is vital to the cells of all mammals. It is a major precursor of reproductive and natural steroid hormones, vitamin D, and digestive bile acids. It forms the "bricks" of the cell membranes and the covering of nerves, and is an important component of the brain. It is important in serotonin receptor function in the brain. Cholesterol maintains the health of the intestinal wall, preventing leaky membranes.

Cholesterol does not attach to healthy vessels. When there is injury to vessels, the body sends out more cholesterol as a repair substance or bandage for the injury. The cholesterol becomes part of the injured area of the vessel (within the intima, not on the lining of the vessel wall). So yes, the elevated cholesterol in the blood is associated with heart disease—but it is not the direct cause. The cholesterol plaques that form within the wall are part of the problem. The causes of vessel injury are the main source of the problem, and they include: genetics, aging, high blood pressure, high blood glucose, inflammation, infections, viruses, stress hormones, deep-fried foods, hydrogenated oils, oxidized fats, lack of antioxidants, excess free radicals, lack of B vitamins, elevated C-reactive protein (CRP), and elevated homocysteine.

The limit on cholesterol intake at 300 milligrams per day is based on the faulty premise that consuming cholesterol is harmful to health. Studies show that at four times the "limit," there is little impact on blood cholesterol. Cholesterol is an important nutrient for the body.

The lower the cholesterol, the better, is not necessarily true. Remembering that cholesterol is necessary for cell membrane structure, it is easy to understand why low cholesterol levels can lead to hemorrhagic (bleeding) strokes. There is solid evidence that as cholesterol levels decline below 180, bleeding strokes increase and cholesterol levels above 240 increase the risk for ischemic (blockage of blood flow) strokes. The levels differ for women.

Low Cholesterol Levels and Autism

Recent studies have found that a subset of children with autism spectrum disorders have a cholesterol level that is *too low*. Some of these children have low cholesterol as part of a defined genetic disorder (described below) while others do not.

Smith-Lemli-Opitz Syndrome (SLOS), is a genetic disorder characterized by low cholesterol levels, other abnormalities of cholesterol pathways (i.e., elevated 7-dehydrocholesterol) and, in many cases, autism symptoms. In this disorder, the low cholesterol level is due to a deficiency of 7-dehydrocholesterol (7-DHC) reductase, the enzyme responsible for the final step in making cholesterol. Blood testing in SLOS shows an elevated 7-DHC and oftern a low total cholesterol. The severity of symptoms in this syndrome seems to correlate with the degree of deficiency in cholesterol.

Recent studies have also shown that a subset of children with autism spectrum disorders have low total cholesterol but not due to SLOS. The cause of low cholesterol is not yet known. Studies are currently being done in an effort to determine the cause.

Dietary cholesterol supplementation in individuals with SLOS and autistic symptoms can result in a decrease in autistic behaviors, irritability, hyperactivity, aggression, self-injury, temper outbursts, and improvements in physical growth, language, sleep, and social interactions. It is possible that increasing cholesterol in individuals with autism who do not have SLOS may also be helpful, according to some studies.

You can increase cholesterol through diet or supplements. Dietary interventions include increasing the intake of egg yolks, either by eating eggs or by hiding additional egg yolks in other foods (such as in pancake batter). In children who are sensitive or allergic to eggs—or who refuse to eat eggs—use of a cholesterol supplement may be necessary.

produces less. In fact, egg intake is associated with increased good HDL cholesterol levels and improved cholesterol ratios.

As long as there are not allergies, eggs are, indeed, incredible and edible! They are an excellent way of increasing good-quality protein and can be "hidden" in many foods.

The Good Egg

Eggs, another item wrongly maligned over time, are not the enemy either, as confirmed by numerous current scientific studies. The egg is a high-protein, nutrient-rich food so beneficial to health that it is considered a healthy food. Because cholesterol production is regulated by the liver, egg intake contributes little to total blood cholesterol levels. Remember, when you consume more cholesterol, the liver

Sugar Blues

Most children with ADHD or autism eat low-protein and low-fiber diets. They crave the "white foods"— refined grains and carbohydrates, pasta, breads, crackers, pretzels, bagels, and sugars. They also crave sugary sweets, sodas, and juices. These foods are glycemic, meaning they raise blood glucose (sugar) too quickly. Whole grains, on the other hand, release their sugars slowly. However, when any whole grain

Glycemic Index vs Glycemic Load

Carbohydrates affect blood glucose depending upon whether they are simple and result in quick elevations of blood glucose or more complex and result in more stable blood glucose. When glucose rises too quickly, there is an excess release of insulin which drives glucose down too rapidly and/or too low. Stability in glucose levels is the key to health, focus, attention, and mood stability as well as hunger and weight control.

- The glycemic index (GI) is a measure of how a food triggers a rise in blood glucose. The higher the number, the greater the blood glucose rise.
- The glycemic load (GL) assesses the impact of carbohydrate consumption accounting for the amount of that carbohydrate in a serving

and the total effect on the blood glucose. It is based on the idea that a high glycemic index food consumed in small quantities would give the same glucose effect as larger quantities of a low glycemic index food.

- For example, the glycemic index of watermelon is high at 72, but due to the high water content, very little of the watermelon contains the carbohydrate. It's GL is low at 3. Spaghetti has a lower GI of 38 but much higher glucose effect because of the high relative amount of carbohydrate. It's GL of 9 is three times that of watermelon.

Resources
www.ajcn.org/cgi/content/full/76/1/5
www.mendosa.com/gilists.htm

is ground into flour, it becomes glycemic, or sugar raising. Whole-grain flours are not whole grains.

This results in the release of too much insulin, which drives the blood sugar down too fast and too low. The brain is the first system affected by rapid changes in glucose. As the glucose drops, there is "brain fog," irritability, hunger headaches, and cravings for a "quick fix"—more sugar. Sugars, sweets, juices, and refined flours on an empty stomach have a much stronger effect on blood glucose. High fructose corn syrup (HFCS) has a double impact on blood glucose and must be avoided. HFCS increases risk for diabetes, obesity, heart disease, and eye and nerve damage

Besides wearing out the body's ability to handle sugar and setting up children for early diabetes, glycemic foods have a serious negative effect on mood stability, focus, and attention. Because children with ADHD or autism already suffer from these problems, it is important to not reward good behavior and attention with sugar treats, candies, and so forth.

There is less negative impact when only a small amount is present among glucose-stabilizing foods such as proteins (fish, poultry, meat, eggs, beans, nuts, and seeds) and fiber (whole grains, beans, nuts, seeds, vegetables, and fruits). The dietary goal is to consume good protein and fiber while significantly reducing the glycemic foods, which raise blood sugar.

Sodas—Don't!

Sodas, both diet and regular, are a problem, and not just because they take the place of drinking more water and nutritional beverages. They are a problem because they are high in phosphorus—a nutrient abundant in any diet. Excess phosphorus can bond with minerals, making them unavailable for use by the body. Phosphorus depletes (drains) calcium, magnesium, potassium, zinc, chromium, manganese, chloride, and water-soluble vitamins such as vitamins C and B. Sodas are the opposite of electrolyte drinks—they are electrolyte "drains." They take nutrients out of the nutrient stores.

Both diet and regular sodas significantly increase risk for obesity and diabetes. Diet sodas are worse because they contain artificial sweeteners. Through human and animal studies, it is clear that artificial sweeteners impair regulation of calorie intake resulting in overeating and the long-term health consequences of overeating. All sodas and artificial sweeteners must be avoided.

Children with ADHD or autism characteristically have low levels of minerals and vitamins. Especially in autism, the nutrient deficiencies are significant, and the nutrient needs are well above what is standard. What these children do not need is a drink that deprives them further and increases their risk for diabetes, obesity, and heart disease. Try a natural soda: flavor seltzer water (it does not contain phosphorus) with a splash of juice.

Salt—Yes!
Sodium Preservatives—No!

A subset of children with ADHD or autism have constant physiologic and physical challenges due in part to inefficiencies in metabolism and poor diet, especially low protein intake. They experience a cluster of symptoms, including generalized physical weakness, low tone, cold extremities, lower body temperatures, and extremely pale skin. Commonly, there is lower blood pressure, poor balance, and dizziness upon standing up too quickly. The symptoms are signs of decreased adrenal function (not adrenal disease). Adrenals require salt. So for these children, salt is important. However, sodium preservatives do not meet this requirement and are additives to be avoided.

Chloride is necessary for cell function, balance, and distribution of body fluids, and a necessary part of digestive acid (hydrochloric acid). It is depleted through sweat, vomit, and diarrhea.

The sodium preservatives (nitrites, benzoates, MSG) are generally not well handled by children on the autism spectrum. The preservatives provide sodium but not the chloride found in salt.

Do not restrict salt for your child, unless your health care provider has instructed you to do so because of a specific medical condition.

It's Not Nice to Fool Mother Nature—Go Organic

This is not fluff or a trendy concept. The U.S. Department of Agriculture (USDA) Organic seal is a certification that mandates specific standards. Organic foods may not be irradiated or produced with genetically modified organisms (GMO). All organic farmers and processors are required to be certified.

According to the USDA and the National Organic Standards Board, organic food and fiber are grown without relying on synthetic chemical pesticides. Techniques must help protect the air, soil, water, and food supply from potentially toxic chemicals and other pollutants. Organic farming conserves natural resources by recycling natural materials and protecting ecosystems and preventing contamination of crops, soil, and water by plant and animal pathogenic organisms, heavy metals, or toxic residues.

The definitions are strict and easy to understand:

- **100% ORGANIC:** 100 percent of all the substances, ingredients, processing aids, additives, coloring, and flavoring are certified organic

- **ORGANIC:** contains at least 95 percent organic ingredients

- **MADE WITH ORGANIC INGREDIENTS:** contains between 70 and 94 percent organic ingredients

Chapter Summary

- Children with ADHD or autism tend to require and benefit from high-nutrient foods.

- Hydrogenated oils are mutant, plastic fatty acids that cause increased risk for many chronic conditions, including problems in brain and neurological functions. They must be avoided.

- Good oils include olive, avocado, almond, safflower, sunflower, flaxseed, peanut, and canola oils. Coconut oil is beneficial and useful in baking.

- Cholesterol is necessary in human health. If high-cholesterol foods are consumed, the liver makes less. If cholesterol intakes are low, the liver makes more.

- A subset of children with autism have cholesterol levels that are too low and require significant increases in the diet or by supplementation.

- Eggs are a high-protein, nutrient-dense food that should be included in the diet if there are not egg allergies, sensitivities, or intolerances.

- Diets high in sugar, refined flour, and refined carbohydrates affect body energy, mood, behavior, attention, and brain function. Good protein and fiber stabilize blood sugar.

- Soda depletes nutrients from the body and is unhealthy for all children, and is especially bad for children with ADHD or autism.

- Salt is beneficial to many children with autism and should not be avoided unless advised by your doctor. Sodium preservatives should be avoided.

- Organic foods are free of harmful additives and pesticides and, therefore, limit the toxic load—especially important for children with ADHD or autism.

As a rule, we recommend using organic foods whenever possible. Some children with ADHD and many children with autism already have inefficiencies in metabolizing, which places a burden on their systems. Ingesting harmful pesticides, additives, contaminants, and toxins can increase that burden. USDA certified organic products are therefore safer to consume. We recognize that organic foods are more expensive, however. When buying organic produce is not possible, make sure to wash it thoroughly before preparing it.

We are not just what we eat; we are what we eat, digest, absorb, and utilize.

CHAPTER 5

Yes—There Is Plenty Left to Eat!!

Life Beyond Gluten, Milk, Soy, Hydrogenated Oils, Soda, and Junk Food

IN ADDITION TO THE NUMEROUS SUBSTITUTES FOR GLUTEN, MILK/CASEIN, and soy, there is an abundance of healthy foods to eat! Remember, early humans ate fish, meats, fruits, vegetables, and nuts and seeds. They did not consume milk, grains, beans, or potatoes, because milk products were not available and the other items could not be eaten raw without causing severe symptoms or illness. Eventually, cooking and domestication brought these foods into the human diet. A GFCF diet returns us to the basic foods, which are easier for the body to digest and handle. So here is the list of choices available (as long as they do not cause allergy or intolerance reactions and/or violate your beliefs):

- Meats—all varieties
- Seafood—fish, shellfish, mollusks
- Fowl—chicken, turkey, hen, duck
- Eggs
- Vegetables—all varieties
- Fruits—all varieties
- Grains—all varieties except for glutens

The Yuck Factor:
Why Children Refuse Foods
They Should Eat

After the shock of being told what the child cannot eat, most parents panic because those are the only foods the child does eat. In fact, the kids refuse the healthy foods, no matter how much they are bribed, begged, or coerced.

The problem is a double whammy:

- The opiate effect from glutens, milk, and soy causes addictions to those foods. The children therefore limit their diet to their favorite, "craved" foods, which make them feel good but unfortunately cause disturbances in brain chemistry and function.

- Zinc deficiency is one of the most common deficiencies we find in the autism population. It is also common in children with ADHD. It usually results from maldigestion, malabsorption, and/or the presence of toxic metals. Beyond many other problems with brain and sensory development, zinc deficiency results in significant problems with taste, taste perception, food-texture issues, and picky or odd appetites. Foods, especially vegetables, seem to have no taste or a foul taste. In the extreme, children may gag at the sight of vegetables, and in some cases refuse protein and fruits as well. If toxic metals are significant, children will exhibit pica and eat nonfood substances such as dirt, clay, and paper.

With the combination of lousy taste perception and the opiate effect on the brain, the opiate-forming foods become the only acceptable foods. The solution is a two-handed approach:

- The "addicting" foods must be removed.

- Zinc and other needed nutrients must be replaced in order to start improving taste perception and appetite.

In chapter 6, "Getting Started and Bumps Along the Way," we describe the easy way to accomplish this removal/replacement process. Although some parents attempt the cold turkey method, we prefer the "Easy Does It" method. Gradually wean the kids off the troubling foods by slowly introducing substitutes and hiding healthy foods within the favorite foods.

Cooking with substitutes and making substitute foods is different but does not have to be difficult. Part II of this book is devoted to recipes that are gluten-free and casein (milk)-free and also free of other problem foods such as soy, egg, corn and nuts.

"Hippocrates said, 'Let thy food be thy medicine and thy medicine be thy food.' Good advice, surely, but it was probably a lot easier to follow in 400 B.C., when he didn't have to contend with three McDonald's, two Starbucks, and a Cinnabon within a five-mile radius of the Parthenon. Overwhelming temptation is one reason it's hard to stay on a restricted diet, but there are plenty of others."

—Kathryn Scott,
in her article
"Flirting with Disaster," from
Living Without, *Spring 2006*

Simplifying the Pyramid— The Kid-Friendly Square Meal

Whether or not certain foods must be avoided, there is still the need to know how to eat healthy foods easily. The previous and current food pyramids include grains and milk products as if they are mandatory separate food groups, when, in fact, they are not. This faulty assumption leads many parents to panic because they can't violate the accepted recommendations. These foods are not food groups; they are foods. Grains are one type of carbohydrate choice, and milk products are one type of protein choice. Any style of recommendations for diet must apply to all people—not just one culture or one diet style. Humans are omnivores—able to eat animal- and vegetable-source foods. Therefore, the diet must apply to all—from vegetarians to those who are more carnivorous (consume more animal-source foods). There are only three mandatory categories of foods:

Protein

- **ANIMAL SOURCES:** Seafood, meats, poultry, eggs, animal milk products
- **VEGETABLE SOURCES:** Beans, nuts, seeds

Fat

- **SATURATED:** More solid at room temperature; manufactured in the body and found in animal- and vegetable-source foods
- **UNSATURATED:** More liquid at room temperature; found in animal- and vegetable-source foods

- **MONOUNSATURATED:** More stable; more prevalent in olive, avocado, almond, safflower, sunflower, peanut, and canola oils
- **POLYUNSATURATED:** More unstable
- **ESSENTIAL OMEGA 3:** From fish, fish oil, nuts, seeds, and breast milk
- **ESSENTIAL OMEGA 6:** From vegetables, seeds, and their oils

Carbohydrate

- Vegetables, fruits, grains, beans, nuts, seeds

We use a Square Meal concept to guide our families toward healthy balanced eating. Picture a square picnic-style plate that has three sections:

- One-half of the plate includes the high-fiber vegetables of all colors and varieties—served in a variety of ways, including raw, steamed, cooked in soups, pureed, and juiced.
- One-quarter of the plate includes protein choices—animal and/or vegetable sources.
- One-quarter of the plate includes starches, grains, and fruits.

Kid-Friendly GFCF Square Meal

AGE	CALORIES/DAY	PROTEIN GRAMS	FIBER GRAMS	WATER OUNCES
2–3	1,000–1,400	24	15	30–35
4–6	1,200–1,800	30–35	15–19	40–45
7–10	1,200–2,000	40–45	15–20	45–50
11–14	1,600–2,400	45–60	20–25	55–60

More Vegetables

HIGH-FIBER VEGGIES

- 1–3 cups a day
- Eat many different colored vegetables (green, orange, red, purple)
- Use these raw, steamed, cooked, or pureed:

Artichokes	Okra
Asparagus	Olives
Avocado	Onions
Beet	Parsley
Bok Choy	Parsnips
Broccoli	Peppers
Brussels sprouts	Pumpkin
Cabbage	Radishes
Carrots	Rhubarb
Cauliflower	Rutabaga
Celery	Shallots
Chard	Snow peas
Chicory	Spinach
Chives	Sprouts
Collards	Squash
Cucumber	String beans
Eggplant	Sweet Potato
Garlic	Swiss Chard
Green leafies	Tomato
Jerusalem artichoke	Turnip
Kale	Turnip greens
Kohlrabi	Water chestnut
Leeks	Watercress
Lettuces	Yam
Mushrooms	Zucchini

Good Protein (24–60g/day)

ANIMAL PROTEIN	VEGETABLE PROTEIN
Seafood	Beans
Poultry	Nuts
Meat	Seeds
Eggs	

- 1 serving = size of each person's palm
- 7–8 grams protein = 1 oz meat = 1 egg = 2 tbs. nut butters, 2 oz. nuts, ½ cup beans, 1 cup milk substitute
- AVOID MILK/CASEIN

Starches & Fruit

EAT LESS		EAT MORE
Refined Grains	**Starch Vegetables**	Whole grains (2–6 oz/day)
Bagels	Beets	Fruit (1–2 cups/day)
Breads	Corn	
Cold Cereals	Popcorn	
Pasta	Potato	
Pancakes		
Muffins		
Other		
Dried fruit		
Fruit juices		

- Not on an empty stomach
- AVOID GLUTENS

AVOID	LIMIT	DRINK	SWEETENERS	OILS (3–5 tsp./day)
Trans fats / Hydrogenated	Sugar	Water	Agave	Olive
Artificial sweeteners	Sweets	Herb teas	Honey	Avocado
High fructose corn syrup	Deli meats	Seltzer	Maple syrup	Almond
Sodas (diet & regular)	Refined foods	Rice milk	Splash of juice	Safflower
Fried Foods	Caffeine	Coconut water	Brown rice syrup	Flaxseed
		Coconut milk kefir	Stevia	

PROTEIN SERVINGS

Each person's animal-protein serving size is equal to his or her own palm (minus fingers and thumb).

Each ounce of an animal protein serving contains approximately 8 grams of protein. The following protein foods have 7 to 8 grams of protein:

- 1 ounce (28 g) meat, fish, or poultry
- 1 egg
- ½ cup (90 g) baked beans, cooked dried peas, cooked lentils
- 2 tablespoons (32 g) peanut butter
- 1.5 ounces (42 g) nuts/seeds
- 1 cup (235 ml) milk

CHILD 2 TO 3 YEARS OLD:

1 serving = 1 ounce = 8 grams protein

CHILD 4 TO 6 YEARS OLD:

1 serving = 1.5 ounces = 12 grams protein

CHILD 7 TO 10 YEARS OLD:

1 serving = 2 ounces = 16 grams protein

CHILD 11 TO 14 YEARS OLD:

1 serving = 2.5 ounces = 20 grams protein

Supplements Make the Difference

With their profound problems in digestion and absorption, limited appetite, and documented presence of toxic metals, it is easy to understand why children with autism exhibit so many severe nutritional deficiencies, including zinc, vitamin A, magnesium, B vitamins, essential fatty acids, vitamin D, vitamin E, amino acids, Coenzyme Q10, and glutathione. These deficiencies are evidenced by sophisticated blood and urine testing. A brief review of symptoms associated with the deficiencies is an overview of autism symptoms as well. The deficiencies are also present in those with ADHD, though less severe.

Mineral deficiencies are very common. For example, zinc deficiency is common in children with ADHD or autism; it is usually much more severe in autism. Zinc deficiency results in problems with growth and development, brain and sensory function, amino-acid metabolism, vitamin A function, and immunity. Zinc is critical in sensory issues such as appetite, taste perception; vision; vision perception; eye contact; hearing and auditory perception; as well as perception of touch, pressure, and pain.

A common symptom for low zinc is altered and limited taste. This is sometimes seen in children with ADHD and is often seen in those with autism. Foods—especially vegetables—taste lousy, even horrible; and of course, the kids do not eat these foods! Until the zinc levels improve, it is difficult to change the eating habits. And the aversions are worse when there is an opiate effect from gluten, milk, and soy. If low zinc is due to the presence of toxic metals, kids may also have pica, or appetites for nonfood substances such as dirt, paint chips, play dough, and paper.

Zinc is necessary for utilization of amino acids (from protein). Even if protein intake is good and it is well digested to amino acids, the amino acids will not be fully functional when zinc is low. The result looks like inadequate protein and may show up as poor tone and muscle planning dysfunction.

Since zinc is critical for vitamin A function, deficiencies of zinc can result in vitamin A deficiency. The most notable symptom is poor eye contact, which often responds readily to supplementation with vitamin A (cod liver oil) and zinc.

Magnesium, so prevalent in dark greens, vegetables, beans, nuts, and seeds, is poorly absorbed in the presence maldigestion/malabsorption problems. Low levels can result in mood disorders, hyperactivity, distractibility, impulsivity, sound sensitivity, irritability, muscle spasms, depression, and poor muscle endurance.

B-vitamin deficiencies are frequent in children with ADHD or autism; however, a subset of these children are intolerant to B vitamins. For those with deficiencies, there can be a wide range of emotional, psychological, neurological, and developmental symptoms.

Essential fatty-acid deficiency is common in both ADHD and autism and shows up as eczema; poor hair quality; and problems with brain and neurological development, vision, immunity, and bowel health.

What is notable in children with ADHD or autism is that the nutrient doses required for optimum function are often significantly higher than standard recommendations. This is due to so many inefficiencies in digestion, absorption, utilization, and need. The more problems and the greater the severity, the higher the nutrient needs. This is like having a "hole in the bucket." To get a full bucket of water from the well requires carrying five buckets. Additionally, when nutrient needs are high, the body quickly uses up what comes, and nutrient stores do not build up. Under these circumstances, the high doses are therefore not toxic. In the body, the supplements get used up by the high demands and many functions improve, but the nutrient stores remain low. It takes a long time to fulfill all the demands and build up nutrient reserves. When higher than standard nutrient doses are used, appropriate monitoring by blood or urine testing is advised.

"After three months on supplements, Jonathan is starting to make progress. He responds more when called. And the other day, when he was watching Elmo on PBS, he counted on his fingers and repeated after him; his speech wasn't clear, but it's still progress."

—Jackie Robinson, *mother of five-year-old Jonathan*

CHAPTER 6

Getting Started and Bumps along the Way

"The person who moves a mountain begins by carrying away small stones."
—Chinese proverb

"My daughter, Cassie, is autistic. She was in early intervention from the time she was eighteen months old. We had every form of therapy, including Applied Behavioral Analysis (ABA), but nothing was helping and, actually, the situation was getting worse. When I first was told about the gluten- and casein-free diet, I was still devastated over the autism diagnosis and praying for a miracle. I couldn't face the fact that my little girl, who was so tiny and underweight to begin with, might have a food restriction. As it was, she barely ate, and every food she was willing to eat would have to be eliminated from her diet. At that time, I was not willing to do this diet. One year later, when the improvements were not happening quickly enough for me, I gave in and told her doctor I was ready to try to get Cassie gluten- and casein-free. This decision changed our lives.

Originally, when I tried to slowly take Cassie off of the offending foods and slowly introduce new, acceptable foods, she would not try one new food. So I had to take drastic measures and go cold turkey. Within a week, we began to see withdrawal symptoms of crying and screaming; this lasted many weeks. Then suddenly one morning, instead of waking up to her crying, we heard little happy sounds coming from her room. We found her with a smile on her face, staring directly into our eyes. You could clearly see that this was a new person.

In the weeks that followed, Cassie showed us that she wanted to be cuddled and kissed and hugged. She smiled all of the time, began to play with select toys appropriately, sought out social interaction from other children, and best of all, she showed interest, for the first time, in her little brother. This diet had lifted a fog that had been clouding Cassie's brain. Now, even her ABA therapy was much more effective because we had broken through such a strong barrier. Cassie today, three years after beginning the diet, is a social being, who loves to play chase, get tickled, and receive love. Her speech improved and so did every aspect of her life. We are a "real" family now and I know that going gluten- and casein-free gave us our little girl.

—Jennifer B., *mother of Cassie,
a five-year-old with autism*

We cannot do everything at once,

but we can do something at once.

—Calvin Coolidge

Getting Started—Easy Does It!

Modifying your child's diet can feel like an overwhelming and almost impossible task. Most parents are already exhausted from the full-time job of seeking appropriate services and therapies for their children. Adding a specialized diet can put some people over the edge. Know that you are not alone in this feeling. Know that, as with most difficult tasks in life, the hardest part is getting started. Often the worry about the challenge of the diet is worse than actually doing it. There is a lot of support available for you in doing an elimination diet. In addition to this cookbook, there are Web sites and parent Listservs that can provide lots of good information. Talk with other parents in your community; there are others who have done this ahead of you, and most are more than glad to make your road easier than theirs was. Most of all, do the best that you can and focus on what you *are* doing for your child rather than what you aren't doing. Some children are easy to get on these diets, but most require time and effort. Even simply decreasing the amount of offending foods can often be helpful. Remember that your child is different from all other children with ADHD or autism. Your family structure is unique, and you need to do what works best for your child and family. This section will provide you with guidelines and helpful hints for starting the diet.

We're Overwhelmed— Where Do We Start?

There are many ways to start the elimination diet. Some practitioners advocate taking the child off the offending foods cold turkey. This approach feels right for some parents, who "want to get it over with." In general, however, this approach results in more significant withdrawal symptoms. For many children, the only foods in their diet are dairy and wheat products, and they will not eat when all of those foods are removed.

For these children, we advocate a gradual removal of offending foods. The rate of removal is dictated by both the ease with which your child accepts the new foods as well as the degree of withdrawal symptoms. Again, the most common offending foods are casein, gluten, and soy, in that order. Casein is the easiest protein to remove, as there are many acceptable substitutes. Often changing the type of milk is the easiest place to start. Casein-free rice, almond, and potato-based milk substitutes are available in both vanilla and chocolate flavors. (See chapter 2 for more details about substitute foods.) These milks provide equivalent calcium to cow's milk. However, they do not contain significant protein. This can be an issue for children whose main protein source is dairy protein in milk. This topic will be addressed in the sections that follow.

An important note about removing casein: We recommend that you do not use soy as a replacement for casein foods, because soy is also such a common offending food. If you replace cow's milk–based products (milk, cheese, yogurt, ice cream) with soy versions, you will be significantly increasing your child's soy intake. For some children, this means you are taking out one problem food and substituting it with another, possibly equally problematic food. This may mask any potential benefit from removing casein, and you will not be able to tell whether casein was a problem. Initially, it may be too difficult to completely remove soy from your child's diet, as soy lecithin is found in many food products. There are options for replacing some cow's milk products with nonsoy alternatives. Unfortunately, there is no commercially available good soy-free substitute for yogurt or cheese. (Rice cheese contains casein.) There are, however, rice-based ice cream alternatives available.

As you remove casein, you will often also be decreasing gluten. All of the recipes in this book are casein- and gluten-free. Many commercially available products are also free of both proteins. Once you have removed casein, you can focus on more completely removing gluten. This is a more challenging task, since gluten is found in so many foods. It is found in a variety of grains, not just wheat. (See chapter 2 for details.) However, again, you will find that there are a variety of recipes and commercially available products that are not just palatable but actually enjoyable.

Variety Is Not Always the Spice of Life

We tend to be fairly routine about what we eat. When we shop, we tend to buy the same foods week after week. And although what we eat on a given day varies, in the bigger picture, we tend to eat the same foods week in and week out. This actually works in your favor when trying to change your child's diet. Your child's main motivation is not that food is good for him or her, but that it tastes good. So if your child loves chocolate chip cookies and you always make or buy one particular type, your challenge is to find a GFCF version of that cookie. Once you find it and your child accepts it, that cookie is the type of cookie you buy or make week in and week out. The same applies to main courses, side dishes, snacks, and desserts. The challenge is starting the diet and finding the substitute foods. Maintaining the diet is much less difficult.

"Denial and anger are bad enough when you're sabotaging yourself, but it's worse when you're facing—or not facing—your child's food issues. Denial allows you to keep feeding your child things that make him or her sick because you're pretending nothing's wrong."

—Kathryn Scott
in "Flirting with Disaster," from Living Without, *Spring 2006*

The Trojan Horse Technique—Sneaky Works!

Remember Odysseus from seventh grade mythology? Seeking to gain entrance into Troy, he cleverly ordered a hollow wooden horse so large that the Greek army could hide inside. What looked like a huge horse was really a disguise to conquer the city. We have used this concept for decades to hide nutritious food to nourish picky eaters.

In the recipe sections, we provide clever ways to introduce and hide new foods, especially vegetables. Years of experience have proven to us and to parents of our patients that this is an easy way to introduce new foods. Mix, blend, or puree a very small amount (1 tablespoon) of the new food with a well-liked food. As the child accepts the taste, more can be included. The key is to start small! Blended foods may also be better tolerated with those children who have oral sensory issues regarding food textures. Their sensory development may be younger than their age. It is better to adapt to the sensory level and return to purees until the sensory issues have improved. It is important to have the child eat rather than encourage progression to foods that are not tolerated because they are "lumpy" or unpleasant to chew.

Assume the new food to be introduced is a vegetable. It must be cooked and pureed well with a food where it will not change the overall color, texture, or taste. If there is nothing but white food in the diet, then start with very light-colored vegetables (squash, cauliflower, corn). If the child likes ketchup or tomato sauce, then you can introduce deeper-colored vegetables (beets, greens, peas, beans). First, the vegetable must be well cooked and pureed completely with the child's favorite food. You can also use baby-food purees. Pureed vegetables can be included in batter for pancakes, muffins, brownies, and cookies or in sauces such as tomato sauce, pizza sauce, and ketchup. Blend pureed vegetables into fruit sauces. You can also add pureed vegetables to meatballs, if they are a favorite food, and even to peanut butter.

Many of our patients' families have developed what we call "muffin casseroles". One child would eat only breads and muffins. His clever, resourceful mother developed a GFCF muffin he liked and then gradually started adding fruit puree to the batter. As that was tolerated, she added vegetable puree, and finally added pureed meat. Until he was able to transition to eating foods in a traditional manner, he had these muffin casseroles at every meal and snack—and loved them!

You can also add a vegetable juice to a fruit juice. The color change will not matter if you serve it in a sippy cup. Try carrot juice with orange juice, and then add a small amount of another vegetable juice. Again, start with only 1 teaspoon (5 ml) or less. Expand as tolerance improves.

There are dried vegetable powders that can be added easily to various foods and dishes. And if none of the above works, consider natural gummy bears made of vegetables and fruits. As your child expands to eating vegetables, try vegetables dipped in honey or GFCF mayo/ketchup mix or hummus. It's a start. But remember to carry out the Trojan Horse technique—out of sight of your child!

If more protein is needed, there are many clever ways to increase it. If eggs are tolerated, add more eggs, especially the high-protein whites, to foods. This works for batters, breads, and meatballs. Rice-protein powders can be added to batters, breads, and smoothies made of rice milk and fruit. Do not add raw eggs to smoothies. Taste and texture determine acceptance.

As your child accepts an increasing number of vegetables, try vegetables dipped in honey, a mayo/ketchup mix, or hummus. It is a start. But remember to carry out the Trojan Horse technique—out of the sight of your child! Keep trying this sneaky manner of introducing new foods, eventually, he or she will accept the food alone—we promise! All it takes is patience, and a lesson from Greek mythology.

How Strict Does an Elimination Diet Have to Be, and How Long Should It Last?

There is no single answer to these questions. It really depends on the individual child. Most books written or lectures given on this subject emphasize the importance of completely and strictly eliminating the problem foods. There is no doubt that this is the purest approach. However, authors and lecturers are generally talking about the "generic" child with ADHD or autism; they are not talking about your child with ADHD or autism. They are also not talking about the family of the child with these disorders. It is important to look at each child as an individual and as a member of a family to determine the best approach for that child. We have never seen a "generic" child. There is a bumper sticker that jokingly says, "I'm unique—just like everyone else." In treatment of children with special needs, this is actually a very serious statement. While children with ADHD or autism can have similar underlying biochemistry, no children are exactly alike in the way symptoms present themselves through behavior and development.

Some children with ADHD or autism truly require a strict elimination diet to show benefit. Even small exposures can result in significant negative behaviors. Other children seem to benefit from even a decrease in the problem foods. Still others require strict elimination initially but are eventually able to loosen up on the diet once the leakiness of their intestine has healed and it has become a good barrier again. The use of digestive enzymes specifically designed to digest casein and gluten has also allowed some children to eventually eat foods they previously needed to avoid completely. While there is no enzyme that can equal the complete elimination of foods, for some children, "mimicking" the elimination diet by use of enzymes can allow some "cheating" on the diet and can even allow some to eat a normal diet. Again, this mostly relates to how well the leaky gut has healed, since this is what allows the problem foods to get into the blood.

In most cultures, much social experience revolves around food. When a child's autism symptoms are severe, he has no awareness that his diet is different from other kids' diets. However, as autism symptoms lessen and awareness improves, a child may start to care that he is different from other children or that he can't eat the same cake as other kids at a birthday party. He may want to eat pizza on "pizza Fridays" at school. These are all good signs, as they show improved social awareness and a desire to be like peers. It would certainly help social development if a child who has been on a strict elimination diet were able to eat "normal" foods in these social situations. For some children, once the intestine has healed sufficiently, and especially with the use of digestive enzymes before meals, broadening the diet to include other foods is possible. For other groups of children, unfortunately, this is not possible, as any intake of problem foods, however small, results in unacceptable side effects on brain functioning. The only way to tell is to try. The ideal timing for reintroduction of foods is best discussed with the health care practitioner (doctor or nutritionist) who is guiding your child's dietary treatment.

What Kind of Improvements Can We Expect?

It is our experience that about two-thirds of children with autism improve when gluten and casein are removed from their diets. With soy removal, there may be even further improvement. Some children have immediate and dramatic improvement, whereas others have slower but steady improvement. Less than one-third of children with autism do not respond to the diet, and the GFCF diet does not appear to be a contributing factor to their symptoms. Remembering that the GFCF diet is not the only diet change recommended for those with autism, the other diet changes can also have an important effect as reported by the "Parental Rating" findings of the Autism Research Institute (updated February, 2008). These improvements are also noted in those with ADHD.

How Long Before We See Results?

It could be days, weeks, or months depending on the:

- Child's age
- Disorder subtype
- Presence of other conditions
- Co-existing additional food allergies or sensitivities
- Health of the gut
- Amount of gluten and dairy previously in the diet
- Degree of elevation of opiates from casein or gluten
- Diet compliance and strictness
- Nutritional supplements used (including digestive enzymes)

Our experience that two-thirds of those with autism spectrum disorder improve on the GFCF diet is consistent with the "Parental Rating" findings of the Autism Research Institute (updated February, 2008). For one third of the children this may not be the issue.

Chapter Summary

- The hardest step is starting the diet and finding substitute foods your child will accept. Maintaining the diet is much easier.

- Gradual rather than abrupt removal of offending foods is often easier on you and on your child, both physically and emotionally.

- When initially removing casein products, do not replace them with soy-based products. Soy is also a common offending food, and you may be substituting one problem for another.

- Each child is unique. The best results come from strict avoidance of offending foods. The outcome depends on the child's age, severity of the condition, digestive health, nutritional supplementation, and the presence of other offending foods.

- Every child is different in terms of how strict an elimination diet needs to be in order to see results.

- Try not to get discouraged. Focus on what you are able to do rather than what you aren't able to do.

- Improvement with casein and soy removal can occur within days or weeks as compared to gluten removal, which may take months. Approximately two-thirds improve when casein, gluten, and soy are eliminated.

- Talk with other parents who are doing the diet. They are often excellent sources of support and information.

CHAPTER 7

Dealing with the Diet and Common Concerns

"He who lives on air alone."

—A parent's description of her autistic child

"MY STOMACH DOES NOT HURT ANYMORE. NOW, I CAN GO places. I love to go places. I made honor roll twice this year. I love to read and I can now do math easier. School is much easier. I am no longer in speech therapy. My teachers are proud of me and say I am a role model. I feel GREAT!"

—*Ashley Stilson*

Right now my life is just one learning experience after another.

By the end of the week, I should be a genius.

—Jeanette Osias

Picky Appetites, Texture Issues, and Odd Food Choices

A common problem in children with ASD is picky eating. This can show itself in a variety of ways. Children may limit themselves to only dairy and wheat foods. They may decide what to eat not based on taste, but by the smell or the look of foods. They may become very brand-specific, eating only one brand of chicken nuggets, for example, but not another, virtually identical brand. They may limit themselves to unusual categories of food, such as eating only food that is white or brown. Some like only crunchy foods, while others like only soft or mushy foods. Some like both types but cannot stand having them mixed together or even on the same plate together. They may be exquisitely sensitive to any change in food or to hiding supplements in food. Children with autism can often detect even the subtlest difference in foods. All of these factors combine to make adequately nourishing these children a potentially very challenging task.

There are many reasons why children develop these picky appetites. Many children, not just children with autism, are deficient in zinc. Zinc is a critically important nutrient in the body. One important consequence of zinc deficiency is a change in taste and smell. The taste of a food is what makes eating

pleasurable. If you are unable to taste or smell a food, the main sensation you would be aware of when eating the food is its texture. You can well imagine that, at best, this would not be as enjoyable, and at worst, this could be unpleasant or intolerable. Many of us have also likely experienced a negative response to a food, such as developing food poisoning. These types of "sense memories" can be strong, resulting in a complete lack of desire for that food for a long time, even if you can logically convince yourself that the reaction was a fluke or the result of a specific situation. This is important to remember because even when zinc deficiencies are corrected and taste normalizes, there may be a strong behavioral component to avoidance of specific foods that may need to be addressed. Often the best treatment is time and patience, though in severe situations, specific feeding therapy interventions may be needed.

As previously described, opiate-like reactions from food can also lead to picky appetites. Children may not know why they are choosing particular foods; they may simply be responding to an awareness that certain foods make their brain feel good. They may then want to eat only those foods, either due to a physically based craving for those foods or to an "addiction" to the pleasurable feelings they get from them. Once this addiction is broken—either by eliminating those foods from the diet or by digesting them more efficiently (through the use of digestive enzymes)—children's dietary choices may broaden.

A large number of children with autism and a subset of children with ADHD also have a condition known as sensory integration dysfunction or sensory processing disorder. This refers to problems handling the variety of sensations that bombard our bodies every day. We sense the environment through touch, sound, smell, taste, and movement. In some children, these senses are heightened, so that sounds that don't typically bother people are too loud, or smells are too strong. If severe enough, this can actually be painful for children. Related to eating, if a child does not process taste or smell or touch normally, foods may be very unpleasant. Mild tastes may seem strong, mild smells may be overwhelming, or particular textures may be intolerable. In these cases, occupational therapy can be helpful to normalize a child's ability to process sensory feelings in a more normal and tolerable way.

Withdrawal Symptoms from Foods—How Can This Be?

Some children, especially those who are making opiate-like peptides from their foods, are actually physically addicted to those foods. When the foods are removed from the diet, they can experience symptoms that are similar to drug withdrawal. The most common symptoms are irritability and sometimes anger or rage. Children may also temporarily regress in their behavior or in their developmental skills. Withdrawal symptoms can actually be viewed as a good sign, as this indicates the foods were having some effect on the child. Anytime there are negative symptoms from removing a food from the diet, the food is a problem. Not having withdrawal symptoms does not necessarily mean the food is not a problem. Some children have resilient personalities and bodies and can tolerate withdrawal symptoms well, without obvious side effects.

Some children can tolerate abrupt removal of the offending foods. However, most do best with gradual removal of the foods, as this allows their body to adjust with fewer side effects. From a practical standpoint, gradual withdrawal is usually a necessity if your child is a picky eater, as you need to find substitute foods your child is actually willing to eat.

What Can Be Done for Withdrawal Symptoms?

The best treatment for withdrawal symptoms is time. Food-withdrawal symptoms often subside within a few days and usually not longer than a week. In some cases, they may last longer, again depending on the particular child. As the body becomes clear of the offending foods, there will be a period of time when the child is actually more sensitive to those foods. If there are unknown dietary infractions during that time, the child's behavior may worsen. If withdrawal symptoms seem prolonged, they may not actually be withdrawal but rather reaction to intake of problem foods.

It is worth then carefully reviewing possible sources of exposure to the eliminated foods in case unknown infractions are occurring. One commonly overlooked source of gluten is play dough at school. Play dough is now often made out of flour at school. One of our patients had prolonged behavioral regression without any obvious cause. The cause of his regression became clear only when he came home from school with flour all over his clothes from the play dough.

Time may seem to pass very slowly as you try to survive your child's withdrawal symptoms, but try to remember that there is a light at the end of the withdrawal tunnel.

Is the Diet Helping?

The best test for determining response to the diet is the change in the child's physical and behavioral symptoms. For some children, this is very easy: Within days or weeks, there is an obvious and dramatic improvement noticed by a variety of people in the child's life. In other children, the response to an elimination diet is more slow and subtle, especially if there are other complicating factors (significant nutritional deficiencies, untreated food allergies/sensitivities, toxic metals). When the total load is great, it takes longer and more effort to overcome it.

Parents often ask if they should keep data in order to tell whether the diet is working. As a general point, it is our opinion that if the only way to tell the diet is working is by minute inspection of data, then it is

probably not worth doing the diet long-term. The goal of the diet is noticeable change that results in an improved quality of life for the child.

Elimination diets result in increased expense and effort, and the benefit needs to be worth that effort. Parents are usually the best people to determine whether the improvements seen are worth the challenge of the diet. That said, there are often already existing sources of outside or objective information. Most children with ASD have multiple adults involved in their care who can provide helpful feedback. Feedback from those who are not aware there has been any change in diet is the most valuable. Their observations are less influenced, consciously or unconsciously, by awareness that something has been changed. This type of feedback may come from relatives or friends who have not seen the child since the elimination diet was started, and who spontaneously comment on positive changes. A school-bus driver may comment on improved behavior. Teachers and therapists often need to be informed about the dietary changes because food is often part of the school day or the therapy sessions. However, they can also provide good feedback on apparent changes. For example, a therapist may comment that prior to the diet, the majority of the hour-long therapy session was spent trying to keep a hyperactive child seated in order to do therapy. After the diet, he or she may be able to spend the majority of the session actually providing therapy. Children receiving ABA or discrete trial training as a therapy will already have data collection as part of that therapy.

Another way to tell if the diet is helping is through dietary infractions. These may be planned but are often unplanned. Children are exposed to foods that are not on their diets. This can occur at home, school, restaurants, and therapy offices. Siblings may leave food out where their brother or sister with ADHD or autism can accidentally get into it. And you can guarantee that if a classmate leaves a gluten-containing snack unattended, your child will be the first one to grab it. This will result in an unplanned "challenge" to your child's system. Often, in the initial months on an elimination diet, these challenges will result in obvious worsening of symptoms. This is evidence that the food is a problem. It often gives parents motivation to continue the diet, as these infractions often occur around the time parents are tiring of these diets, especially if there has not been convincing improvement by that point. When the child is further along in the healing process, these accidental dietary infractions also provide information. If digestion has improved and/or the intestine has healed enough and is no longer leaky, the same infractions that caused significant symptoms in the past may no longer cause the same degree of symptoms. This is evidence that less of the bothersome food peptides are reaching the brain and causing it problems.

In general, the timing of planned food challenges is best discussed with the practitioner who is guiding your child's care. Some individuals believe that it is best to challenge the body with a large amount of the offending food so that any reactions will be obvious. We would not recommend that approach because some children are exquisitely sensitive and may be miserable for a significant period of time after a large challenge. Rather, we would suggest an initial challenge with a single serving of one type of offending food (such as casein). For example, we would suggest a challenge with a single slice of cheese rather than an unlimited amount. In addition, we would not recommend a combination food such as pizza, since this contains both casein and gluten. The single serving should be given and no further offending foods given over the next three days. The child's behavior should then be monitored over these three days, remembering that food sensitivity reactions can occur anytime within seventy-two hours of eating the food. Reactions most commonly appear the next day or two days after eating the offending food. If no reaction is obvious, a second challenge can be done with a larger serving of the food, again with monitoring of behavior for three days. If still no reaction, servings can be given every two days, then every day, until you are sure there is no negative reaction. Most common negative reactions are irritability or regression in behavior or development (such as reappearance of ADHD or autism symptoms, decrease in language, etc.). There are many fine points to food challenges and interpretation of reactions, and these challenges are best done under the guidance of a knowledgeable practitioner (functional medicine physician, nutritionist).

There is also debate about how long of an elimination period is necessary to determine whether particular foods are a problem. There seems to be general agreement that casein clears out of the system more rapidly than gluten. Recommendations regarding casein elimination have ranged from five days to three weeks; however, in children with autism, longer elimination trials are usually necessary because of the combinations of offending foods and the complexity of all of the other nutritional and medical factors affecting the brain. Some say that gluten can take six to twelve months to completely clear the system and that one cannot say a gluten elimination trial has failed until it has been done for that period of time. Again, a knowledgeable practitioner can discuss this with you as part of your child's overall treatment plan.

"As a mother to several special-needs children, I have been completely thrilled with the unbelievable progress my eldest son, Dorian, has made since going on the gluten-free, casein-free diet with added supplements. In fourth grade, he was floundering to just stay afloat in school and was completely antisocial. He couldn't focus in class because he was too busy using all of his mental energy to keep his involuntary body movements [tics] from being so noticeable. At lunchtime, he would sit alone with his head down. His typical recess routine was to walk the perimeter of the playground and try to be invisible. His grades were suffering even though all of his teachers said, and testing showed, that he was incredibly bright.

After he was evaluated and diagnosed with Asperger's syndrome, he went on the gluten-free, casein-free diet and supplements. Within a month, we began noticing changes. By three to six months later, he was a different child. He was able to focus and participate in class so well that his teachers were amazed. His playground activities were astonishing—he was playing basketball with the other kids and was chosen team captain! He was even chosen for the starring role in his school play. I can proudly say that Dorian has become an honor-roll student who has a fun group of close friends he has hung out with through middle school and now into high school. He is well known at school and well liked everywhere. Granted, he does still have some quirkiness and his special interests but he has been able to transform all of these points into assets rather than liabilities!

Had anyone ever told me that having an autistic child would be the least of my concerns as a parent of special-needs children, I would have never believed them. But last year when we went to adopt in Ukraine, they were amazed that we were willing to take on a child that had gluten-free, casein-free dietary needs. We said, 'No problem, we know all about it.'

—**Natalie Sirota,** *mother of Dorian, who has Asperger's syndrome*

Common Concerns
THE PICKY APPETITE

My child is an extremely picky eater. I'm afraid he'll starve if I take away casein and gluten foods.

This is a very real concern. Some children will go on "hunger strikes" when their preferred foods are removed. But it is absolutely not an option to starve your child's brain. It will not matter that casein and gluten have been removed if your child's brain is not otherwise being nourished. Because of this, despite your best intentions and efforts, some children will just not be able to do a full elimination diet initially.

Because of this obstacle, there needs to be a variety of approaches to implementing the diets. One way to think about this is "going in the front door" versus "sneaking in the back door." For some children, you can walk through the front door of the diet elimination house and simply substitute foods without much negative effect. However, for a significant number of children, you need to sneak in the back door and make some other changes before you can come through the front door again. Coming in the back door involves looking at the possible causes of your child's extreme reluctance or inability to try new foods. As previously discussed, there are several reasons why children may have picky appetites, including zinc deficiency, opiate-based addictions to foods, and sensory sensitivities. Back-door approaches involve correcting these problems. Often when this is done, children's diets will expand, and it is much easier to substitute healthier food choices. While working on these issues, slowly introduce new GFCF and soy-free foods mixed in with the old foods.

Here is one potential back door approach:

- Introduce zinc supplements. There are commercially available "taste tests" as well as blood tests that can indicate whether your child is zinc deficient. Zinc deficiency results in abnormal taste and smell. Giving zinc supplements improves zinc levels and normal taste returns; eating then becomes a more pleasurable experience again.

- Use digestive enzymes first. If children have a very strong addiction to certain foods, it can be nearly impossible to get them to take foods that do not make the brain feel as good. Sometimes it is necessary to give digestive enzymes that have been specifically designed to break down these opiate-like products. This substitution, in effect, mimics doing the diet to some degree and helps decrease the amount of opiates. The addictive type of response to foods lessens and often dietary choices expand.

- Occupational therapy may be necessary to help address extreme sensitivities to food textures, tastes, or smells so that the experience of eating is not unpleasant.

Individual children may have any or all of these factors contributing to their picky appetites, and sometimes a back-door approach is the place to start. It is often helpful to have a knowledgeable health professional guide these treatments.

IS THE GFCF DIET HEALTHY?

My child's doctor is concerned that the GFCF diet is not healthy.

Your physician's goal is to make sure your child is healthy. Your doctor is right to raise the question of whether your child is being adequately nourished. The concern is usually that two "essential food groups" are being removed from the diet. What is factual, but not well known, is that milk products and grains are not mandatory food groups for human survival. There are only three essential food groups for humans: proteins, fats, and carbohydrates. Milk products are a choice in the protein group. Grains are a choice in the carbohydrate group. For over 200,000 years of human history, milk products and grains have been present since the beginning of domestication, which is only 0.05 percent of that time (5,000 to 10,000 years). Hence, it is not a surprise to find that many humans are predisposed to negative reactions to "newer foods" in human history.

What most physicians do not realize is that children on the GFCF diet often eat much healthier diets than those who eat "regular" diets. Children on the GFCF diet eat much less fast food and processed food, which often contain casein or gluten. In addition, not much attention is paid to what typical children are getting in their diets, other than ensuring they get enough calcium for bone health. Given the pace of today's lifestyle, many children eat too much in the way of processed food or fast food, and often eat in ways that do not support healthy digestion (such as eating in the car on the way to classes or sports practices).

When removing milk products from the diet, there is always the concern that calcium, vitamin D, and protein will be inadequate. As described in chapter 5, there are other sources of protein, calcium, and vitamin D in addition to dietary supplements, which can be used as needed.

The true miracle for most of us, children and adults alike, is that our brains continue to function adequately in spite of being poorly nourished. For children on elimination diets, it is just as important to pay attention to what is being put back into the diet as it is to what is being taken out. When this is done, children's diets are healthy, and often more healthy than that of their typically developing peers.

ELIMINATION DIET—WORTH IT OR NOT?

My child's doctor feels the elimination diet is a waste of time.

Again, a pediatrician's responsibility is to make sure that your child is healthy. Physicians are also concerned that parents of children with special needs do not get taken advantage of in their desire to help their children. They are concerned that parents may have false hope or undertake treatments that are harmful or expensive. These can be positive qualities in a physician. However, most physicians did not receive much education about nutrition during their formal training. They may only hear that you are removing foods from your child's diet and may not be aware of the potential health benefits. An elimination diet, done correctly, will not be harmful to your child and will hopefully be helpful. All physicians take the Hippocratic Oath, which states, "First do no harm." It may help to tell your physician that you are aware of this and that you will be pursuing the diet in a way that "does no harm." Even if your physician feels the diet may not help, at least you can make him or her aware that it will not harm your child if done thoughtfully.

GETTING SUPPORT FROM FAMILY AND THE SCHOOL TEAM

What can we do to get more support from family and the school?

It is very important that all caregivers involved in the child's life be aware of the diet and be committed to supporting it. Especially when starting the diet, it is important to be as strict as is reasonably possible so that you can feel you've given the diet an adequate trial. Again, some children improve simply with a decrease in the amount of offending foods. However, other children need to be taken completely and strictly off the offending foods before improvement is seen. If other adults involved with a child give nonpermitted foods, this may sabotage the elimination trial.

Some people, such as grandparents, teachers, or other family members, may think a small amount of a prohibited food couldn't hurt. In this case, it may help to compare the GFCF diet to a diet for a child with diabetes or a life-threatening peanut allergy. In those situations, no adult would contemplate giving just a little bit of an impermissible food. Similarly, while food infractions on the GFCF diet are not life-threatening, they can have serious negative effects on brain functioning. The adults in your child's life who know and love your child and want the best for him or her may be better able to support the diet if they understand what problems the foods can cause in the brain.

One additional challenge in convincing other caregivers about the consequences of cheating on the diet is that the effects of the cheat often do not occur immediately. Effects of infractions often occur the next day or two days later, when the adult who gave your child the food is no longer present. Some parents have jokingly told their child's grandparents that they were welcome to give the child an offending food but then they would have to keep the child for the weekend. Many a grandparent has probably become aware of the reactions to food when babysitting a grandchild for the weekend.

Chapter Summary

- Causes of picky appetites include zinc deficiency, opiate-like addiction to craved foods, and sensory sensitivities. Addressing these factors often helps expand dietary choices.

- Many children will experience withdrawal symptoms such as irritability or regression when foods are eliminated. This is a temporary effect.

- The trial elimination approach is effective and safe in that it includes foods from the three essential food groups: protein, fat, and carbohydrate. Milk is not an essential food group, it is a protein choice. Gluten is not an essential food group, it is a family of grains within the carbohydrate group. There are many other grains available. To assure adequate nutritional status, supplements usually include calcium, magnesium, vitamin D, and GFCF fiber as needed.

- For the diet to be successful, other adults in your child's life (teachers, family members) need to be educated about the need for compliance with the diet. Even small infractions may affect your ability to tell whether the elimination trial is working or may result in significant negative behavioral effects.

- Elimination trials and dietary challenges provide helpful information. Due to the complexities of administering and interpreting the results of these tests, guidance by a knowledgeable practitioner is recommended.

> "Another barrier when it comes to putting children on a restricted diet, according to Ms. Laake, involves the belief system of the parents. 'If there are doubts, or a trusted physician has said that a diet is unhealthy and/or does not work, there will be reluctance to try it.' This is more common when the parents are faced with a diagnosis such as autism, where the mainstream medical community views the gluten-free, casein-free dietary intervention with great skepticism. In that case, a limited trial period may help resolve doubts that one or both parents have. Not only will it tell you whether or not the diet will help but, as Ms. Laake points out, 'It is truly a *do no harm* and non-invasive approach that has the potential for profound improvement.'"
>
> —Kathryn Scott,
> *"Flirting with Disaster,"*
> from Living Without, *Spring 2006*

I think a hero is an ordinary individual
who finds strength to persevere and endure
in spite of overwhelming obstacles.

—Christopher Reeve

CHAPTER 8

A Complete Guide to Making Breakfast and Packing Lunches

THE MEAL TO FOCUS ON FIRST IS BREAKFAST. STUDIES HAVE SHOWN THAT THE FIRST FOOD or drink of the day is the most important. It sets the pattern of eating for the day. Typical breakfast foods include too many refined carbohydrates, which raise blood sugar too quickly: breads, bagels, muffins, cold cereals, and instant hot cereals. This results in a pattern throughout the day of mood swings, frequent hunger, and cravings for more sweets and refined carbohydrates. Studies on the effect of breakfast quality on children's performance repeatedly reveal that the sweet and sugared breakfasts impair focus, attention, and performance.

Breakfast Like a King

The ideal breakfast should start with a protein or mix of proteins such as fish, poultry, meat, eggs, beans, nuts, and seeds. Protein is critical for making brain neurotransmitters, strengthening immunity, and maintaining lean muscle mass and good muscle tone. Lunch and dinner leftovers are perfect choices for breakfast and certainly Quick N Easy. There are no "Breakfast Police"; you can improve the quality of breakfast by moving toward non-typical breakfast foods. Make a little extra at dinner and refrigerate enough for a serving at breakfast.

Eggs are the most nutrient-dense food available and have the highest-quality protein. Do not use egg substitutes. Humans have enjoyed and benefitted from eggs over 400,000 years. It is only in the last fifty years that they have been incorrectly vilified. Please read "The Good Egg" in chapter 4. As long as there are no allergies, include eggs!

BREAKFAST IDEAS

Hardboiled eggs + fruit
Christina's Delicious Deviled Eggs
   (p. 177)

Egg salad on tomato slice or egg salad + fruit
Simple Egg Salad (p. 264)

Scrambled eggs with or without vegetables + fruit
Scrambled Veggie Eggs (p. 173)

Vegetable omelet + fruit
Ground Vegetable Omelet (p. 174)
Mexican Breakfast Pizza (p. 175)

GFCF Quiche + fruit
Crustless Spinach Quiche (p. 172)

Hearty soup + fruit
Erika's Chicken Noodle Soup (p. 288)
Turkey Noodle Soup (p. 276)
Jane's Lentil Vegetable Soup (p. 274)
Best Beef Soup Ever (p. 277)

Breakfast sausage + fruit
Breakfast Sausage (p. 171)
Best's Kosher Sausage Links
   (www.bestskosher.com)

Other meat dishes + fruit
Shepherd's Pie (p. 200)
GFCF Chicken Nuggets (p. 178)
Fruit Rice Chicken or Turkey (p. 185)
Chicken Puree (p. 184)
Nutritious Delicious Meatballs in
   Sauce (p. 204)
Meatballs with Vegetables (p. 203)

Waffles, bars, granola, or oatmeal + additional protein (nuts, egg, GFCF sausage)
High-Protein Waffles (p. 158)
Crispy Breakfast Bars (p. 159)
Tracy Smith's Granola (p. 159)
Hot Oatmeal (p. 167) + additional
   protein (1–2 ounces of nuts or
   1 hardboiled egg)

Nuts and other options
Peanut butter on apple slices
Lentil Loaf (p. 216) + fruit
Dahl (Vegetarian or With Chicken)
   (p. 217)

Packing School Lunches

THE CHALLENGE

With only twenty minutes to eat, kids with autism spectrum disorder should be given "fast" foods that are not only easy to eat, but healthy, tasty, loaded with nutrients, and free of the culprits that are common problems: gluten, milk products, soy, and artificial additives and coloring. Compounding the time challenge are sensory issues involving food texture, color, and taste along with unusually picky appetites so common in ASD. Now the task seems insurmountable. Beyond the challenges with foods themselves are the safety issues concerning the food containers, especially plastics containing phthalates and bisphenyl A (BPA). And, of course, there is the "cool," factor which affects preschoolers through high schoolers. Food that is different is totally uncool for kids who already face so many social and learning stigmas.

Knowing the challenges, we can now focus on the solutions.

THE SOLUTIONS

Basics—As is the case with any meal, there are some basics to follow. Protein, fiber, and good fats are needed to stabilize blood sugars. Blood-sugar control is critical. All people are affected by rapidly rising blood sugar which then cascades down too quickly and too low. The most noticeable effects are on brain function especially mood and attention. When the blood sugar drops too quickly, there can be irritability, hunger headaches, lack of focus, behavior problems, and cravings for a "quick sugar fix" which keeps the cycle going. This interferes with learning and can be disruptive to the class.

Avoid—Glycemic foods, which raise blood sugar (glucose) quickly, including sugars, sodas (see below), candy, sweets, juices, and any refined grains (e.g., pretzels, bread, crackers, bagels, chips) on an empty stomach. Limit the sugars and keep the refined carbohydrates limited. If small amounts are consumed at the end of the meal, the negative effect is less.

Below is a summary of the basic rules for any meal, but especially helpful when preparing school lunches.

Stay away from sodas, both regular and diet. (See chapter 4, Eater Beware). They have no place in a healthy diet. They are high in phosphorus, which depletes healthy nutrients. Consider them removers of vitamins and minerals, not drink options. Water is best, but other good choices include: diluted juices, seltzer water with juice to flavor, vegetable juices.

Promote protein. Smart protein-packed choices include fish, poultry, meat, eggs, beans, nuts, and seeds. Remember, the serving size for protein for each person is the size of the palm. A child's may be 1 to 2 ounces and a teen and adult may be 3 to 5 ounces. For beans, however, the serving size is two cupped palms.

Include fabulous fiber. High-fiber options include fruits, beans, nuts, seeds, and grains. These are especially important if your child eats very few vegetables. Fiber as pure guar gum is easy to add to any recipe and also to drinks. It is GFCF and more fine than sugar, mixing completely in water or juice.

Toss in a favorite food. Promote more interest in the meal by including at least one food that your child considers "a favorite."

Add to the fun-factor. Take a tip from the fast-food marketers and include a surprise gift in the lunch. It might be a small collectable such as a car, baseball card, character, hair clip, sticker, or ring or bracelet. Homemade "giftlets" (tiny gifts) are perfect.

Go organic as frequently as possible. The "USDA Organic" label means the food is produced without the use of harmful pesticides, artificial fertilizers, antibiotics, growth hormones human waste, or sewage sludge, and that they were processed without ionizing radiation or food additives. Children with ASD are already coping with their own excess metabolites and really can not handle the burden of harmful chemicals in the environment and foods. The less the exposure the better. Anything you can do for your child is a benefit.

Seek GFCF foods and give them a test run. There are numerous resources for GFCF foods and recipes online and in many books. Use all of these to find the commercially available foods your child will eat as well as recipes that are not just GFCF, they are nutritious and delicious. There are GFCF juice boxes, pretzels, breads, wraps, and snacks.

Test them at home, however, not in the school lunch.

Also: Establish three to five basic lunches that work. If your child is willing and interested, engage him or her in the process. Use freezer packs for keeping foods cold and thermos for hot foods. Include non-toxic hand sanitizers which are commercially available (avoid the commercial sanitizers). You can also send two paper towel pieces— one moistened with soap and one moistened with water.

Packaging: A Good Opportunity to Go Green

Again, follow the marketer's lead—jazz it up! Select a lunch container your child loves. Young children love to decorate a lunch box with stickers and paints. Make the lunch box the child's own work of art, personalized with a name. Reusable containers and boxes are the green way to go. Older children will definitely want to select whatever is considered cool. The most cool may be a paper bag or small recycled bags carried in a back pack. Go with the trend and your child's own choice. There are companies who make safe, BPA-Free, safe lunch box sets with inserts for the different foods.

Avoid plastic wraps and sandwich bags for sandwiches, instead use wax paper or parchment paper. Avoid containers with BPA by avoiding items with the recycle number 7. There are many BPA-free containers which can be washed and reused. Your child will need to be reminded to bring these back home rather than throw them away.

For napkins, use washable cloth napkins or dishcloths, or choose processed chlorine-free (PCF), post-consumer-waste (PCW) paper napkins available in stores and online. If utensils are needed, use stainless steel appropriate to the child's skill level and age.

Nutritious Can Be Delicious

Recall what we discussed in chapter 6, and use the Trojan Horse concept as a way to sneak nutrition into your child's lunches. Disguise the new foods within the usual, well-liked foods. We can't emphasize enough the importance of matching the color and texture, mixing vegetable juice with fruit juice, and including muffin "casseroles" that mask pureed fruits, vegetables, and even meat. Your goal is to get a child to eat nutritious food, however you can.

Assuming the new food is a vegetable, use organic baby food purees or make your own. Puree the vegetable into an established food in such a fashion that it does not change the overall color, texture, smell, or taste of the well-liked food. If a child eats nothing but white food, start with very light-colored vegetables such as squash, cauliflower, and corn. If the child likes ketchup or tomato sauce, then introduce deeper-colored vegetables such as beets, greens, peas and beans. Pureed vegetables can be beaten into batter for pancakes, muffins, brownies, and cookies or into tomato and other pasta and pizza sauces, and even into ketchup.

Six Simple and Delicious Lunch Suggestions

Use the following six lunch suggestions (on pages 99–103) as they are written or feel free to mix and match the pieces to find the perfect lunchtime combination for your little one.

Drinks: All of these lunches should be accompanied by either water, GFCF vegetable juice, GFCF juice box, or fortified organic rice-milk drink box.

Containers: Use BPA-free containers to store foods whenever possible.

Lunch #1: BBQ Chicken for Champions

- **Chicken strips**
- **BBQ dipping sauce**
- **Steamed vegetables**
- **Veggie dipping sauce**

Snack, if needed: GFCF chips and 1 cup (260 g) Fruity Salsa (recipe below)

Toy surprise ideas: yarn bracelet, miniature toy character figure

Chicken Breast

- $^1/_2$ chicken breast

Add salt and pepper to taste and pan fry in olive oil on medium-high heat for six minutes on each side. Cut into strips. Serve with $^1/_4$ cup (65 g) serving of BBQ Sipping Sauce.

Steamed Vegetables

- 1 broccoli stock (or frozen single-serving package)

Steam broccoli florets for 7 minutes. Run cold water over them.

BBQ Sipping Sauce

- 1 cup (240 g) organic ketchup
- 1 tablespoon (6 g) lemon juice
- 1 teaspoon Worchestershire sauce (GFCF)
- 1 tablespoon (20 g) honey
- Dash of black pepper

Blend all of the above until smooth

YIELD: *$1^1/_4$ cup (300 g)*

Fruity Salsa

- 1 cup (250 g) salsa
- $^1/_4$ cup (80 g) grape, blueberry, or raspberry fruit spread

Mash the fruit spread into the salsa.

YIELD: *$1^1/_4$ cup (330 g)*

Lunch #2: DLT ("Deli" meat, lettuce, and tomato sandwich)

- **DLT sandwich**
- **GFCF Potato Salad, ¹/₃ cup (85 g) from recipe, below**
- **Fruit (e.g., apple or grapes)**

Snack, if needed: Peanut butter on rice crackers

Toy surprise ideas: hair scrunchie, baseball card

DLT ("Deli" meat, lettuce, and tomato sandwich)

- 2 slices of turkey or chicken GFCF preservative-free organic lunch meats (by Boar's Head, Applegate, or Shelton)
- 2 slices of GFCF bread, toasted
- 1 tablespoon (14 g) GFCF mayonnaise
- Lettuce and tomato

Spread the mayonnaise on a slice of bread. Cover with 2 slices of GFCF lunch meat and top with lettuce and a slice of tomato. Cut into 4 squares and wrap in wax paper.

GFCF Potato Salad

- 3 pounds (1.4 kg) potatoes, cooked until just tender, cubed, cooled
- 5 or 6 hard-cooked eggs, cooled, coarsely chopped, optional
- ¹/₄ (40 g) to ¹/₂ cup (80 g) chopped red onion
- ¹/₄ (25 g) to ¹/₂ cup (50 g) chopped celery, optional

For the dressing:

- ³/₄ cup (175 g) mayonnaise
- 1 (14 g) to 2 (28 g) tablespoons prepared GFCF mustard
- Salt and pepper to taste

Prepare the dressing, combining the mayonnaise, mustard, and salt and pepper to taste. Combine potatoes, egg, onions, and celery and stir in the dressing.

YIELD: *6 to 8 servings*

Lunch # 3 Kids Favorite Chicken Salad and Deviled Eggs

- **Chicken Salad ($^1/_3$ to $^1/_2$ cup) (70 to 100 g)**
- **Deviled Eggs (two halves)**
- **Carrot sticks wrapped in wax paper and served with applesauce**

Snack, if needed: GFCF chips & hummus

Toy surprise ideas: mini toy car, hair clip

Chicken Salad

- 3 cups (420 g) cooked chicken, diced
- 2 ribs celery, thinly sliced
- 1 cup (150 g) seedless green grapes, halved
- $^3/_4$ cup (175 g) mayonnaise
- 2 tablespoons (12 g) finely minced green onions
- 1 teaspoon (5 ml) lemon juice
- $^1/_4$ teaspoon ground ginger
- Salt and pepper, to taste

Combine chicken, celery, and grapes in a large bowl; set aside. In a small bowl, whisk together remaining ingredients. Then, combine with chicken mixture, using as much or as little as necessary to moisten as desired. You may add a little more mayonnaise if you like a creamier salad. Chill and stir again before serving.

YIELD: *4 to 6 servings*

Deviled Eggs

- 6 hard-boiled eggs, cooled, shelled, cut in half, yolks removed and set aside
- $1^1/_2$ tablespoons (21 g) mayonnaise
- 1 teaspoon (4 g) prepared mustard
- $^1/_2$ teaspoon salt
- 2 tablespoons (30 g) sweet pickle relish, or to taste
- Paprika

Mash yolks and combine with mayonnaise, mustard, salt, and relish. Refill centers of the egg whites with the mixture. Garnish with ground paprika.

YIELD: *6 servings (2 halves per person)*

Lunch # 4 Meatballs in Spaghetti Sauce

- **Meatballs in Spaghetti Sauce, (1 cup or 140 g) served warm in thermos**
- **Wonderful Waldorf Salad ($^1/_3$ to $^1/_2$ cup or 90 to 130 g)**
- **Broccoli trees, asparagus, or carrot strips with Russian Dressing ($^1/_4$ cup) dipping sauce or honey**
- **Fruit Smoothie**

Snack, if needed: Organic GFCF "O"s cereal

Toy surprise ideas: stickers, appropriate to the child

Meatballs in Spaghetti Sauce

- 1 small yellow onion
- 1 slice GFCF rice bread
- 1 teaspoon salt
- $^1/_2$ teaspoon oregano
- 1 pound (455 g) ground beef
- 2 jars (16 oz or 475 ml) GFCF pasta sauce

Put onion in food processor and mince. Add bread, 2 tablespoons water, salt, and oregano and mix again. Pour mixture into a mixing bowl. Knead by hand together with ground beef until thoroughly mixed. Shape into desired meatball size. Put meatballs into a slow cooker with spaghetti sauce and cook on high for 4 hours. Refrigerate.

YIELD: *4 to 6 servings*

Wonderful Waldorf Salad

- 1 cup (165 g) pineapple chunks (fresh or unsweetened, canned)
- 3 cups (450 g) apples, peeled and cut in $^1/_2$-inch cubes
- $^1/_3$ cup (50 g) raisins
- 1 cup (130 g) carrots, thinly sliced
- $^1/_2$ cup (60 g) walnut pieces, optional
- 1 cup (225 g) GFCF mayonnaise

Combine all ingredients in a large bowl and mix thoroughly. Chill before serving.

YIELD: *4 to 6 servings*

Russian Dressing

- 1 cup (225 g) GFCF mayonnaise
- 1 cup (240 g) GFCF ketchup

Combine in a bowl.

YIELD: *8 servings*

Fruit Smoothie

- $1^1/_4$ cup (295 ml) rice milk
- 4 ice cubes, crushed
- 1 tablespoon (5 g) rice powder
- 1 tablespoon (15 g) coconut milk, optional

Add one of the following with the above in a blender and blend at high speed until smooth and thick.

- 1 sliced medium banana
- 1 cored and chopped medium pear
- $^1/_2$ cup (75 g) berries (strawberries, blueberries, raspberries, or combination)

YIELD: *1 serving*

Lunch #5: Chicken, Apple Salad, and Magical Veggie Muffins

- **Baked or grilled chicken leftovers from dinner, approximately $1/2$ chicken breast**
- **Apple Salad, packed in a cold thermos**
- **1 to 2 Magical Veggie Muffins**

Snack, if needed: Carrots and Bean Dip

Toy surprise ideas: hand stamp or mood ring

Apple Salad

- 2 large Red Delicious apples, unpeeled, cored, and cut into 1-inch chunks
- $2/3$ cup crushed and drained pineapple or fresh minced pineapple (reserve juice for dressing)
- $1/3$ cup diced celery
- 2 tablespoons raisins

For the dressing:
- 3 tablespoons soy yogurt
- 2 teaspoons GFCF mayonnaise
- 1 tablespoon pineapple juice
- $1/8$ teaspoon cinnamon

In a medium bowl, combine the salad ingredients. In a small bowl, whisk the dressing ingredients together and pour the dressing over the salad. Toss to combine.

YIELD: *2 servings*

Magical Veggie Muffins

- 1 box (14.8 ounces) store-bought GFCF cake mix
- 1 cup puréed vegetables (use one or more of the following: carrots, squash, peas, or green beans)
- $1/2$ cup applesauce
- 1 cup GFCF chocolate chips, optional

In a large bowl, prepare cake mix batter according to package directions. Add puréed vegetables and applesauce and mix to combine. Stir in chocolate chips (if using).

Lightly grease a muffin tin or line with paper liners. Spoon the batter into the muffin cups, filling each about two-thirds full. Bake at 375° F for 25 to 30 minutes, or until a toothpick inserted in the center of a muffin comes out clean. (Do not overcook, as this will result in dry muffins.)

Once cooled, store the muffins in an air-tight container or freeze for later use.

YIELD: *24 muffins*

Lunch #6: Sensory Sensible Pot Pie Muffins and Dip (for those who avoid "lumps and bumps")

- **1 to 2 Sensory Sensible Protein Muffins**
- **Hummus dip (with carrots or GFCF crackers, if tolerated)**
- **Applesauce or other fruit**

Toy surprise ideas: festive pencil/penn

Snack, if needed: Organic apple chips

Sensory Sensible Pot Pie Muffins

- 1 box (14.8 ounces) store-bought GFCF muffin or quick bread mix
- 1 cup puréed vegetables (use one or more of the following: carrots, squash, peas, or green beans)
- $1/2$ cup applesauce
- $1/2$ cup puréed chicken*

In a large bowl, prepare cake mix batter according to package directions. Add puréed vegetables , applesauce, and chicken and mix to combine.

Lightly grease a muffin tin or line with paper liners. Spoon the batter into the muffin cups, filling each about two-thirds full. Bake at 375° F for 25 to 30 minutes, or until a toothpick inserted in the center of a muffin comes out clean. (Do not over-cook, as this will result in dry muffins.)

Once cooled, store the muffins in an air-tight container or freeze for later use.

*To purée chicken, combine cooked, chopped chicken with a bit of chicken broth or water (or even white grape juice) in a blender, and blend until desired consistency is reached.

YIELD: *24 muffins*

CHAPTER 9

Introduction to Recipes

From Yucky to Yummy: Finding the Right Kid-Friendly Foods

*You don't have to cook fancy or complicated masterpieces—
just good food from fresh ingredients.*

—Julia Child

BEYOND OUR OWN RECIPES AND ADAPTED RECIPES, MANY HAVE BEEN GRACIOUSLY CONTRIBUTED by the parents of our patients and by some of the children themselves. There are also recipes inspired by others who have expertise in cooking for special children.

We are grateful for the collective wisdom of those who have been through the journey that so many are now beginning, including: Lisa Barnes, Lizzie Vann, Lori Skalitzky, Joyce Mulcahy, Jeannie Fritz Godbout, Michael Thurmond, Elaine Gottschall, Linda and Bill Schmidt, Iris, Bette Hagman, Tracey Smith, Lori Brown Tremper, Travis Martin, Lisa Lewis, Pauline McFadden, Marie Donadio, Jody Cutler, Sue Chubb, Angela Lowry, Nicole Young, Diana Hann, Kathy Rivers, Bobby Warfield, Sue and Dick Redding, Leonardo Hosh, Mollie Katzen, Jennifer Richardson, Sally Fallon, Jeanne Wilson, Barbara Rees, Glenda Ingham, Colleen Godbout, Bonnie Gutman, Anne Evans, Jane Ruane, Doug and Jeannette DeLawter, Lisa Compart, Marilyn Lammers, Vivian Cavalieri, Maria Ribaya Than, Wendy Higgins, Carla and Aidan Hancock, Sharon Dahn, Vivian Duckett, Erika Melton, Melissa Kemp, Elynn Demattia, Sueson Vess, Christina Godbout, Welby Griffin and Julie Matthews.

We, as authors, have tried to provide recipes that can meet differing needs from Quick N Easy to gourmet and take into account the variation in appetite and food tolerances within families. There are Quick N Easy recipes for those who want to provide their families with healthy food and still juggle the extremely stressful demands of everyday schedules. The more complex recipes may appeal to those with the culinary skills and desire to create interesting dishes. For many of the complex recipes, we have offered Quick N Easy alternatives as well.

There are recipes throughout the book that attempt to accommodate the unique appetite and feeding problems so common to children with autism. There are also many children with ADHD and those without developmental and behavioral issues who share one or more of the issues regarding appetite and food acceptance.

This is why we repeatedly hear parents describe their children's appetite changes as follows: "He ate all kinds of foods as a baby and when we moved to more solid foods, he developed an extremely picky appetite." The food needs to be adapted to the child's preferences until the child is ready to advance to the next stage. Limited appetites and food aversions are not behavioral choices; they result from the way a food's appearance, smell, color, taste, and texture are perceived.

One Person's Yummy Food Is Another Person's Yucky Food

Vegetables and protein (fish, poultry, meats, and beans) are the most common food aversions.

Some children even reject fruits. The diet becomes extremely restricted to bland, white foods, including sweets, breads, pasta, crackers, pretzels, chips, and macaroni and cheese. These foods are glycemic and raise blood glucose, quickly increasing the demand for insulin production. Zinc is part of the insulin molecule and is depleted, resulting in abnormal taste and taste perception. What develops is an aversion to the flavors in natural foods and increased cravings for highly sweetened foods and those foods containing MSG. (MSG affects the brain's perception of flavor.) The diet becomes more narrow, and nutritional status declines, resulting in more limited food choices. The white diet and vegetable aversions are common among children in Western cultures due to the high exposure to processed and sweet foods. For children with sensory and developmental issues, the aversions are much more pervasive and serious.

There are three potential contributors that lead to the limited appetite, cravings, and food aversions:

1. The formation of opiate-like peptides from gluten and milk products, resulting in cravings for the foods that are the sources.

2. Zinc deficiency or deficiencies in zinc metabolism and function. Zinc is responsible for sensory development and function, including taste and taste perception.

3. The presence of toxic metals that can interfere with sensory development and function.

The negative effect of this combination can result in faulty messages from the sensory receptors to the brain and dysfunctional interpretation of those messages by the brain. Perception is the "truth" for that person. This is why begging, bribing, and punishing do not and will not work.

The solution is multifaceted. Correction of nutritional deficiencies, especially zinc, is necessary. Identification of potential interfering toxic metals and subsequent treatment if needed is also important. Foods that cause reactions and/or opiate-like peptides need to be eliminated as healthy, safe foods are introduced and accepted.

How to Go from Yucky to Yummy—The Trojan Horse Technique

For those with texture issues, it is important to adapt the diet to the child's oral and food developmental stage. If textures are a sensory issue, no matter how tasty the food, it will not be consumed. By providing the food in a sensory-pleasing form, the child benefits nutritionally and begins to find mealtime more pleasant and rewarding. Purees are generally helpful. They are better tolerated and can open the door for getting more types of foods into the diet. Many family dishes, including soups, casseroles, or the meat and vegetable main dish, can also be served pureed for the child who has sensory texture issues. In this way, the whole family is enjoying the same meal.

Many of the recipes in this book have been selected to expand nutritional intake, especially using the Trojan Horse Technique—hiding a small amount of the new food (especially vegetables and proteins) within a very well tolerated and acceptable food. Each child differs and, therefore, it is important to identify what foods will work as "carriers" to get the new foods in.

Purees can be made from cooked fresh or frozen vegetables and/or purchased baby foods. If your child is offended by being served baby food, simply keep it well hidden. Create interesting new names for the foods and see that others in the family join in consuming them. The secret to success in introducing these new foods is to combine a small amount with the food the child already likes. For many children, this is the only way new foods can be introduced.

Start with 1 tablespoon (15 g) or less—and then increase when tolerated. Hide the cooked vegetable purees anywhere you can, selecting colors that are not obvious when added to the carrier food. The carrier food needs to be one that the child enjoys. It may even be a food that is being slowly eliminated.

Include pureed fruits to improve the taste. Here are some examples of places to hide foods (and even supplements):

- **SPAGHETTI SAUCE.** Blend the pureed vegetables thoroughly with at least three times as much spaghetti sauce; then hand-mix the new blend in with the rest of the sauce. Carrots, beets, sweet potatoes, turnips, squash, green beans, and peas are easy to hide in spaghetti sauce. Watch the amount of green if it is a food color that your child rejects.

- **MUFFINS, CAKES, AND BROWNIES.** Well-pureed foods are easy to hide in these batters, including pureed chicken and turkey. A chicken/vegetable/fruit muffin becomes a healthy meal!

- **PANCAKES.** Not only can pureed vegetables and fruits hide well in the batter, but they are also a good hiding place for supplements such as protein powders (if heat-stable), calcium, magnesium, and zinc.

- **PEANUT BUTTER.** If a child likes peanut butter, it is an excellent medium for adding small amounts of protein and nutritional supplements.

- **MEATBALLS**. If these are well liked, especially with spaghetti sauce, the job becomes a whole lot easier. Well-pureed vegetables and fruits are an excellent thickener/filler for meatballs. Make many and freeze them, and then bring them out for snacks.

- **JUICES.** Juices with a strong flavor, such as pineapple juice, grape juice, nectars, apple cider, and orange juice, are particularly good for hiding supplements.

- **SMOOTHIES, FRUIT PUREES, AND APPLE-SAUCE.** These offer an unlimited opportunity for expanding nutrition and an excellent way to hide supplements. Protein powders can be included to expand protein intake, especially for those with texture issues who avoid meat, beans, and other sources of protein. Always start with the fruit your child favors and then expand.

- **CHOCOLATE.** Let chocolate be your friend. There are sources of GFCF chocolate chips, sauces, powders, and so forth. Check the product search section of the GFCF Diet site (www.gfcfdiet.com/directory.htm).

Feeding a Child Who Won't Eat
Rules to Make

- Turn off phones, cell phones, and unpleasant noise or upsetting programs.
- Put a note on the front door that you are not available.
- Keep the mealtime pleasant and happy.
- Allow no one at the table to speak negatively about the food or meal.
- Prohibit any gross talk at the table.
- Always have a favorite food as part of the child's meal.
- Provide a small portion of the favorite food to be followed by new or less-liked foods.
- Finish the meal with the favorite food.
- Provide a reward for any effort toward eating or participating. Be casual about this—parent anxiety undermines success.
- If one parent is more effective with feeding, have that parent do the feeding.
- If there is a well-liked sitter or relative, have that person participate.
- There are no "breakfast police"! Start serving lunch and dinner foods for breakfast.

A Rule to Break

Allow a child to watch TV or a favorite tape during mealtime. This results in a positive association with the meal and eating. The attention to the show reduces the sensory focus on the food. It can allow for more food consumption and slipping in the well-disguised new foods. It is temporary—it's not forever—and it works!

Gelatin

As stated several times in this book, gelatin itself is a health food. The presence of gelatin in foods improves digestion by attracting digestive juices to the surface of food particles. According to Sally Fallon and Mary Enig in *Nourishing Traditions,* gelatin has been used throughout history in the treatment of many digestive and intestinal disorders.

Include it in meat broths, soups, stews, vegetable purees, fruit salads, vegetable salads and gelatin desserts. The vegetarian gelatin source, carrageenan, does not have the same healthy effect and can hinder the actions of digestive enzymes. The recipes in this book use only unflavored gelatin.

Substitutions: What to Use and How to Do It

SUBSTITUTES FOR SUGAR AND GUIDELINES ON SWEETENERS

The natural sweeteners are preferred over table sugars (sucralose). Some of the substitutes are too acidic and require the addition of baking soda to compensate. The information that follows comes from multiple sources, two of which are Sally Fallon's and Mary Enig's *Nourishing Traditions,* which provides excellent information, and Carol Fenster's *Special Diet Celebrations,* which also provides detailed information for food substitutions.

SWEETENERS	EQUIVALENT TO 1 CUP SUGAR	INFORMATION
Brown Rice Syrup	1 1/3 cups (425 g) Add 1/4 teaspoon baking soda per cup. Reduce liquid by 1/4 cup (60 ml) per cup.	Less sweet than sugar, it is excellent for baking. Be certain it is GF.
Agave Nectar	3/4 cup (255 g) Reduce liquid by 1/4 cup (60 ml) per cup.	Sweet liquid from the cactus plant. The texture is similar to honey. It has a lower glycemic index and less effect on blood glucose. It works well in baked goods, puddings, and beverages.
Raw Honey	1/2–3/4 cup (170–255 g) Add 1/4 teaspoon baking soda per cup of honey. Reduce liquid by 1/4 cup (60 ml) per cup.	Honey should not be heated above 117°F (47°C). It is loaded with beneficial enzymes that digest carbohydrates, including grains. Local honey is best. When used in heated recipes, it will not have the enzyme activity. Lower oven temperature 25°F (4°C) to prevent overbrowning. Avoid honey in any form in babies up to age 1.
Maple Syrup, Maple Sugar	2/3–3/4 cup (160–175 ml) Add 1/4 teaspoon baking powder. Reduce liquid by 1/4 cup (60 ml) per cup.	This syrup (distilled sap) from deciduous maple trees is rich in trace minerals. The sugar is dehydrated syrup. Both have a distinct flavor and are best used in creamy desserts and baked goods. Use organic only.
Fruit Juice Concentrate (Liquid)	2/3 cup (160 ml) Add 1/4 teaspoon baking soda. Reduce liquid 1/3 cup (80 ml) per cup juice.	This has a negative impact on glucose control in the same way sugar does. Avoid high-fructose corn syrup (HFCS) in foods. Reduce oven temperature 25°F (4°C) and adjust baking time for slightly longer period. Orange juice is more acidic.

SWEETENERS	EQUIVALENT TO 1 CUP SUGAR	INFORMATION
Fruit Juice Concentrate (Frozen)	**1/2 cup (140 g)** Add 1/8 teaspoon baking soda. Reduce liquid 1/2 cup (120 ml) per cup juice.	Frozen concentrate must be 100 percent pure juice whether one juice or a combination. Use less than when using the liquid juice concentrate. See information above.
Fruit Puree	**1 cup**	A good way to provide nutritional sweetener in baked goods. Works best if used to replace only 1/4 to 1/2 of the sugar in the recipe.
Molasses	**1/2 cup (170 g)** Reduce liquid by 1/4 cup (60 ml) per cup.	This "waste" product from the production of refined sugar has a strong, moderately sweet taste and is rich in minerals.
Brown Sugar	**1 cup**	Refined cane or beet sugar with molasses still on the sugar crystals. It is no healthier than white sugar.
Date Sugar	**2/3 –1 cup (150–220 g)**	Made from dehydrated dates, this sweetener is nutritious but does not dissolve easily. It is best sprinkled on a food or used in combination with other sugars. Dissolve in hot water before using in batters. Lower baking temperature 25°F (4°C).
Fructose	**1/2 cup (100 g)**	Refined simple sugar made from fruit juices, corn, or corn syrup. Know the source! Less glycemic (sugar-raising) than sucrose and glucose. Avoid HFCS.
Sucanet	**1 cup (200 g)**	Dehydrated cane sugar juice that is rich in nutrients. Most similar to sugar.
Stevia Powder or Liquid	**1 teaspoon** May need to increase dry ingredients. **1 teaspoon sugar = 2–4 drops liquid stevia or pinch stevia powder.**	A little bit goes a long way. This sweet-tasting herb is 30 times sweeter tasting than sugar (and has an aftertaste). It does not affect blood glucose. Substitution is not easy. Baked items with stevia do not brown well. It is best used in recipes requiring very little sugar or as part of the sugar replacement.

SUBSTITUTES FOR WHEAT FLOUR

SUBSTITUTE	EQUIVALENT TO 1 CUP (125 G) WHEAT FLOUR
Buckwheat flour	7/8 cup (1 cup – 2 tablespoons [105 g])
Corn flour	1 cup (120 g)
Cornmeal, cornstarch	3/4 cup (105 g cornmeal, 98 g cornstarch)
Chickpea flour	3/4 cup (105 g)
Nut flours (ground fine)	1/2 cup (60 g)
Potato flour	1 cup (160 g)
Potato starch	3/4 cup (105 g)
Rice flour, sorghum	7/8 cup (140 g rice flour, 125 g sorghum)
Tapioca flour or starch	1 cup (120 g)

SUBSTITUTE THICKENERS

SUBSTITUTE	EQUIVALENT TO 1 TABLESPOON (8 G) WHEAT FLOUR
Arrowroot	1 ½ teaspoons
Bean flours	1 tablespoon (9 g)
Cornstarch	1 ½ teaspoon
Gelatin powder (unflavored)	1 ½ teaspoons dissolved in water
Guar Gum	1 ½ teaspoons mixed in liquid
Potato starch	½ tablespoon (5 g)
Tapioca flour	1 ½ tablespoons (12 g)

SUBSTITUTES FOR MILK PRODUCTS

MILK PRODUCT	SUBSTITUTE
1 cup (235 ml) milk	1 cup (235 ml) milk substitute: rice, coconut, soy, nut, hemp
1 cup (230 g) yogurt	1 cup (230 g) yogurt substitute: coconut, soy
1 cup (235 ml) light cream	¾ cup (175 ml) milk substitute + ¼ cup (55 g) butter substitute, melted
1 cup (235 ml) heavy cream	⅔ cup (160 ml) milk substitute + ⅓ cup (75 g) butter substitute, melted
1 cup (225 g) cottage cheese	1 cup (250 g) crumbled tofu (better flavored with dressing)
1 cup (235 ml) buttermilk	2 tablespoons (28 ml) lemon juice in 1 cup (235 ml) milk substitute

SUBSTITUTES FOR BUTTER

- Earth Balance Whipped Spread 100% vegan, nonhydrogenated (no trans-fat)
- GFCF, organic, non-GMO expeller-pressed oils, no artificial flavor or color
- Lard (excellent in baking, 4 parts lard for 5 parts butter)
- Coconut Butter/Coconut Oil (excellent for baking), heathly, non-hydrogenated unrefined good vegetable fat
- Spectrum Palm Shortening (excellent in baking and ice creams)
- For melted butter, substitute oil (safflower, almond, avocado, coconut) or melted ghee

SUBSTITUTES FOR EGG

SUBSTITUTE	EQUIVALENT TO 1 EGG
Unflavored gelatin 1 envelope (1 tablespoon or 7 g) unflavored gelatin in 1 cup (235 ml) boiling water	3 tablespoons
Pureed fruits, mild flavors only—apple or pear	3 tablespoons (45 g)
Ener-G Egg Replacer (egg-free)	2 teaspoons (10 ml) + 2 tablespoons (28 ml) water
Cornstarch	2 tablespoons (16 g)
Arrowroot flour	2 tablespoons (16 g)
Potato starch	2 tablespoons (20 g)
Soy milk powder	1 tablespoon (8 g)
Banana (good in cakes)	¼ cup (60 g)
Tofu naturally fermented	¼ cup (60 g)
Flaxseeds	Egg White Substitute: ½ cup flaxseeds + ¾ cup water Blend for 2-3 minutes. Refrigerate for ½ hour

GENERAL SUBSTITUTES

ITEM	SUBSTITUTE
1 clove garlic	⅛ teaspoon garlic powder
1 cup (240 g) ketchup	1 cup (245 g) tomato sauce + ¾ cup (255 g) agave + 2 tablespoons (28 ml) vinegar
1 medium lemon	3 tablespoons (45 ml) lemon juice
1 tablespoon (15 g) mustard	1 teaspoon dry mustard
1 small onion	2 tablespoons (20 g) fresh chopped or minced
1 medium onion	4 tablespoons (40 g) fresh chopped or minced
2 cups (300 g) chopped tomatoes	1 (16-ounce [455 g]) can chopped tomatoes, drained
1 cup (235 ml) wine	1 cup (235 ml) apple juice, apple cider, or chicken or beef broth
1 cup (330 g) corn syrup	1 cup (235 ml) maple syrup or 1 cup (340 g) honey

Hemp Milk

Organic hemp milk is a perfectly legal. It is produced from the seeds of the hemp plant and contains no THC. It is a healthy alternative for vegetarians or nonvegetarians. It is not SCD compliant. It contains the following nutrients:

Omega 3 essential fatty acids
Omega 6 essential fatty acids .
All 10 essential amino acids
Protein
Vitamins A, D, E, B12, B2, folic acid
Minerals: calcium, magnesium, potassium, phosphorus, iron, and zinc

Quick Online Resources

- GFCF product finder:
  www.gfcfdiet.com/directory.htm

- Baking with Substitutes—
  Troubleshooting:
  Miss Roben's site:
  www.missroben.com/id1171.htm

Play Dough Recipe

From the Autism Recovery Network

gluten   milk   soy   egg   corn   nuts

Because kids do touch it, and some will eat the dough.

- 2 cups (320 g) white rice flour
- 4 teaspoons (12 g) GFCF cream of tartar
- ¹/₄ cup (75 g) salt
- 2 teaspoons xanthan gum
- ¹/₄ cup (60 ml) oil
- Natural organic food coloring

Place all ingredients into a food processor. Slowly add ¹/₂ cup (120 ml) boiling water and stir until mixture forms a ball. If the dough is crumbly, add more water, 1 tablespoon (15 ml) at a time, until dough is soft and firm. Let cool. Knead on a floured board for 10 minutes. Separate into 4 small balls of dough and add 8 drops of food coloring to each. Store in sealed containers

"Up until Tim was five, he would put everything in his mouth. When it came to the regular play dough, there was no way I could give it to him. The edible version allowed him his play dough and he could eat it too!"

—**Sue**, *mother of Tim*

Throughout our recipes section we use icons as an easy reference to signal what potential problem foods and ingredients it contains.

 A solid circle and slash means the recipe is free of that ingredient

 A dashed circle and slash indicates that the problem ingredient is included in the recipe's optional ingredients or that one of the ingredients could potentially be linked to a problem food, as in the case of xanthan gum, which is sometimes corn-derived.

 No circle or slash of any kind indicates that the recipe calls for a problem ingredient

Beverages and Healthy Shakes

QUICK N EASY

Wonderful Water

gluten   milk   soy   egg   corn   nuts

It is the only beverage that is essential for human life on Earth.

- Water (filtered, bottled, carbonated)

This should be the first and last beverage of every day.

Drink half the body weight in ounces of water.

Drink most between meals, sipped throughout the day.

Drink $1/2$ to 1 glass with meals.

Enjoy.

YIELD: *Unlimited*

 QUICK N EASY

Rice Milk #1

gluten   milk   soy   egg   corn   nuts

It is best to use warm water and warm rice.

- 4 cups (940 ml) hot/warm water
- 1 cup (160 g) cooked rice (white or brown)
- 1 teaspoon (5 ml) vanilla

Place all ingredients in a blender until smooth. Let the milk set for about 30 minutes. Pour the milk steadily into another container (an old honey jar can be used), leaving most of the sediment in the first container. It can be stored in the refrigerator for up to five days.

YIELD: *About 4-4$1/2$ cups (940 ml-1 L)*

Calories (kcal): 63; **Total fat:** trace; **Cholesterol:** 0mg; **Carbohydrate:** 13g; **Dietary fiber:** trace; **Protein:** 1g; **Sodium:** 8mg; **Potassium:** 18mg; **Calcium:** 10mg; **Iron:** trace; **Zinc:** trace; **Vitamin A:** 0IU

Rice Milk #2

gluten milk soy egg corn nuts

- 4 cups (940 ml) boiling water
- 2 cups (370 g) rice (white or brown)
- Oil (high-oleic safflower, avocado)—for texture (optional)
- Pure vanilla flavor to taste (optional)
- Salt to taste (optional)

Rinse rice to clean. Pour 4 cups (940 ml) boiling water over rice and let soak for 1 to 2 hours. Blend 1 cup (185 g) soaked rice with 2¹/₂ cups (590 ml) water (can be cold water.) Blend rice to a slurry (textured liquid), pour into a pot, and repeat with rest of rice. Bring to a boil and then reduce heat and simmer for 20 minutes.

Line a colander with a nylon tricot or a few layers of cheesecloth. Put a bowl under colander. Pour rice mix in colander; another 1 cup (235 ml) water (or less or more) can be poured over the rice to get out more milk. Press with the back of a spoon, twist nylon, and squeeze out as much milk as possible. This milk is very plain and can be flavored with oil, vanilla, salt, etc.

YIELD: *4 cups (940 ml)*

Calories (kcal): 351; Total fat: 2g; Cholesterol: 0mg; Carbohydrate: 74g; Dietary fiber: 1g; Protein: 7g; Sodium: 78mg; Potassium: 106mg; Calcium: 31mg; Iron: 4mg; Zinc: 1mg; Vitamin A: 0IU

Rice Milk #3

gluten milk soy egg corn nuts

- 2 cups (370 g) rice (white or brown)
- 10 cups (2.4 L) water
- 1 coconut
- 1 quart (9,464 ml) water
- 1 teaspoon (5 ml) GFCF vanilla
- Honey, maple syrup, Stevia, or sugar to taste

Boil rice in water for 15 to 18 minutes (cook to taste). Drain rice and save liquid (rice may be eaten or refrigerated).

Crack coconut shell open. The coconut meat may be shredded, grated, or minced. Add 1 quart (9464 ml) water to coconut and place in a blender.

Strain the liquid (grated coconut can be mixed with a sweetener for use as a topping for cakes).

Mix the quart of rice milk with the quart of coconut milk. Add the GFCF vanilla and sweeten to taste.

YIELD: *2 quarts (1.9 L)*

Calories (kcal): 346; Total fat: 17g; Cholesterol: 0mg; Carbohydrate: 45g; Dietary fiber: 5g; Protein: 5g; Sodium: 21mg; Potassium: 230mg; Calcium: 26mg; Iron: 3mg; Zinc: 1mg; Vitamin A: 0IU

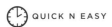 QUICK N EASY

Dana's Drink

gluten   milk   soy   egg   corn   nuts

My favorite flavoring juice is white grape juice. This drink is named by my neighbors because I always serve it as a "soft drink" when we have parties, and it was the official drink of the Garret Park Swim Team for years.

- 1 (liter) bottle seltzer (not soda water)
- 4–6 tablespoons (2–3 ounces [55–85 g]) 100% frozen fruit juice concentrate, thawed (avoid any juice that is not 100% fruit juice)

  Best juice choices:
  - White grape juice plus squeeze of lemon and lime
  - Orange juice

Pour a small amount of seltzer out of the bottle and slowly add the thawed fruit juice concentrate. Do this slowly so the contents don't fizz out of the bottle. Use just enough to flavor the drink. Leave this in the refrigerator so your family can enjoy this natural soda. Serve over ice, in a pitcher, or in a punch bowl.

When weaning children off sodas, it may be helpful to make the drink slightly sweeter at first.

To make a party punch that is nonalcoholic sangria, add a variety of juices and cut-up fruits. This is a definite crowd-pleaser.

YIELD: *1 liter*

Calories (kcal): 97; **Total fat:** 0g; **Cholesterol:** 0mg; **Carbohydrate:** 22g; **Dietary fiber:** 0g; **Protein:** 1g; **Sodium:** 25mg; **Potassium:** 277mg; **Calcium:** 35mg; **Iron:** 0mg; **Zinc:** 0mg; **Vitamin A:** 0IU

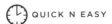 QUICK N EASY

Agave-Sweetened Lemonade or Spritzer

gluten   milk   soy   egg   corn   nuts

An extract of the wild agave cactus from Mexico, agave nectar is a sweetener similar to honey. It has less of an effect on blood glucose compared to sugar. And is quite versatile and works well in baked goods, puddings, and beverages. Less agave nectar is needed compared to sugar, but that is a matter of taste. Approximately 3/4 cup (255 g) of agave is equal to 1 cup (200 g) of sugar.

- 1/2 medium lemon, squeezed
- 1 cup (235 ml) water or seltzer water (unflavored GFCF)
- 2 teaspoons agave nectar (to taste)
- Ice cubes

Squeeze fresh lemon into glass of water. Add agave nectar and ice cubes. Stir and enjoy.

YIELD: *1 tall glass (about 12 ounces [355 ml])*

Calories (kcal): 46; **Total fat:** trace; **Cholesterol:** 0mg; **Carbohydrate:** 14g; **Dietary fiber:** trace; **Protein:** trace; **Sodium:** 8mg; **Potassium:** 42mg; **Calcium:** 12mg; **Iron:** trace; **Zinc:** trace; **Vitamin A:** 9IU

Soymilk Made Easy

gluten   milk   soy   egg   corn   nuts

- 2 cups (370 g) soybeans
- 12 cups (2.8 L) water

Rinse and soak the beans overnight (or at least 10 hours) in refrigerator. When ready, drain and rinse the beans.

Grind the beans into a paste using a blender or food processor with boiling water ($^3/_4$ cup [140 g] beans to $1^3/_4$ cups [410 ml] boiling water at a time). Pour into a large, heavy pot. (**NOTE:** Do not overestimate the blender's abilities. Be careful to not burn out the blender while grinding beans. A food processor offers better results [with sharp blades].)

Bring the resulting milky substance to a boil while stirring over medium to high heat. Turn down immediately after it starts to boil. Simmer (no stirring necessary) for 20 to 30 minutes.

Meanwhile, line a colander with a thin cloth and set it over a big bowl or another pot. When the soymilk is cooked, ladle it into the colander, straining the pulp in the cloth and allowing the milk to collect in the bowl. Make sure to squeeze all the milk from the pulp before transferring it into a jug or two to cool. Taste and add water, sweetener, vanilla, GFCF chocolate, carob, or sea salt as desired. This can be stored in the refrigerator for up to five days.

YIELD: *2 quarts (1.9 L)*

Calories (kcal): 193; **Total fat:** 9g; **Cholesterol:** 0mg; **Carbohydrate:** 14g; **Dietary fiber:** 4g; **Protein:** 17g; **Sodium:** 12mg; **Potassium:** 836mg; **Calcium:** 136mg; **Iron:** 2mg; **Zinc:** 2mg; **Vitamin A:** 11IU

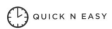

Blueberry Blend

gluten   milk   soy   egg   corn   nuts

This purple-blue shake is inspired by Lisa Barnes in The Petit Appetit Cookbook. *Blueberries contain a number of vitamins, including A, C, and E, as well as antioxidants that improve immunity. It is better to serve the blueberries blended as a shake as they can be a choking hazard to young children. This also hides the milder-tasting supplements.*

- 1¹/₂ cups (235 g) frozen blueberries
- ¹/₄ cup (60 g) vanilla soy or rice yogurt
- ¹/₄ cup (60 ml) coconut milk
- 1 cup (235 ml) unfiltered pasteurized organic apple juice

Combine all ingredients in a blender and process until smooth. Strain through a mesh strainer for the smoothest texture.

YIELD: *About 3 servings of 1 cup (235 ml) each*

Calories (kcal): 134; **Total fat:** 6g; **Cholesterol:** 0mg; **Carbohydrate:** 21g; **Dietary fiber:** 3g; **Protein:** 2g; **Sodium:** 6mg; **Potassium:** 193mg; **Calcium:** 15mg; **Iron:** 1mg; **Zinc:** trace; **Vitamin A:** 64IU

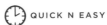

Melon Mango Smoothie or Cold Soup

gluten   milk   soy   egg   corn   nuts

According to Lisa Barnes (The Petit Appetit), *this makes a great breakfast soup. Packed with vitamins A and C and calcium, this soup makes a great alternative to a plain piece of fruit or a morning shake. Mangoes are grown throughout the tropics and are often called "the peach of the tropics." This recipe will hide some of the milder-tasting supplements.*

- ¹/₂ large cantaloupe
- ¹/₂ large mango
- ³/₄ cup (175 g) plain soy yogurt or ¹/₂ cup (120 ml) rice milk or coconut milk

Cut cantaloupe in half and remove seeds. Cut flesh away from skin and cut into 1-inch (2.5 cm) cubes. Peel mango and remove flesh from pit. Cut into 1-inch (2.5 cm) cubes. Put cantaloupe and mango into food processor or blender and process until smooth, about 20 seconds. Pour mixture into a large glass or plastic bowl. Stir yogurt or rice milk into mixture. Cover and chill for 1 hour before serving.

YIELD: *About 3 servings of 1 cup (235 ml) each*

Calories (kcal): 84; **Total fat:** 2g; **Cholesterol:** 0mg; **Carbohydrate:** 15g; **Dietary fiber:** 2g; **Protein:** 3g; **Sodium:** 9mg; **Potassium:** 338mg; **Calcium:** 14mg; **Iron:** trace; **Zinc:** trace; **Vitamin A:** 4310IU

QUICK N EASY

Fruity Good Shakes

gluten   milk   soy   egg   corn   nuts

There are so many varieties of this recipe that there is bound to be one suitable to each child. Children with sensory issues will appreciate the smooth texture, without any lumps or pieces. The addition of coconut milk provides taste, variety, and healing nutritional qualities. According to Sally Fallon and Mary Enig, Ph.D. (Nourishing Traditions), the principal fatty acid in coconut milk is lauric acid, which is antiviral, antifungal, and antimicrobial. This is another good food source for hiding nutritional supplements.

- 1¼ cups (295 ml) rice milk or nonmilk toddler formula
- ½ glass crushed ice
- 1 tablespoon (3 g) protein powder
- 1 tablespoon (15 ml) coconut milk (optional)
- **FOR BANANA SHAKE:** add 1 sliced banana
- **FOR PEAR SHAKE:** add 1 cored and chopped pear
- **FOR BERRY SHAKE:** add 1 handful strawberries, raspberries, blackberries, or blueberries, or a combination
- **FOR PEACH SHAKE:** add 1 pitted and chopped ripe peach or nectarine

Blend the milk, crushed ice, rice powder, and coconut milk (if desired) in a blender. Add the fruit or fruits. Blend the mixture at high speed until smooth and thick (no lumps or pieces).

Pour into glasses and serve immediately.

YIELD: *2 to 3 child-sized servings*

Calories (kcal): 75; **Total fat:** 2g; **Cholesterol:** 0mg; **Carbohydrate:** 13g; **Dietary fiber:** trace; **Protein:** 1g; **Sodium:** 8mg; **Potassium:** 35mg; **Calcium:** 9mg; **Iron:** trace ; **Zinc:** trace ; **Vitamin A:** 0IU

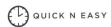

Connor's Peanut Butter Blast Shake

gluten   milk   soy   egg   corn   nuts

Lori Skalitzky offers this delicious recipe, which also is perfect for hiding supplements, especially those with a strong taste.

- $^1/_4$ cup (60 ml) milk substitute
- 2 tablespoons (32 g) creamy GFCF peanut butter
- 1 tablespoon (15 ml) 100% maple syrup or 1 tablespoon (20 g) honey
- 3–4 scoops vanilla-flavored ice cream substitute

In a blender, mix the milk substitute, peanut butter, and maple syrup or honey at medium speed until smooth. Add the ice cream substitute and pulse until combined.

YIELD: *1$^1/_2$ to 2 cups (355 to 475 ml)*

Calories (kcal): 789; **Total fat:** 46g; **Cholesterol:** 116mg; **Carbohydrate:** 85g; **Dietary fiber:** 2g; **Protein:** 18g; **Sodium:** 366mg; **Potassium:** 786mg; **Calcium:** 373mg; **Iron:** 1mg; **Zinc:** 3mg; **Vitamin A:** 1080IU

"Our son, Connor, who is now five and a half years old, has been gluten-free and casein-free now for over three years. He is also mostly soy-free, though not 100 percent. Connor was minimally verbal before we started the diet—he said some words but didn't even put two words together for a statement yet. We took him off of milk products first and began to see some improvement; he seemed much more with it. But the most mind-boggling thing for us was when we took him off of gluten. Three days later, our boy was singing full versions of songs, something he had never done before. And now, after many years on the diet and many other interventions, many people tell us that other than a few self-stimming behaviors, he looks just like any other five year old around."

—Lori Skalitzky, *mother of Connor, a five-year-old with autism*

QUICK N EASY

Blueberry Flax Smoothie

gluten   milk   soy   egg   corn   nuts

Flaxseed is a great source of omega-3 fatty acids and dietary fiber. To get the omega-3 fatty acid benefit of flaxseeds, they need to be ground and used within 2 days. You will get this benefit if you add unground flaxseeds to the blender. Using already ground flaxseeds older than 2 days will get you the benefit of fiber but not the maximum omega-3 benefit.

- 1 cup (155 g) frozen blueberries
- 1/4 cup (60 ml) unsweetened concentrated cranberry juice
- 3/4 cup (175 ml) water
- 2 tablespoons (14 g) freshly ground flaxseed, or 1 heaping tablespoon (14 g) whole flaxseeds
- 1/2 teaspoon stevia

Blend all ingredients in a blender until smooth, adding more water if necessary. Serve immediately.

NOTES: *1 cup of regular cranberry juice can be substituted for the unsweetened cranberry juice, water, and stevia.*

YIELD: *2 servings*

Calories (kcal): 98; **Total fat:** 3g; **Cholesterol:** 0mg; **Carbohydrate:** 16g; **Dietary fiber:** 4g; **Protein:** 2g; **Sodium:** 4mg; **Potassium:** 48mg; **Calcium:** 9mg; **Iron:** trace; **Zinc:** trace; **Vitamin A:** 64IU.

Creamy Custard Drink

gluten   milk   soy   egg   corn   nuts

Adapted from Welby Griffin

This thick, creamy beverage is perfect for those who don't like to eat eggs otherwise. It is also a great place to sneak in all sorts of vitamins and supplements.

- $^1/_3$ cup (43 g) cornstarch
- $^1/_2$ cup (50 g) sugar
- 1 quart (950 ml) rice milk
- 6 large eggs
- 2 teaspoons GFCF vanilla extract

In a large sauce pan, whisk together cornstarch and sugar to eliminate any lumps. Add rice milk and cook over medium high heat until warm and slightly thickened, but not boiling.

Meanwhile, beat eggs together in a medium bowl. Slowly pour half of warmed milk mixture into the eggs, stirring constantly. Then transfer the egg mixture into the remaining milk mixture in the pan, stirring well to combine. Cook the mixture over medium heat, stirring constantly, until it reaches 175°F. Add the vanilla and allow to cool to room temperature before transferring the custard to the refrigerator to chill completely. Store in a covered container up to 3 days.

NOTE: *If custard becomes too thick or lumpy, pulse in a blender a few times until smooth, while adjusting the consistency by adding more rice milk.*

VARIATION: *Add up to one-half pound of boiled, mashed carrots to the custard after cooking. You may want to add a teaspoon more vanilla or a pinch of nutmeg for flavor, and some extra rice milk to adjust the consistency.*

YIELD: *4 to 6 servings*

Calories (kcal): 250; **Total fat:** 6g; **Cholesterol:** 229mg; **Carbohydrate:** 43g; **Dietary fiber:** trace; **Protein:** 7g; **Sodium:** 128mg; **Potassium:** 116mg; **Calcium:** 40mg; **Iron:** 1; **Zinc:** 1; **Vitamin A:** 247IU.

Ginger Soda

gluten   milk   soy   egg   corn   nuts

From Lisa Barnes of Petit Appetit

Ginger has such a pleasant aroma and taste, besides helping upset tummies. Here's a natural and refreshing ginger ale drink without any of the high fructose corn syrups and added colorings of storebought.

For Syrup

- ¹/₂ cup (170 g) agave nectar
- 1 (3-inch, or 7.5 cm) piece fresh ginger, peeled and finely chopped
- 1 cup (235 ml) water

For Soda

- 1 recipe Ginger Syrup
- 3¹/₂ cups (825 ml) sparkling water
- Ice cubes

To make the syrup: Place agave nectar, ginger, and water in a small saucepan and bring to a boil over medium-high heat. Reduce heat to simmer, cover, and cook until ginger aroma and flavor is strong, about 1 hour. Let cool. Strain and refrigerate for up to one week; should yield ²/₃ cup (160 ml).

To make the soda: In a pitcher, combine syrup with the water. Pour over ice to serve.

TIP: *To choose good-quality, fresh ginger, look for smooth light brown skin with a light sheen and white flesh. Pick the roots with the least number of knots and/or branching.*

YIELD: *4 servings*

Calories (kcal): 111; **Total fat:** trace; **Cholesterol:** 0mg; **Carbohydrate:** 30g; **Dietary fiber:** 2g; **Protein:** trace; **Sodium:** 2mg; **Potassium:** 2mg; **Calcium:** 1mg; **Iron:** trace; **Zinc:** trace; **Vitamin A:** 0IU.

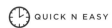

QUICK N EASY

Great Grape Slush

gluten   milk   soy   egg   corn   nuts

From Lisa Barnes of Petit Appetit

This is a healthy improvement over the brightly colored slushies with fake flavors and colorings from the fast food and convenience stores. You can add ice cubes for older children, which will increase the yield.

- ³/₄ cup (112.5 g) frozen organic seedless purple grapes, see note below
- 1 organic apple (150 g), peeled, cored, and chopped
- ¹/₂ cup (120 ml) organic unfiltered apple juice

Add all ingredients to a blender and blend until slushy.

NOTE: *Spread individual grapes on a pan and freeze. Then transfer to a freezer bag or container to have available for kids to eat alone as a frosty snack, or to make this tasty slush.*

YIELD: *1¹/₂ cups (355 ml)*

Calories (kcal): 185; **Total fat:** 1g; **Cholesterol:** 0mg; **Carbohydrate:** 48g; **Dietary fiber:** 4g; **Protein:** 1g; **Sodium:** 5mg; **Potassium:** 444mg; **Calcium:** 28mg; **Iron:** 1; **Zinc:** trace; **Vitamin A:** 146IU.

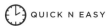

QUICK N EASY

Popeye Smoothie

gluten   milk   soy   egg   corn   nuts

This smoothie recipe is another way to get a vegetable into kids. It's hard to believe, but you can't taste the spinach in this smoothie. However, the smoothie is bright green, so would need to be hidden in a covered cup, like a Sippy cup.

- 2 cups (60 g) baby spinach
- ¹/₂ banana, very ripe
- 1 cup (235 ml) water
- 4 to 6 ice cubes (about 4 ounces, or 112 g)

Combine all the ingredients in a blender. Blend on high until smooth. Serve immediately.

YIELD: *2 servings*

Calories (kcal): 34; **Total fat:** trace; **Cholesterol:** 0mg; **Carbohydrate:** 8g; **Dietary fiber:** 2g; **Protein:** 1g; **Sodium:** 28mg; **Potassium:** 284mg; **Calcium:** 34mg; **Iron:** 1; **Zinc:** trace; **Vitamin A:** 2018IU.

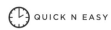 QUICK N EASY

Popeye Smoothie II

gluten   milk   soy   egg   corn   nuts

Another variation on the spinach smoothie where, again, you would never know the spinach is in there! Feel free to leave the peel on the apple, but be sure to wash it well.

- 2 cups (60 g) baby spinach
- 1 kiwi, peeled and chopped
- 1 sweet apple, cored and sliced
- 1 to 2 teaspoons lime juice
- $^1/_2$ cup (120 ml) water
- 4 to 6 ice cubes (about 4 ounces, or 112 g)

Combine all the ingredients in a blender. Blend on high until smooth. Serve immediately.

YIELD: *2 servings*

Calories (kcal): 72; **Total fat:** 1g; **Cholesterol:** 0mg; **Carbohydrate:** 18g; **Dietary fiber:** 4g; **Protein:** 1g; **Sodium:** 27mg; **Potassium:** 378mg; **Calcium:** 46mg; **Iron:** 1; **Zinc:** trace; **Vitamin A:** 2118IU.

Dairy-Free Delicious Hot Cocoa

gluten   milk   soy   egg   corn   nuts

GFCF Chocolate Syrup

- $^1/_2$ cup (40 g) GFCF unsweetened cocoa powder
- $^3/_4$ cup (255 g) agave nectar
- $^1/_4$ cup (60 ml) water
- $^1/_2$ teaspoon vanilla extract
- Pinch salt

Combine cocoa powder, agave nectar, and water in a small saucepan, and bring to a boil. Add vanilla and salt and cool to room temperature. Store in an airtight container in the refrigerator for up to 5 days.

YIELD: *1 cup, 8 servings*

Hot Cocoa

- 2 tablespoons (30 ml) GFCF chocolate syrup
- $^3/_4$ cup (180 ml) soy, almond, or other dairy-free milk of choice

Heat milk in a saucepan or in the microwave until very hot but not boiling. Whisk syrup into milk to combine. Serve.

YIELD: *1 serving*

Calories (kcal): 157; **Total fat:** 4g; **Cholesterol:** 0mg; **Carbohydrate:** 28g; **Dietary fiber:** 6g; **Protein:** 6g; **Sodium:** 23mg; **Potassium:** 341mg; **Calcium:** 14mg; **Iron:** 2; **Zinc:** 1; **Vitamin A:** 60IU.

Nut Milk and Nut Yogurt

gluten

milk

soy

egg

corn

nuts

From Karyn Seroussi and Lisa Lewis from The Encyclopedia of Dietary Interventions (Autism Network for Dietary Intervention) *and Julie Mathews in* Cooking To Heal (Nourishing Hope).

Nut milk and nut yogurt are alternatives to dairy-based milk and yogurt. They can be made from a variety of nuts, and you can experiment with adding your favorite sweetener and flavorings. Nut yogurt contains far more beneficial bacteria than you can get from a capsule, and has a mild pleasant flavor.

Nut Milk

- 2 cups (270 g) nuts (macadamia nuts, raw almonds, and/or walnuts) soaked overnight (8 to 12 hours)
- 4 cups (946 ml) cold water
- 2 tablespoons (40 g) honey or 2 pitted dates (optional)

Combine drained, soaked nuts, and honey or pitted dates (if using) in a blender with cold water, at low speed, and then increase speed to high for 10 to 15 seconds. Then strain (see note below) and serve.

NOTE: *A "nut milk bag" makes it easy to squeeze out the liquid when making nut milk and nut yogurt. You can order one at www.purejoyplanet.com.*

TIP: *You may also sweeten the milk with rice syrup, vegetable glycerin, or stevia; or flavor it with some natural vanilla extract. Some nuts have a slight sweetness on their own and the addition of fruit for a smoothie may add all the flavor and sweetening needed. The residual nuts can be saved and used in muffins or cookies or as a "breading" or filler in meatballs or loaves. If unsweetened, or sweetened with honey, nut milk*

is perfect for monosaccharide diets such as the SCD™ (although not good for a low oxalate diet).

YIELD: *4 cups (946 ml) nut milk*

Using honey: Calories (kcal): 450; **Total fat:** 37g; **Cholesterol:** 0mg; **Carbohydrate:** 23g; **Dietary fiber:** 8g; **Protein:** 14g; **Sodium:** 8mg; **Potassium:** 525mg; **Calcium:** 189mg; **Iron:** 3mg; **Zinc:** 2mg; **Vitamin A:** 0IU.

Using dates: Calories (kcal): 430; **Total fat:** 37g; **Cholesterol:** 0mg; **Carbohydrate:** 18g; **Dietary fiber:** 8g; **Protein:** 14g; **Sodium:** 8mg; **Potassium:** 547mg; **Calcium:** 190mg; **Iron:** 3mg; **Zinc:** 2mg; **Vitamin A:** 2IU.

Nut Yogurt

- 2 cups (270 g) nuts (macadamia are best), soaked overnight (8 to 12 hours)
- 4 cups (946 ml) hot water
- 1/8 teaspoon yogurt starter (GI ProStart from GI ProHealth)

Combine drained, soaked nuts and water in a blender, at low speed, and then increase speed to high for 10 to 15 seconds. (Julie suggests the milk then be heated to 160°F [71°C] to prevent the yogurt from separating.) Strain through a fine sieve or nut bag and cool to between 105°F to 110°F (40.5°C to 43°C), then whisk in yogurt starter. Place in a yogurt maker (at 95°F to 105°F) for at least 8 hours (if using individual containers, leave the lids off during fermentation to avoid condensation). Place in refrigerator for at least 5 hours. It will separate somewhat, but do not throw away the liquid—it is rich in probiotics. You can drink it, or stir it back in to make a yogurt smoothie. Additional straining of the yogurt is optional and will result in a thicker yogurt.

TIP: *You may add any one or combination of the following to the yogurt:*
- *Cinnamon*
- *Natural GFCF vanilla extract*
- *Cut up fruit, stirred into the yogurt*

YIELD: *4 cups*

Calories (kcal): 470; **Total fat:** 49g; **Cholesterol:** 0mg; **Carbohydrate:** 9g; **Dietary fiber:** 6g; **Protein:** 6g; **Sodium:** 10mg; **Potassium:** 247mg; **Calcium:** 52mg; **Iron:** 2mg; **Zinc:** 1mg; **Vitamin A:** 0IU.

CHAPTER 11

Condiments, Dressings, and Sauces

Condiments are like old friends—
highly thought of, but often taken for granted.

Butter Substitute

gluten milk soy egg corn nuts

- 6 tablespoons (85 g) Omega Nutrition coconut oil (room temperature)
- 2 tablespoons (28 ml) flax oil
- 2 tablespoons (28 ml) sunflower oil

Place ingredients in a blender and mix until integrated. Do not overmix. Place in an opaque container with a lid to protect the delicate oils from the light.

YIELD: *10 tablespoons (140 g)*

Calories (kcal): 119; **Total fat:** 14g; **Cholesterol:** 0mg; **Carbohydrate:** 0g; **Dietary fiber:** 0g; **Protein:** 0g; **Sodium:** trace; **Potassium:** 0mg; **Calcium:** trace; **Iron:** trace; **Zinc:** 0mg; **Vitamin A:** 0IU

Good Mayonnaise

gluten milk soy egg corn nuts

- 1 egg
- $1/2$ teaspoon dry mustard
- $1/2$ teaspoon sugar
- $1/4$ teaspoon paprika
- 2 tablespoons (28 ml) white wine vinegar
  (or Ener-G yeast-free vinegar powder, reconstituted)
- $1/2$ teaspoon arrowroot
- 1 cup (235 ml) oil (corn, avocado, soybean, or safflower), divided

Use a blender and combine all of the ingredients except $1/2$ cup (120 ml) of the oil. After all the other ingredients are blended, slowly add the remaining oil and blend until the mixture is smooth and thick. If a blender is not available, use a hand whisk (and a lot of elbow grease).

YIELD: *1 1/2 cups (360 g)*

Calories (kcal): 201; **Total fat:** 223g; **Cholesterol:** 187mg; **Carbohydrate:** 6g; **Dietary fiber:** trace; **Protein:** 6g; **Sodium:** 56mg; **Potassium:** 104mg; **Calcium:** 27mg; **Iron:** 1mg; **Zinc:** 1mg; **Vitamin A:** 631IU

Even Better Mayonnaise

gluten   milk   soy   egg   corn   nuts

- 1 egg
- $1/8$ teaspoon salt
- $1/4$ teaspoon pepper
- 2 tablespoons (28 ml) vinegar or lemon juice (or Ener-G yeast-free vinegar powder, reconstituted)
- 1 teaspoon mustard
- $1/2$ teaspoon arrowroot
- 1 cup (235 ml) sunflower oil, soy bean oil, or avocado oil

Whisk egg, salt, pepper, vinegar or lemon juice, mustard, and arrowroot together. Very slowly add sunflower oil (or any mild-tasting tolerated oil) while stirring, until it becomes the right consistency.

It won't be as thick as mayo from a jar, but it tastes quite good. It must be refrigerated, and shelf life is limited because there are no preservatives. Be sure eggs are fresh and not contaminated with salmonella or antibiotics. Free-range eggs from a reputable health food store are best.

YIELD: *1¹/₂ cups (360 g)*

Calories (kcal): 200; **Total fat:** 223g; **Cholesterol:** 187mg; **Carbohydrate:** 4g; **Dietary fiber:** trace; **Protein:** 6g; **Sodium:** 385mg; **Potassium:** 97mg; **Calcium:** 33mg; **Iron:** 1mg; **Zinc:** 1mg; **Vitamin A:** 280IU

Miracle Spread

gluten   milk   soy   egg   corn   nuts

- 2 tablespoons (16 g) GFCF flour
- $1/2$ teaspoon xanthan gum
- 2 tablespoons (26 g) sugar
- $1/2$ teaspoon dry mustard
- $1/8$ teaspoon cayenne pepper
- 2 eggs
- 1 cup (235 ml) water
- $1/3$ cup (80 ml) GFCF vinegar or lemon juice
- 3 tablespoons (45 ml) almond, safflower, avocado, or corn oil

Put dry ingredients in a small saucepan.

In a bowl, whisk eggs and water. Add to dry ingredients. Stir until smooth. Add vinegar or lemon juice. Stir again until smooth.

Cook over medium heat until very thick, stirring constantly. Remove from heat and add oil. Stir until smooth. Put into a bowl or jar and refrigerate. It only lasts a day or two until it starts to separate.

YIELD: *2 cups (480 g)*

Calories (kcal): 666; **Total fat:** 50g; **Cholesterol:** 374mg; **Carbohydrate:** 44g; **Dietary fiber:** 1g; **Protein:** 13g; **Sodium:** 119mg; **Potassium:** 215mg; **Calcium:** 59mg; **Iron:** '. 3mg; **Zinc:** 1mg; **Vitamin A:** 654IU

Dana's Simple Dressing

gluten   milk   soy   egg   corn   nuts

- 1 cup (240 g) GFCF mayonnaise
- 1/2 cup (120 g) GFCF ketchup (see recipe on page 135 or purchase)

Combine mayonnaise and ketchup in a small bowl until blended.

YIELD: *1 1/2 cups (360 g)*

Calories (kcal): 170; **Total fat:** 187g; **Cholesterol:** 77mg; **Carbohydrate:** 33g; **Dietary fiber:** 2g; **Protein:** 4g; **Sodium:** 2674mg; **Potassium:** 652mg; **Calcium:** 62mg; **Iron:** 2mg; **Zinc:** 1mg; **Vitamin A:** 1835IU

Simple Thousand Island Dressing

    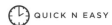

gluten   milk   soy   egg   corn   nuts

- 1 1/2 cups (360 g) Dana's Simple Dressing (above)
- 1/4 cup (60 g) GFCF sweet pickle relish
- 1 hard-boiled medium egg, chopped
- 1 tablespoon (10 g) chopped or minced onion (optional)

Combine all ingredients until blended.

YIELD: *2 cups (480 g)*

Calories (kcal): 1862; **Total fat:** 193g; **Cholesterol:** 289mg; **Carbohydrate:** 56g; **Dietary fiber:** 3g; **Protein:** 11g; **Sodium:** 3231 mg; **Potassium:** 746mg; **Calcium:** 91mg; **Iron:** 3mg; **Zinc:** 1mg; **Vitamin A:** 2210IU

Simple Russian Dressing

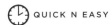   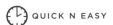

gluten   milk   soy   egg   corn   nuts

- 1 cup (240 g) GFCF mayonnaise
- 1/4 cup (60 g) GFCF ketchup (see recipe on page 110 or purchase)
- 1/4 cup (60 g) GFCF chili sauce
- 1/4 cup (60 g) GFCF sweet pickle relish
- 1 hard-boiled medium egg, chopped
- 1 tablespoon (10 g) chopped or minced onion (optional)

Place all ingredients in a medium bowl; mix until blended.

YIELD: *2 cups (480 g)*

Calories (kcal): 1812; **Total fat:** 193g; **Cholesterol:** 289mg; **Carbohydrate:** 42g; **Dietary fiber:** 4g; **Protein:** 10g; **Sodium:** 2534mg; **Potassium:** 796mg; **Calcium:** 83mg; **Iron:** 3mg; **Zinc:** 1mg; **Vitamin A:** 6082IU

Ranch Dressing/Mayo

gluten milk soy egg corn nuts

This recipe is a modification from the Yeast Connection Cookbook *by Crook and Jones.*

- ¹/₂ cup (65 g) hulled sunflower seeds
- 1 tablespoon (8 g) arrowroot starch or potato starch
- 1 teaspoon sea salt
- 1 tablespoon (15 ml) oil (corn, safflower, soy, or avocado)
- 1 teaspoon unbuffered, corn-free vitamin C crystals
- 1 cup (235 ml) water
- ¹/₂ teaspoon garlic power

Blend seeds in a blender on highest speed for 1 to 2 minutes until they become a fine powder. Stop at least once to scrape sides and bottom of blender jar. Do not overmix or you will create a butter. If needed to make it smoother, add flour or starch and blend on highest speed 1 minute longer.

Add remaining ingredients. Blend on highest speed for a minute longer, stopping once or twice to scrape sides and bottom of blender jar.

Pour mixture into a small saucepan. Add desired seasoning. Cook over medium heat, stirring constantly with whisk until mixture is thick yet smooth.

Chill the mixture. If too thick, add 1 tablespoon (15 ml) more water. Taste and add more seasoning if desired. (Add 1 teaspoon basil and 2 teaspoons leaf oregano to make Creamy Italian.)

Limiting the garlic powder to ¹/₄ teaspoon makes a nice mayonnaise. For those on a rotation diet or who have allergies to sunflower seeds, this recipe can be made using almonds, filberts, macadamia nuts, or unsalted cashews. Flour and starch also can be rotated.

YIELD: *1¹/₂ cups (330 g)*

Calories (kcal): 564; **Total fat:** 49g; **Cholesterol:** 0mg; **Carbohydrate:** 22g; **Dietary fiber:** 8g; **Protein:** 17g; **Sodium:** 1890mg; **Potassium:** 512mg; **Calcium:** 93mg; **Iron:** 5mg; **Zinc:** 4mg; **Vitamin A:** 36IU

Lemon Vinaigrette

gluten   milk   soy   egg   corn   nuts

- $^1/_4$ cup (60 ml) lemon juice
- 2 tablespoons (20 g) finely chopped shallots, mild onion, or scallions
- 1 tablespoon (15 ml) GFCF cider vinegar or white wine vinegar
- 2 tablespoons (28 ml) olive oil
- $^1/_2$ teaspoon GFCF Dijon mustard
- Salt and pepper to taste

Combine lemon juice, shallots, and vinegar. Let stand 5 minutes.

Whisk in oil, mustard, salt, and pepper.

YIELD: *$^2/_3$ cup (160 ml)*

Calories (kcal): 273; **Total fat:** 27g; **Cholesterol:** 0mg; **Carbohydrate:** 10g; **Dietary fiber:** trace; **Protein:** 1g; **Sodium:** 301 mg; **Potassium:** 164mg; **Calcium:** 18mg; **Iron:** 1mg; **Zinc:** trace; **Vitamin A:** 2510IU

Tangy Vinaigrette

gluten   milk   soy   egg   corn   nuts

Jeannie Fritz Godbout offers this quick version.

- $^1/_2$ cup (120 ml) balsamic vinegar
- $^1/_4$ cup (60 g) GFCF regular or Dijon mustard

Blend ingredients well in a blender (medium-high speed).

YIELD: *3/4 cup (175 ml)*

Calories (kcal): 64; **Total fat:** 3g; **Cholesterol:** 0mg; **Carbohydrate:** 12g; **Dietary fiber:** 2g; **Protein:** 3g; **Sodium:** 753mg; **Potassium:** 211mg; **Calcium:** 58mg; **Iron:** 2 2mg; **Zinc:** 1mg; **Vitamin A:** 0IU

Really Quick N Easy Raspberry Vinaigrette

gluten   milk   soy   egg   corn   nuts

- 1 cup (235 ml) GFCF oil-and-vinegar dressing—Italian or Balsamic
- $^1/_8$ cup (60 g) raspberries (fresh or defrosted frozen)

Place ingredients in a blender. Blend on medium.

YIELD: *1 $^1/_8$ cups (260 ml)*

Calories (kcal): 1130; **Total fat:** 125g; **Cholesterol:** 0mg; **Carbohydrate:** 8g; **Dietary fiber:** 1g; **Protein:** trace; **Sodium:** 1mg; **Potassium:** 43mg; **Calcium:** 3mg; **Iron:** trace; **Zinc:** trace; **Vitamin A:** 21IU

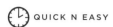

Herb-Mustard Vinaigrette

gluten   milk   soy   egg   corn   nuts

This Joyce Mulcahy dressing is adapted from a Southern Living *recipe.*

- 1 (4-ounce [115 g]) jar pear baby food
- 3 tablespoons (45 ml) white grape juice (100%) concentrate
- 3 tablespoons (45 ml) GFCF white wine vinegar
- 1 teaspoon GFCF Dijon mustard
- 1/4 teaspoon GFCF hot sauce (optional)
- 2 teaspoons fresh tarragon
- 2 teaspoons fresh basil
- 1 tablespoon (15 ml) olive oil
- Salt and pepper to taste

Combine all ingredients except olive oil, salt, and pepper. Whisk in olive oil. Salt and pepper to taste.

YIELD: *1 cup (235 ml)*

Calories (kcal): 217; **Total fat:** 14g; **Cholesterol:** 0mg; **Carbohydrate:** 25g; **Dietary fiber:** 6g; **Protein:** 1g; **Sodium:** 368mg; **Potassium:** 315mg; **Calcium:** 86mg; **Iron:** 2mg; **Zinc:** trace; **Vitamin A:** 335IU

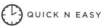

Sweet and Tangy Vinaigrette

gluten   milk   soy   egg   corn   nuts

Expanding on the Tangy Vinaigrette (page 107), we offer the following sweet version. We also added olive oil, especially for those who need more of the good fats and oils.

- 1/2 cup (120 ml) balsamic vinegar
- 1/4 cup (60 g) GFCF regular or Dijon mustard
- 1/4 cup (85 g) honey
- 2 tablespoons (28 ml) light olive oil

Blend ingredients well in a blender (medium-high speed).

YIELD: *1 1/8 cups (260 ml)*

Calories (kcal): 560; **Total fat:** 30g; **Cholesterol:** 0mg; **Carbohydrate:** 82g; **Dietary fiber:** 2g; **Protein:** 3g; **Sodium:** 756mg; **Potassium:** 255mg; **Calcium:** 64mg; **Iron:** 2 2mg; **Zinc:** 1mg; **Vitamin A:** 0IU

QUICK N EASY

Sweet Versatile Cucumber Vinaigrette

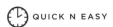

gluten milk soy egg corn nuts

This versatile, delicious recipe is inspired by Michael Thurmond's recipe in the 6 Week Body Makeover, brought to our attention by Suzi Gifford. Originally fat-free, we have added healthy oil, so needed by growing children. It can be used as a salad dressing or a sauce on fish or chicken.

- 2 cucumbers, peeled, seeded, and sliced
- 1/8 teaspoon lemon juice or GFCF vinegar
- 1/2 tablespoon (8 ml) oil (olive, high oleic safflower, avocado, almond)
- 1/3 teaspoon honey
- 1/4 teaspoon GFCF Dijon mustard
- 2 sprigs or 1/8 teaspoon dried dill, parsley, or cilantro
- Salt and pepper to taste

In blender, process (at medium speed) cucumbers; lemon or vinegar; oil; honey; mustard; and dill, parsley, or cilantro. Add salt and pepper to taste.

Additional herbs can expand the flavor of this dressing. Try adding garlic, onion, or ginger.

YIELD: *1 cup (235 ml)*

Calories (kcal): 148; **Total fat:** 8g; **Cholesterol:** 0mg; **Carbohydrate:** 19g; **Dietary fiber:** 5g; **Protein:** 4g; **Sodium:** 295mg; **Potassium:** 878mg; **Calcium:** 91mg; **Iron:** 2mg; **Zinc:** 1mg; **Vitamin A:** 1302IU

 QUICK N EASY

Lemon Tahini Salad Dressing

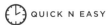

gluten milk soy egg corn nuts

Provided by Seven Oaks Restaurant. This dressing can be used on more than just salad. Try it over a baked potato, in a pasta salad, or over steamed vegetables. It also makes a great dip.

- 1/4 green pepper
- 1/4 large Spanish onion (yellow)
- 1 stalk celery
- 3/4 cup (180 g) tahini
- 1 1/2 cups (355 ml) olive oil
- 1/2 cup (120 ml) lemon juice (bottled)
- 1/4 cup (60 ml) tamari
- 1 teaspoon minced garlic (jarred)
- 1/4 teaspoon black pepper

In food processor, add the first three ingredients and process. Then add the rest of the ingredients and process again.

YIELD: *3 cups (710 ml)*

Calories (kcal): 4071; **Total fat:** 424g; **Cholesterol:** 0mg; **Carbohydrate:** 61 g; **Dietary fiber:** 20g; **Protein:** 40g; **Sodium:** 4267mg; **Potassium:** 1297mg; **Calcium:** 824mg; **Iron:** 18mg; **Zinc:** 9mg; **Vitamin A:** 388IU

Easy-to-Make Ketchup

gluten milk soy egg corn nuts

Adapted from Elaine Gottschall's Breaking the
Vicious Cycle.

- 2 cups (470 ml) tomato juice
- 1–3 tablespoons (15–45 ml) white vinegar
- 1 bay leaf (optional)
- Salt and pepper to taste
- Honey to taste
- GFCF (soy-free) fish sauce to taste (optional)
  *(Thai Kitchen fish sauce [www.thaikitchen.com]
  or A Taste of Thai fish sauce.)*

Mix all ingredients except honey and fish sauce
and simmer on stove until thick, stirring with a
slotted spoon to prevent sticking.

When almost the desired thickness, remove bay
leaf and add honey and optional fish sauce to taste.

Pour or ladle into sterilized jars and seal immediately or place in small containers and freeze.

YIELD: *1 to 1 1/2 cups (240 to 360 g)*

Calories (kcal): 91; **Total fat:** trace; **Cholesterol:** 0mg; **Carbohydrate:**
23g; **Dietary fiber:** 6g; **Protein:** 4g; **Sodium:** 2029mg; **Potassium:**
1108mg; **Calcium:** 50mg; **Iron:** 3mg; **Zinc:** 1mg; **Vitamin A:** 2720IU

Homemade Mustard

gluten milk soy egg corn nuts

*For those who want to make their own GFCF mustard,
here is a good recipe.*

*The Quick N Easy version is, of course, store-bought
GFCF (French's, Ener-G Foods, Inc.). Check out sources
at www.gfcfdiet.com/directory.htm.*

- 3 tablespoons (25 g) tapioca flour
- 2/3 cup (160 ml) water, divided
- 1/4 cup (40 g) dry mustard
- 1/3 cup (80 ml) vinegar
- 2 tablespoons (40 g) honey
- 1/2 teaspoon salt
- 2 tablespoons (30 g) fresh grated horseradish
- 1/4 teaspoon ground turmeric
- 1/8 teaspoon paprika

Mix tapioca flour in 1/4 cup (60 ml) of the water to
form a paste and set aside.

In a small saucepan over medium-low heat, mix
together dry mustard, vinegar, honey, salt, and
remainder of water. Gradually whisk in tapioca-
flour paste until well blended. Bring to boil, stirring
constantly, until mixture thickens.

Remove from heat and stir in horseradish, turmeric, and paprika. Refrigerate in an air-tight container for up to one week.

Dry mustard can be made by grinding mustard
seed in a small coffee grinder.

YIELD: *1/2 to 3/4 cup (120 to 180 g)*

Calories (kcal): 340; **Total fat:** 5g; **Cholesterol:** 0mg; **Carbohydrate:**
73g; **Dietary fiber:** 2g; **Protein:** 6g; **Sodium:** 1109mg; **Potassium:** 400mg;
Calcium: 106mg; **Iron:** 3mg; **Zinc:** 2mg; **Vitamin A:** 243IU

Sunflower Seed Healthy Spread

gluten　milk　soy　egg　corn　nuts

This mild-tasting spread is loaded with vitamins. It can be used on crackers and bread or as a dip with chips or veggies.

- 1 cup (135 g) sunflower seeds, ground
- $^1/_2$ cup (55 g) nutritional yeast or ground flaxseed
- $^1/_4$ cup (35 g) brown rice flour
- Basil, to taste
- Thyme, to taste
- 1 tablespoon (8 g) soy protein powder
- 2 cloves garlic
- 1 carrot, shredded
- 1 onion, chopped
- 1 stalk celery, chopped
- $^1/_4$ –$^1/_2$ cup (60–120 ml) olive oil
- 2 tablespoons (28 ml) lemon juice
- 2 tablespoons (28 ml) tamari
- 1 cup (235 ml) hot water

Blend the first seven ingredients in a food processor (with $^1/_4$ cup [60 ml] olive oil), then add vegetables and blend, then add liquids and blend. If too thick, add more olive oil. If too thin, may adjust with brown rice flour. Bake 55 minutes at 350°F (180°C, or gas mark 4) in a 9 x 9-inch (22.5 x 22.5 cm) pan. (Should be about 1-inch [2.5 cm] thick in pan.)

YIELD: *3 cups (675 g)*

Calories (kcal): 234; **Total fat:** 186g; **Cholesterol:** 0mg; **Carbohydrate:** 121g; **Dietary fiber:** 50g; **Protein:** 81g; **Sodium:** 2139mg; **Potassium:** 3837mg; **Calcium:** 334mg; **Iron:** 29mg; **Zinc:** 15mg; **Vitamin A:** 20416IU

Cranberry Sauce

gluten

milk

soy

egg

corn

nuts

Yes, there is a way to have this holiday favorite without all the corn syrup, and it tastes better, too.

- 4 cups (380 g) fresh cranberries (2 bags)
- 2$^1/_2$ cups (590 ml) water, divided
- 3–4 packets gelatin
- 1$^3/_4$ cups (595 g) honey

Sort through berries, discarding the really light ones and any spoiled fruit. Freeze any amount exceeding 4 cups (380 g). Wash berries and place in a saucepan. Add 2 cups (475 ml) water and place on medium heat, uncovered. Once the berries begin boiling, cover and reduce the heat to continue to simmer. Simmer for 10 minutes.

Meanwhile, pour $^1/_2$ cup (120 ml) water in large bowl. Sprinkle 3 to 4 packets of gelatin over water—3 will give softer set; if a firmer set is desired, use 4 packets. Do not stir the gelatin; just let it sit a few minutes.

Using a strainer, pour berry mixture into the strainer above the bowl of gelatin. Push the juice and pulp through with a spoon, stirring inside the strainer. Work it through, as the skins will stay behind even with aggressive stirring. Scrape the outside of the strainer into the bowl with a spatula to get all of the pulp. Set aside strainer and skins.

Stir to dissolve gelatin. Add honey, starting with 1$^1/_2$ cups (510 g) and adding 1 tablespoon (20 g) at a time until it reaches desired sweetness. Place in a serving dish. Cover and refrigerate. It will take several hours to set.

YIELD: *2 cups (550 g)*

Calories (kcal): 230; **Total fat:** 1g; **Cholesterol:** 0mg; **Carbohydrate:** 613g; **Dietary fiber:** 17g; **Protein:** 10g; **Sodium:** 272mg; **Potassium: Calcium:** 584mg 85mg; **Iron:** ', 3mg; **Zinc:** 2mg; **Vitamin A:** 175IU

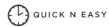
Sassy Salsas

gluten   milk   soy   egg   corn   nuts

There are numerous wonderful recipes for salsa. This is one of our favorites because the basic recipe is as delicious as the three additional versions. Salsas are versatile and can be used for more purposes than as a snack with corn chips. They are excellent used on top of potatoes, fish, pasta, or eggs.

- 1¼ cups (about 8 ounces [225 g]) seeded and chopped firm, ripe tomatoes
- 1 minced fresh jalapeño peppers to taste (optional)
- ⅓ cup (55 g) minced red onion
- ¼ cup (15 g) chopped fresh cilantro
- 2 tablespoons (28 ml) fresh lime or lemon juice
- ½ teaspoon minced garlic (optional)
- ½ teaspoon salt
- ½ teaspoon black pepper

Variations:

- **AVOCADO SASSY SALSA:** add 1 cup (225 g) peeled, chopped avocado
- **BEAN SASSY SALSA:** add 1 cup (225 g) black beans, rinsed, well drained
- **MANGO SASSY SALSA:** add 1 cup (175 g) peeled, chopped mango

Mix tomatoes, peppers, onion, and cilantro in a bowl. Add lime or lemon juice and garlic. Mix together gently. Add salt and pepper to taste.

For variations, add either avocado, black beans, or mango and mix gently. A combination of beans and avocado is also delicious.

NOTES: *The recipe can be made from very mild to very hot, depending on how much jalapeno pepper is used. Use no jalapeno if you like it very mild; use up to 2 tablespoons (20 g) minced jalapeno pepper for a hotter salsa.*

Salsa stores well for up to three days in the refrigerator. It can also be frozen.

YIELD: *2½ cups (500 g)*

Calories (kcal): 82; **Total fat:** 1g; **Cholesterol:** 0mg; **Carbohydrate:** : 19g; **Dietary fiber:** 4g; **Protein:** 3g; **Sodium:** 1091mg; **Potassium:** 660mg; **Calcium:** 42mg; **Iron:** 2mg; **Zinc:** trace; **Vitamin A:** 1674IU

Linda's Salsa

gluten   milk   soy   egg   corn   nuts

Here is a favorite salsa.

- 1 can (28 ounces, or 785 g) whole tomatoes, chopped
- 4 large fresh tomatoes, chopped
- 2 cans (3 ounces, or 85 g, each) diced green chilies
- 1 large bunch scallions, cut up finely
- 2 tablespoons (12 g) ground black pepper
- 2 tablespoons (28 ml) apple cider vinegar
- ¹/₂ cup (30 g) chopped fresh parsley
- ¹/₂ teaspoon lemon juice
- 2 teaspoons (10 ml) GFCF soy sauce
- 2 teaspoons sugar
- ¹/₄ cup (60 ml) light olive oil
- 1 teaspoon dried oregano
- 1 tablespoon (4 g) chopped fresh cilantro (optional)

Mix all ingredients together. Store any leftovers in a sealed container in the refrigerator. Serve with GFCF tortilla chips.

YIELD: *1¹/₂ quarts (1.4 L) salsa*

Calories (kcal): 854; **Total fat:** 59g; **Cholesterol:** 0mg; **Carbohydrate:** 86g; **Dietary fiber:** 20g; **Protein:** 15g; **Sodium:** 825mg; **Potassium:** 3361 mg; **Calcium:** 209mg; **Iron:** 13mg; **Zinc:** 2mg; **Vitamin A:** 9855IU

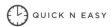 QUICK N EASY

Really Easy Salsa Dip

gluten   milk   soy   egg   corn   nuts

- 1 jar (16 ounces, or 455 g) GFCF Thick and Chunky Salsa (Pace)
- 1 teaspoon chopped fresh cilantro

Mix the cilantro in the salsa and serve.

NOTE: *For a tasty fruit twist on this popular recipe, add ¹/₄ cup (80 g) GFCF natural fruit spread— mixed berry, grape, or apricot (Whole Foods, Cascadian Farms, Harvest Moon).*

YIELD: *2 cups (480 g)*

Calories (kcal): 127; **Total fat:** 1g; **Cholesterol:** 0mg; **Carbohydrate:** 28g; **Dietary fiber:** 7g; **Protein:** 6g; **Sodium:** 1969mg; **Potassium:** 968mg; **Calcium:** 136mg; **Iron:** 4mg; **Zinc:** 1mg; **Vitamin A:** 2752IU

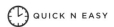

Easy Bean Salsa Dip

gluten　　milk　　soy　　egg　　corn　　nuts

- 1 can (16 ounces, or 455 g) GFCF refried black beans (Eden)
- 2 cups (480 g) Really Easy Salsa Dip (page 114)

Spread refried beans on a plate—approximately $^1/_2$ inch (1.25 cm) deep.

Spread Really Easy Salsa Dip over the refried beans. Serve with GFCF corn chips or taco chips

YIELD: *4 cups (935 g)*

Calories (kcal): 511; **Total fat:** 5g; **Cholesterol:** 0mg; **Carbohydrate:** 88g; **Dietary fiber:** 32g; **Protein:** 30g; **Sodium:** 3364mg; **Potassium:** 968mg; **Calcium:** 136mg; **Iron:** 4mg; **Zinc:** 1mg; **Vitamin A:** 2752IU

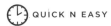

Sofrito

gluten　　milk　　soy　　egg　　corn　　nuts

- $^3/_4$ bunch cilantro
- 3 medium Spanish onions
- 1 head garlic
- 1 green pepper, preferably cubanelle, seeded

Wash cilantro. Peel onions and garlic. Put everything in a tenfood processor and pulse until minced but not liquid.

This will keep in refrigerator for up to 10 days. Freeze in ice cube trays and use to flavor soups and stews and to make taco recipes.

YIELD: *1$^1/_2$ cups (225 g)*

Calories (kcal): 223; **Total fat:** 1g; **Cholesterol:** 0mg; **Carbohydrate:** 51g; **Dietary fiber:** 11g; **Protein:** 7g; **Sodium:** 20mg; **Potassium:** 1037mg; **Calcium:** 129mg; **Iron:** 2mg; **Zinc:** 1mg; **Vitamin A:** 1014IU

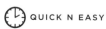

 QUICK N EASY

Thai Peanut Sauce

gluten   milk   soy   egg   corn   nuts

This a great dipping sauce. Serve alongside broiled or grilled chicken breasts.

- ¹/₂ cup (130 g) smooth peanut butter
- ¹/₄ cup (60 ml) warm water
- 2 tablespoons (30 ml) lime juice
- 1 tablespoon (15 g) brown sugar
- 1 tablespoon (15 ml) GFCF tamari sauce
- 1 small garlic clove, minced
- Pinch of cayenne pepper

Whisk peanut butter and water together. Stir in the remaining ingredients, cover, and refrigerate for 20 minutes, until chilled.

TIP: *Use ¹/₂ to 1 cup (120 to 235 ml) of GFCF chicken broth instead of the water, and use as a sauce for stir-fry.*

YIELD: *1 cup (235 ml), or 6 to 8 servings*

Calories (kcal): 103; **Total fat:** 8g; **Cholesterol:** 0mg; **Carbohydrate:** 5g; **Dietary fiber:** 1g; **Protein:** 4g; **Sodium:** 107mg; **Potassium:** 127mg; **Calcium:** 8mg; **Iron:** trace; **Zinc:** trace; **Vitamin A:** trace.

 QUICK N EASY

Spinach Hummus

  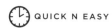

gluten   milk   soy   egg   corn   nuts

Adapted from Lisa Barnes of Petit Appétit

Is your family ho-hum for hummus? Try this variation using spinach. It goes great on a crudités platter, or even just as a snack.

- 1 (8 ounce, or 400 g) can chickpeas, drained and rinsed
- 1 clove garlic
- 1 cup (30 g) packed organic spinach leaves
- 1 tablespoon (15 ml) freshly squeezed lemon juice
- ¹/₂ teaspoon ground cumin
- 1 teaspoon kosher salt
- ¹/₂ teaspoon freshly ground black pepper
- ¹/₄ cup (60 ml) extra-virgin olive oil

In a blender or food processor, combine chickpeas and garlic and puree until smooth. Add spinach, lemon juice, cumin, salt, and pepper, and blend thoroughly. With motor running, gradually add olive oil and process until smooth and creamy. Taste and adjust seasoning as needed.

YIELD: *Makes about 1¹/₂ cups, or 10 servings*

Calories (kcal): 77; **Total fat:** 6g; **Cholesterol:** 0mg; **Carbohydrate:** 6g; **Dietary fiber:** 1g; **Protein:** 1g; **Sodium:** 284mg; **Potassium:** 62mg; **Calcium:** 14mg; **Iron:** 1mg; **Zinc:** trace; **Vitamin A:** 209IU.

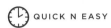 QUICK N EASY

White Bean and Walnut Spread

gluten   milk   soy   egg   corn   nuts

This is a great spread for GFCF crackers or served with a crudités platter.

- 1 can (15 ounces, or 420 g) cannellini beans
- $1/2$ cup (60 g) chopped walnuts, toasted
- 2 tablespoons (30 ml) olive oil
- 3 tablespoons (45 ml) water
- 1 tablespoon (15 ml) lemon juice
- 1 small garlic clove, minced
- $1/2$ teaspoon salt
- $1/8$ teaspoon ground black pepper
- $1/4$ teaspoon paprika

Combine all ingredients in a food processor, pulse until smooth, and serve.

YIELD: *8 servings*

Calories (kcal): 255; **Total fat:** 8g; **Cholesterol:** 0mg; **Carbohydrate:** 33g; **Dietary fiber:** 8g; **Protein:** 14g; **Sodium:** 142mg; **Potassium:** 999mg; **Calcium:** 134mg; **Iron:** 6; **Zinc:** 2; **Vitamin A:** 24IU.

Plenty O' Pesto

gluten   milk   soy   egg   corn   nuts

Pesto is a versatile condiment, and can be made out of any number of combinations of herbs and nuts. It can be used as a sauce for pasta or pizza, a garnish for soup, a topping for grilled or sautéed chicken or fish, or even a flavoring for steamed or mashed vegetables.

- 3 cups (60 g) arugula or basil leaves, or 1 cup (60 g) parsley or cilantro leaves
- 3 cloves garlic
- $1/2$ cup (75 g) nuts (pecans, walnuts, almonds, unsalted pistachios, or pine nuts)
- $1/2$ teaspoon salt
- $1/4$ teaspoon ground black pepper
- $1/2$ cup (120 ml) extra-virgin olive oil
- Water

In a food processor or blender, pulse herbs or greens, garlic, nuts, salt, and pepper until finely chopped. With machine running, slowly add the oil. Add water (if needed), 1 tablespoon (15 ml) at a time, until a smooth paste is formed. Store in an airtight container in the refrigerator for up to 3 days (cover surface of pesto with a thin layer of oil to avoid discoloration).

YIELD: *6 servings*

Calories (kcal): 224; **Total fat:** 24g; **Cholesterol:** 0mg; **Carbohydrate:** 3g; **Dietary fiber:** 1g; **Protein:** 1g; **Sodium:** 178mg; **Potassium:** 82mg; **Calcium:** 21mg; **Iron:** trace; **Zinc:** 1mg; **Vitamin A:** 341IU.

QUICK N EASY

Spinach Pesto

    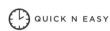

| gluten | milk | soy | egg | corn | nuts |

This spinach pesto is a great way to quickly flavor foods and add a nice boost of vegetables. Try it with pasta, meat, fish, or rice.

- 6 cups (180 g) fresh baby spinach, washed and dried
- $1/2$ cup (75 g) pine nuts, almonds, or walnuts
- 3 large cloves garlic, chopped
- $1/2$ to $3/4$ cup (120 to 175 ml) extra virgin olive oil (or $1/2$ cup oil [120 ml] and $1/4$ cup [60 ml] water as needed to thin pesto)
- 2 teaspoons dried basil
- Salt and ground pepper to taste

Process all ingredients and $1/2$ teaspoon salt in a food processor until smooth, starting with $1/2$ cup olive oil and adding more oil (or water) as needed until desired consistency is reached. Season with salt and pepper to taste, and enjoy! Store in airtight container in refrigerator for up to 1 week.

YIELD: *8 servings*

Calories (kcal): 235; **Total fat:** 25g; **Cholesterol:** 0mg; **Carbohydrate:** 3g; **Dietary fiber:** 1g; **Protein:** 3g; **Sodium:** 18mg; **Potassium:** 194mg; **Calcium:** 34mg; **Iron:** 2mg; **Zinc:** trace; **Vitamin A:** 1549IU.

CHAPTER 12

Breads, Muffins, Waffles, and Pancakes

OUR DAUGHTER WAS ADDICTED TO WHITE PASTA AND cereal. We didn't know how to break the cycle. Once we reduced sugar, increased protein, and eliminated dairy and gluten from her diet, the whole picture changed. We began to offer healthier replacement foods like greens, protein-rich foods, and alternative grains. Now, at dinnertime she normally cleans her plate. We see her eating vegetables like green beans, spinach, zucchini, and broccoli in greater variety and greater quantities. She stays energetic throughout the day and does not have the highs and lows she once did. She seems to understand that our new way of eating is healthier and makes her feel better.

—MARIE, *mother*

Introduction

Using prepared organic flours or mixes helps make a recipe Quick N Easy.

Pancakes, waffles, breads, muffins, and buns are wonderful places to sneak in better nutrition by substituting some of the liquid ingredients with cooked and pureed vegetables. If your child refuses to eat anything green, select vegetables whose colors will not be obvious (cauliflower, carrot, sweet potato, and squash). If color is not a problem, expand to the greens. Pureed fruits can also be included.

The amount of protein can be increased by adding one or more of the following: extra egg whites, nut flours, or rice protein powder (add $1/8$ to $1/4$ cup [15 to 30 g] as a replacement for an equal amount of flour). Favorites include almond flour and hazelnut flour. See the resource product listing in the appendix.

In pancakes, there is room for hiding supplements in what we call the Trojan Horse Technique. Add powdered supplements such as calcium and magnesium here.

What Can Be Hidden in a Muffin?

- Eggs (added protein, amino acids)
- Nuts (added protein)
- Dried fruit, molasses (added iron)
- Flax (linseed) (added omega 3s, fiber)
- Protein powder (if heat stable)
- Calcium powder

Bette Hagman's All-Purpose Flour Substitute

gluten milk soy egg corn nuts

This formula is found in the many Gluten-Free Gourmet *books by Bette Hagman. This combination has become the standard mix for replacing all-purpose flour.*

- 2 parts white rice flour
- $^2/_3$ part potato starch flour
- $^1/_3$ part tapioca flour

Combine all ingredients. Blend with a whisk and store, ready for use any time a recipe calls for all-purpose flour.

Calories (kcal): 4890; **Total fat:** 15g; **Cholesterol:** 0mg; **Carbohydrate:** 1101g; **Dietary fiber:** 40g; **Protein:** 78g; **Sodium:** 103mg; **Potassium: Calcium:** 5496mg 191mg; **Iron:** 55mg; **Zinc:** 12mg; **Vitamin A:** 0IU

White Bread—Bread Machine

 gluten milk soy egg corn nuts

The kids will never know it's healthy!

- 1 cup (235 ml) water
- 3 tablespoons (45 ml) oil
- 1 teaspoon salt
- 1 cup (140 g) brown rice flour
- ³/₄ cup (105 g) garbanzo bean flour
- ¹/₂ cup (80 g) potato starch
- ¹/₄ cup (30 g) tapioca starch
- 4 egg whites
- 2 teaspoons xanthan gum
- 1 teaspoon yeast

Place ingredients in a bread machine in the order listed. Select setting and start. Store in freezer and slice and toast as needed.

YIELD: *1 loaf (12 slices)*

Calories (kcal): 134; **Total fat:** 4g; **Cholesterol:** 0mg; **Carbohydrate:** 21g; **Dietary fiber:** 1g; **Protein:** 4g; **Sodium:** 201 mg; **Potassium:** 109mg; **Calcium:** 6mg; **Iron:** 1mg; **Zinc:** 1mg; **Vitamin A:** 2IU

Banana Bread

 gluten milk soy egg 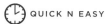 corn nuts

- ¹/₂ cup (120 ml) canola oil
- 2 large eggs
- 1 teaspoon vanilla
- ¹/₂ cup (115 g) dairy-free vanilla pudding mixed with 1 teaspoon xanthan gum
- 1 ripe banana, mashed
- 1 package (15 ounces, or 420 g) Old Fashioned Cake and Cookie Mix from Gluten Free Pantry or 1 package (21 ounces, or 588 g) Miss Roben's Yellow Cake Mix

Grease a loaf pan. Preheat oven to 350°F (180°C, or gas mark 4). Mix the first five ingredients. Fold in cake mix. Pour into 6-cup (1.4 L) loaf pan. Bake 50 minutes or until middle is cooked.

YIELD: *1 loaf (12 slices)*

Calories (kcal): 187; **Total fat:** 10g; **Cholesterol:** 32mg; **Carbohydrate:** 22g; **Dietary fiber:** trace; **Protein:** 2g; **Sodium:** 112mg; **Potassium:** 63mg; **Calcium:** 16mg; **Iron:** trace; **Zinc:** trace; **Vitamin A:** 75IU

Donuts

gluten milk soy egg corn nuts

These are delicious, especially when hot out of the oven.

- $^1/_2$ cup (80 g) white rice flour
- $^2/_3$ cup (80 g) tapioca flour
- $^1/_3$ cup (50 g) potato starch or (40 g) cornstarch
- $^1/_2$ teaspoon salt
- 2 teaspoons baking powder
- 2 teaspoons guar or xanthan gum
- 1 egg, beaten
- $^1/_3$ cup (80 ml) oil (olive, canola, safflower, or vegetable)
- $^1/_2$ cup (120 ml) milk (almond, rice, or potato)
- $^1/_3$ cup (80 ml) club soda or sparkling water

Combine all dry ingredients, mix together. Combine beaten egg, oil, and milk. Add slowly to dry mix. Beat well.

Add sparkling water or club soda very gradually. Beat well.

With floured hands, pull off 4 pieces of dough, each the size of a plum. Roll each piece quickly between your hands to make a strip, then form a ring, pinching the ends of the dough together. Heat one inch of oil in a deep heavy frying pan to 375°F (190°C). Fry donuts a few at a time. Cook on each side until golden brown, then remove to drain on paper towels.

YIELD: *8 to 12*

Donut Glaze

- 1 cup (100 g) powdered sugar
- $^1/_3$ cup (80 ml) boiling water
- $^1/_4$ teaspoon vanilla

Mix together the powdered sugar, vanilla, and boiling water. Dip the hot donuts in the glaze and set on cooling rack to allow the excess to drip off.

Homemade Hamburger or Hot Dog Buns

gluten milk soy egg corn nuts

This recipe is adapted from the Northern Texas Gluten Intolerance Group (GIG) and is available on their Web site, www.northtexasgig.com/recipes/breads/ hamburgerhotdogbuns.htm.

- 1¹/₂ cups (240 g) rice flour
- 1¹/₂ cups (180 g) tapioca starch
- 2 tablespoons (26 g) sugar
- 1 tablespoon (12 g) active dry yeast
- 1 tablespoon (8 g) xanthan gum
- 1 teaspoon salt
- 1 large egg
- ³/₄ cup (175 ml) rice, almond, or soy milk (room temperature or warm)
- 2 tablespoons (28 ml) oil
- 1 teaspoon (5 ml) apple cider vinegar
- ¹/₂ cup (120 ml) plus 1 tablespoon (15 ml) warm water

Combine rice flour, tapioca starch, sugar, yeast, xanthan gum, and salt in a heavy-duty mixer.

In a separate bowl, beat egg. Mix in milk substitute, oil, vinegar, and water. Add wet ingredients to the dry ingredients and beat on high speed for 3 to 5 minutes.

Spoon dough into an oil-sprayed hamburger or hot dog bun pan.

Let dough rise in a warm oven (about 170°F, or 77°C) for 20 minutes or until doubled in size. Remove buns from oven and preheat oven to 350°F (180°C, or gas mark 4).

Brush buns with melted GFCF butter substitute or melted ghee and bake in the oven for 20 to 25 minutes.

YIELD: *8 to 12 hot dog or hamburger buns*

Calories (kcal): 195; **Total fat:** 4g; **Cholesterol:** 19mg; **Carbohydrate:** 39g; **Dietary fiber:** 1g; **Protein:** 3g; **Sodium:** 220mg; **Potassium:** 49mg; **Calcium:** 8mg; **Iron:** trace ; **Zinc:** trace ; **Vitamin A:** 28IU

Gingerlicious Gingerbread

gluten milk soy egg corn nuts

Sorghum flour is similar to rice flour but makes a much better bread than rice flour does. Sorghum flour is not easy to find, but it is available from Twin Valley Mills and can be shipped (www.twinvalleymills.com).

Dry Ingredients

- ¹/₄ cup (50 g) sugar
- 1²/₃ cups (235 g) sorghum flour
- ¹/₂ cup (60 g) tapioca starch
- ¹/₄ teaspoon xanthan gum
- 1 teaspoon ground ginger
- 1 teaspoon cinnamon
- ¹/₄ teaspoon ground nutmeg
- ¹/₄ teaspoon ground cloves
- 3 tablespoons (24 g) chopped fresh ginger or 1 tablespoon (6 g) dried ground ginger
- ¹/₂ teaspoon salt

Wet Ingredients

- ¹/₂ cup (120 ml) CF milk (rice, almond, soy)
- ¹/₂ cup (170 g) light molasses
- ¹/₄ cup (55 g) ghee or Earth Balance Whipped Spread, melted
- ¹/₄ cup (85 g) honey
- 2 eggs
- 1 teaspoon vanilla

Whisk dry ingredients together, and set aside.

Heat the milk and molasses together in a small saucepan over medium heat until warm enough for the molasses to dissolve into the milk when well stirred.

Mix all of the remaining wet ingredients. Add the dry ingredients and mix well.

Pour into a 9 x 9-inch (22.5 x 22.5-cm) cake pan or divide into muffin tins. Bake for 20 to 30 minutes at 350°F (180°C, or gas mark 4), until done. Test for doneness by inserting a knife or toothpick into the center.

YIELD: *8 to 10 pieces or muffins*

Calories (kcal): 357; Total fat: 9g; Cholesterol: 64mg; Carbohydrate: 67g; Dietary fiber: 6g; Protein: 6g; Sodium: 161mg; Potassium: 477mg; Calcium: 66mg; Iron: 3mg; Zinc: trace; Vitamin A: 327IU

"My name is Travis Martin. I am eleven years old and go to a school in Washington, DC. I am on the school's swim team and have a blue belt in Tae Kwan Do. I really enjoy school and my friends. My favorite subjects are dance and drama. I have been on a gluten-free/casein-free diet since I turned five years old in 1999. From 2000 to 2004, I had to avoid eleven other foods, including soy, eggs, tomatoes, yeast, peanuts, banana, and coconut. I was really happy to have eggs, peanut butter, and ketchup added to my diet. I have to avoid gluten and dairy because they make me very tired and spacey and upset my digestive system. I have been helping my mom make GFCF food since I was little, and now I really love cooking. If I do not become a pale-ontologist, I might become a chef."

—**Travis,** *an 11-year-old from Washington, D.C.*

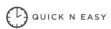 QUICK N EASY

Pecan Bread

gluten milk soy egg corn nuts

Specific Carbohydrate Diet (SCD) compatible

This recipe was adapted from the book Breaking the Vicious Cycle: Intestinal Health Through Diet, *by Elaine Gottschall.*

- 2^1/$_2$ cups (300 g) pecan meal
- ^{1}/$_4$ teaspoon salt
- ^{1}/$_2$ teaspoon baking soda
- ^{1}/$_4$ teaspoon cinnamon
- 4 eggs
- ^{1}/$_2$ cup (170 g) honey
- 1 tablespoon (15 ml) olive oil

Mix the dry ingredients, set aside. Break eggs into a separate bowl and whisk in honey. Add dry ingredients to egg mixture and stir. Add olive oil and mix thoroughly. Pour into 8 x 4-inch (20 x 10-cm) loaf pan that is completely lined (even up the sides) with kitchen parchment paper. Bake at 350°F (180°C, or gas mark 4) for 45 minutes. Once removed from the oven, allow the bread to cool for 5 minutes. Then lift the loaf out of the pan by the ends of the paper and gently roll it out of the parchment onto a cooling rack.

NOTE: *The parchment paper will wrinkle when used to line the pan and the loaf will not necessarily be symmetrical, but without it the bread sticks too much to the baking pan.*

YIELD: *1 loaf (12 slices)*

Calories (kcal): 161; **Total fat:** 3g; **Cholesterol:** 62mg; **Carbohydrate:** 25g; **Dietary fiber:** 2g; **Protein:** 10g; **Sodium:** 116mg; **Potassium:** 112mg; **Calcium:** 17mg; **Iron:** 1mg; **Zinc:** 2mg; **Vitamin A:** 125IU

Pumpkin Bread

gluten milk soy egg corn nuts

This bread freezes really well, if it lasts that long!

- 3^1/$_2$ cups (490 g) GF flour blend of choice
- ^{1}/$_2$ teaspoon xanthan gum
- 3 cups (600 g) sugar
- 2 teaspoons cinnamon
- 2 teaspoons nutmeg
- 1^1/$_2$ teaspoons salt
- 2 teaspoons baking soda
- 1 cup (235 ml) canola oil
- ^{2}/$_3$ cup (160 ml) water
- 1 can (15 ounces, or 420 g) pumpkin puree
- 2 eggs, beaten
- 6–12 ounces (170–340 g) GFCF semisweet chocolate chips (optional)

Preheat oven to 350°F (180°C, gas mark 4). Combine flour blend, xanthan gum, sugar, cinnamon, nutmeg, salt, and baking soda in a large bowl. In a separate bowl, combine oil, water, pumpkin, and eggs. Combine the dry and wet mixtures thoroughly. Add the chocolate chips, if using.

Divide the batter equally among three 8 x 4-inch (20 x 10-cm) loaf pans or two 12-compartment muffin pans that have been sprayed with nonstick spray. Bake loaves for 45 to 50 minutes; bake muffins for 40 minutes. When toothpick in the center comes out clean, the loaves/muffins are done. Cool completely before cutting and serving.

YIELD: *3 loaves or 24 muffins*

Calories (kcal): 342; **Total fat:** 14g; **Cholesterol:** 16mg; **Carbohydrate:** 54g; **Dietary fiber:** 2g; **Protein:** 3g; **Sodium:** 246mg; **Potassium:** 112mg; **Calcium:** 17mg; **Iron:** 1mg; **Zinc:** 1mg; **Vitamin A:** 3962IU

All-Purpose Buns

gluten   milk   soy   egg   corn   nuts

- 2 teaspoons yeast
- 1^1/$_2$ cups (355 ml) water
- 1^1/$_4$ cups (175 g) brown rice flour
- ^{3}/$_4$ cup (105 g) garbanzo bean flour
- ^{3}/$_4$ cup (120 g) potato starch
- ^{1}/$_3$ cup (40 g) tapioca starch
- 1 tablespoon (8 g) xanthan gum
- ^{1}/$_2$ tablespoon (9 g) salt
- 6 egg whites
- ^{1}/$_4$ cup (60 ml) oil (safflower, canola)

Mix yeast and water and let sit until foamy. Place remaining ingredients in a mixer bowl and add yeast mixture. Blend on low speed to incorporate, then on medium-high speed for 2 minutes. The dough will be sticky. Lightly oil bun pans or cookie sheets and top with parchment paper. Use an ice cream scoop to transfer dough. Cover and let the dough rise for 1 hour. Bake in a 350°F (180°C, gas mark 4) oven for 30 to 35 minutes. Store in freezer until needed.

YIELD: *12 buns*

Calories (kcal): 173; **Total fat:** 5g; **Cholesterol:** 0mg; **Carbohydrate:** 27g; **Dietary fiber:** 2g; **Protein:** 4g; **Sodium:** 300mg; **Potassium:** 133mg; **Calcium:** 8mg; **Iron:** 1mg; **Zinc:** 1mg; **Vitamin A:** 2IU

Soda Buns

gluten   milk   soy   egg   corn   nuts

- 1 cup (140 g) brown rice flour
- ^{2}/$_3$ cup (95 g) garbanzo bean flour
- ^{2}/$_3$ cup (80 g) tapioca starch
- ^{2}/$_3$ cup (100 g) potato starch
- 1 tablespoon plus 1 teaspoon (10 g) xanthan gum
- 1 tablespoon plus 1 teaspoon (6 g) baking powder
- 2 teaspoons (12 g) salt
- 8 egg whites
- ^{2}/$_3$ cup (160 ml) oil
- ^{2}/$_3$ cup (160 ml) club soda or sparkling mineral water

Preheat oven to 400°F (200°C, or gas mark 6). Combine all of the ingredients well, except club soda. Add club soda to the mix. Batter will be thick and lumpy. Scoop the dough onto a parchment paper–covered baking sheet. Bake 40 minutes at 400°F (200C, or gas mark 6), until golden brown. The crust will be hard out of the oven, but will soften when cool.

YIELD: *1 dozen buns*

Calories (kcal): 235; **Total fat:** 13g; **Cholesterol:** 0mg; **Carbohydrate:** 27g; **Dietary fiber:** 1g; **Protein:** 4g; **Sodium:** 561 mg; **Potassium:** 114mg; **Calcium:** 98mg; **Iron:** 1mg; **Zinc:** trace; **Vitamin A:** 2IU

Yeast-Free Sweet Potato Buns

    egg   corn nuts

gluten   milk   soy   egg   corn   nuts

Tracey Smith provides a tasty recipe that is perfect for children who love breads and dislike vegetables.

- 1¹/₄ cups (175 g) garbanzo bean flour
- 1¹/₄ cups (150 g) quinoa flour
- 1¹/₄ cups (175 g) brown rice flour
- 1 cup (120 g) tapioca starch
- 4 teaspoons xanthan gum
- 2 teaspoons salt
- 1 teaspoon baking powder
- 8 egg whites
- ¹/₃ cup (80 ml) oil (safflower, canola, avocado)
- 8 ounces (225 g) pureed sweet potatoes
- 1 cup (235 ml) water

Combine the dry ingredients in a mixer bowl. Add liquid ingredients and mix on low to incorporate. Mix on medium-high speed for 1 to 2 minutes, until a smooth dough forms. Dough will be sticky.

Lightly oil bun pans or cookie sheets and top them with parchment paper. Use an ice cream scoop to transfer dough. Bake in a 350°F (180°C, gas mark 4) oven for 30 to 45 minutes. May be stored in the freezer until needed.

YIELD: *12 buns*

Calories (kcal): 248; Total fat: 8g; Cholesterol: 0mg; Carbohydrate: 40g; Dietary fiber: 2g; Protein: 6g; Sodium: 439mg; Potassium: 221 mg; Calcium: 40mg; Iron: 2 2mg; Zinc: 1mg; Vitamin A: 967IU

Better-Than-Bisquick Pancakes

gluten   milk   soy   egg   corn   nuts

- 2 cups (240 g) quinoa flour
- 2 tablespoons (10 g) baking powder
- ¹/₄ teaspoon baking soda
- 2 tablespoons (28 ml) light-flavored oil, such as sunflower
- ¹/₂ cup (75 g) raw cashews
- 2 cups (475 ml) warm water
- 1 teaspoon (5 ml) vanilla extract
- 1 teaspoon (5 ml) lemon juice or ¹/₄ teaspoon ascorbic acid crystals dissolved in 2 tablespoons (28 ml) warm water
- 1 teaspoon (5 ml) maple syrup

In a mixing bowl, whisk together quinoa flour, baking powder, and baking soda. In a blender, grind nuts to a fine powder, pausing to scrape under the blades 2 to 3 times. Add water, vanilla extract, lemon juice, and maple syrup to blender and blend 3 to 4 minutes. Pour liquid over dry ingredients and whisk a few times, eliminating lumps. If batter is too thick, add water as necessary.

Pour a scant ¹/₄ cup (60 g) batter onto hot nonstick griddle (heated until water dances on it) for each pancake. Serve with fruit sauce or applesauce.

VARIATIONS: *Add 1–2 tablespoons (10–20 g) flaxseed to blender with the cashews. For a heartier, buckwheat sourdough pancake, replace up to 1 cup (120 g) quinoa flour with buckwheat flour.*

Yield 12 to 14 pancakes

Calories (kcal): 161; Total fat: 7g; Cholesterol: 0mg; Carbohydrate: 22g; Dietary fiber: 2g; Protein: 5g; Sodium: 278mg; Potassium: 240mg; Calcium: 156mg; Iron: 3 3mg; Zinc: 1mg; Vitamin A: trace

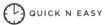 QUICK N EASY

Joe's "Veggies in Disguise" Nutritious Muffins

gluten   milk   soy   egg   corn   nuts

Another great trick for getting a picky eater to eat some veggies!

- 1 cup (120 g) carrots, finely chopped
- 1 cup (120 g) zucchini, finely chopped
- 1 cup (175 g) GFCF chocolate chips, finely chopped
- 1 cup (125 g) walnuts or pecans, finely chopped
- 1 store-bought GFCF cake mix, prepared according to package directions, but not baked

Add carrots, zucchini, chocolate chips, and nuts to prepared cake batter; stir to combine.

Transfer the mixture to a muffin pan, filling each cup about two-thirds of the way. Bake at 375°F (190°C, or gas mark 5) for 20 minutes or until a toothpick inserted in the center of a muffin comes out clean. Do not overcook, as this will result in dry muffins. Once cooled, these muffins can be frozen to be eaten later.

This clever recipe can also incorporate extra protein by adding ⅛ to ¼ cup pureed chicken.

YIELD: *12 muffins*

Calories (kcal): 285; **Total fat:** 15g; **Cholesterol:** 0mg; **Carbohydrate:** 38g; **Dietary fiber:** 2g; **Protein:** 5g; **Sodium:** 204mg; **Potassium:** 218mg; **Calcium:** 74mg; **Iron:** 1mg; **Zinc:** 1mg; **Vitamin A:** 3084IU

Cinnamon Pancakes

gluten · milk · soy · egg · corn · nuts

- 2 cups (280 g) sorghum or rice flour
- $2/3$ cup (100 g) potato starch
- $1/3$ cup (40 g) tapioca flour
- 3 tablespoons (40 g) sugar
- 2 teaspoons xanthan gum
- 1 tablespoon (5 g) baking powder
- 1 teaspoon cinnamon
- $1/8$ teaspoon salt
- 2 cups (475 ml) water
- 1 cup (235 ml) milk substitute (rice, almond, coconut)
- 3 eggs
- 3 tablespoons (45 ml) oil
- $1/2$ teaspoon vanilla

Combine the dry ingredients and set aside. In a separate bowl mix wet ingredients. Add the dry ingredients to the wet ingredients and cook on a griddle until done.

VARIATION: *Fold $1/2$ cup (75 g) fresh or frozen (thawed) blueberries into the batter.*

YIELD: *12 to 14 pancakes*

Calories (kcal): 200; **Total fat:** 5g; **Cholesterol:** 47mg; **Carbohydrate:** 36g; **Dietary fiber:** 1g; **Protein:** 3g; **Sodium:** 160mg; **Potassium:** 36mg; **Calcium:** 80mg; **Iron:** trace; **Zinc:** trace; **Vitamin A:** 70IU

Honey Vanilla Pancake Recipe

gluten · milk · soy · egg · corn · nuts

These really cook up well the next day too. They are light and fluffy.

- 1 large egg
- $3/4$ cup (175 ml) milk substitute (rice, soy, almond, or coconut)
- 1 tablespoon (20 g) honey
- $1/2$ teaspoon vanilla
- 1 cup (140 g) GF flour
- $1/4$ teaspoon xanthan gum
- $1/4$ teaspoon salt
- 1 tablespoon (5 g) baking powder

Combine egg, milk substitute, honey, and vanilla in a bowl. In a separate bowl, combine flour, xanthan gum, salt, and baking powder. Add the dry mixture to the wet mixture and blend well. Cook on a hot, greased griddle, using about $1/4$ cup of batter for each pancake. Cook until brown on one side and around edge; turn and brown the other side.

VARIATION: *Fold $1/2$ cup (75 g) fresh or frozen (thawed) blueberries into the batter.*

YIELD: *4 to 6 pancakes*

Calories (kcal): 161; **Total fat:** 1g; **Cholesterol:** 47mg; **Carbohydrate:** 32g; **Dietary fiber:** 1g; **Protein:** 5g; **Sodium:** 915mg; **Potassium:** 54mg; **Calcium:** 218mg; **Iron:** 2mg; **Zinc:** trace; **Vitamin A:** 70IU

Sunday Morning Pancakes

gluten   milk   soy   egg   corn   nuts

- 1¹/₂ cups (210 g) brown rice flour
- 2¹/₄ cups (270 g) quinoa flour
- ³/₄ cup (90 g) tapioca starch
- 6 eggs
- ¹/₂ tablespoon salt
- 1¹/₈ teaspoons baking soda
- ¹/₃ cup (80 ml) oil (safflower, canola)
- 1²/₃ cups (395 ml) rice milk

Combine all ingredients with mixer on medium-high speed for 2 minutes. Cook on a lightly oiled griddle over moderate heat.

VARIATION: *Fold ¹/₂ cup (75 g) blueberries into the batter.*

YIELD: *12 to 14 pancakes*

Calories (kcal): 286; **Total fat:** 11g; **Cholesterol:** 94mg; **Carbohydrate:** 39g; **Dietary fiber:** 3g; **Protein:** 9g; **Sodium:** 422mg; **Potassium:** 322mg; **Calcium:** 35mg; **Iron:** 4mg; **Zinc:** 2mg; **Vitamin A:** 140IU

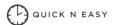 QUICK N EASY

Low-Carb, No-Sugar Pancakes

gluten   milk   soy   egg   corn   nuts

- 1 egg
- 1 cup (235 ml) liquid (water, rice milk, or juice)
- 1 tablespoon (15 ml) oil
- 1 teaspoon (5 ml) vanilla
- 1 cup (140 g) GF flour mixture (almond, buckwheat, and rice or millet)
- 1 teaspoon baking powder

Combine the wet ingredients. In a separate bowl, combine the dry ingredients. Add the dry mixtures to the wet mixture. Blend thoroughly. Batter should be thin. Cook on heated skillet, flipping once.

VARIATIONS: *Add Stevia, cinnamon, coconut, almonds, sliced bananas, walnuts, or blueberries. These ingredients can be added to the pancake as it cooks on the pan or blended into batter before pouring onto pan. Serve with almond butter, jam, and/or stewed fruit.*

YIELD: *4 to 6 pancakes*

Calories (kcal): 211; **Total fat:** 5g; **Cholesterol:** 47mg; **Carbohydrate:** 36g; **Dietary fiber:** 1g; **Protein:** 4g; **Sodium:** 138mg; **Potassium:** 48mg; **Calcium:** 79mg; **Iron:** trace; **Zinc:** 1mg; **Vitamin A:** 70IU

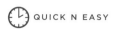

QUICK N EASY

Pecan Meal Pancakes

gluten   milk   soy   egg   corn   nuts

SCD compatible

This recipe was adapted from the book Breaking the Vicious Cycle: Intestinal Health Through Diet, *by Elaine Gottschall.*

- 2^1/$_2$ cups (300 g) pecan meal
- ^{1}/$_2$ teaspoon baking soda
- ^{1}/$_4$ teaspoon salt
- ^{1}/$_3$ cup (115 g) honey
- 7 large eggs or 8 medium eggs
- 1 teaspoon (5 ml) vanilla (be sure it does not have corn syrup)

Combine the dry ingredients in a bowl, and set aside. In a separate bowl, whisk honey into eggs, then add vanilla extract. Whisk the dry mixture into the wet mixture.

Spray a nonstick, electric frying pan with olive oil to lightly coat, and set the temperature to 200°F (95°C). It is best to let the pan preheat; otherwise, the first pan of pancakes may get too dark.

NOTE: *A nonstick electric frying pan is highly recommended for this recipe. Honey causes the pancakes to stick, and pecan meal can cause them to brown quickly. A thermostat-controlled temperature will help to prevent headaches.*

YIELD: *15 to 18 pancakes*

Calories (kcal): 127; **Total fat:** 3g; **Cholesterol:** 100mg; **Carbohydrate:** 17g; **Dietary fiber:** 1g; **Protein:** 10g; **Sodium:** 108mg; **Potassium:** 102mg; **Calcium:** 19mg; **Iron:** 1mg; **Zinc:** 1mg; **Vitamin A:** 174IU

GFCF "No Yolking Around" Pancakes

gluten   milk   soy   egg   corn   nuts

For those allergic to eggs, this adaptation of Lisa Barnes's recipe in The Petit Appetit Cookbook *is an excellent option.*

- 1 cup (140 g) GF flour
- ^{1}/$_2$ tablespoon (6 g) cane sugar
- 2 teaspoons baking powder
- ^{1}/$_4$ teaspoon salt
- ^{1}/$_2$ teaspoon baking soda
- ^{1}/$_2$ teaspoon ground cinnamon
- 1 cup (235 ml) organic milk substitute (rice, almond)
- 1 tablespoon (15 g) applesauce or pearsauce
- 2 tablespoons (28 ml) safflower, almond, or avocado oil

In a medium mixing bowl, stir together flour, sugar, baking powder, salt, baking soda, and cinnamon. In a separate bowl, whisk together milk, applesauce, and oil. Add milk mixture to flour mixture all at once. Stir with a rubber spatula until just blended. If batter is too thick, thin with milk substitute.

Heat a large nonstick skillet or griddle over medium heat. Lightly grease skillet with cooking spray.

VARIATION: *Pureed vegetables (carrots, sweet potato) can replace some of the liquid (1 to 2 tablespoons [15 to 30 ml]). Add fruits, fruit spread, or fruit purees on top.*

YIELD: *About 8 (5-inch, or 13-cm) pancakes*

Calories (kcal): 115; **Total fat:** 4g; **Cholesterol:** 0mg; **Carbohydrate:** 19g; **Dietary fiber:** 1g; **Protein:** 1g; **Sodium:** 268mg; **Potassium:** 19mg; **Calcium:** 73mg; **Iron:** trace; **Zinc:** trace; **Vitamin A:** trace

Wonderful Waffles

gluten　　milk　　soy　　egg　　corn　　nuts

This recipe was modified from a recipe that came with the waffle maker itself. Our waffle maker is nonstick and calls for 2/3 cup (80 g) batter per waffle. Modify this recipe to suit your waffle maker's size and shape.

- 1 cup (140 g) GF flour blend of choice
- 3 teaspoons baking powder
- 1/4 teaspoon salt
- 1 tablespoon (13 g) sugar
- 1/2 teaspoon guar gum or xanthan gum
- 3 eggs, separated
- 1 cup (235 ml) milk substitute (rice, soy, almond)
- 1/4 cup (60 ml) canola oil
- 1 teaspoon (5 ml) vanilla

Preheat a waffle maker and spray with nonstick spray. Whisk together the flour blend, baking powder, salt, sugar, and guar or xanthan gum in a large bowl. Separate the eggs—the whites go into a large mixing bowl and the yolks go into the flour mixture. Add the milk substitute to the flour mixture and whisk well. Beat the egg whites until stiff. Meanwhile, add the oil and vanilla to the batter and mix well. Pour the batter over the stiff egg whites and whisk. Pour 2/3 cup (80 g) of batter onto the waffle maker and cook for 7 minutes each.

YIELD: *4 to 6 waffles*

Calories (kcal): 347; **Total fat:** 18g; **Cholesterol:** 140mg; **Carbohydrate:** 40g; **Dietary fiber:** 1g; **Protein:** 7g; **Sodium:** 543mg; **Potassium:** 75mg; **Calcium:** 226mg; **Iron:** 1mg; **Zinc:** 1mg; **Vitamin A:** 210IU

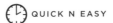 QUICK N EASY

High-Protein Waffles

gluten　　milk　　soy　　egg　　corn　　nuts

This high-protein waffle mix can sneak in some mineral supplements.

- 1³/4 cups (245 g) brown rice flour
- 2³/4 cups (330 g) quinoa flour
- 3/4 cup (90 g) tapioca starch
- 1/2 tablespoon baking soda
- 1/2 tablespoon salt
- 6 eggs
- 1/3 cup (80 ml) oil
- 3¹/2 cups (830 ml) rice milk

Combine all ingredients with a mixer on low-medium speed for 2 minutes. Lightly oil waffle iron. Pour batter onto waffle iron and cook.

VARIATION: *For a sweeter waffle, replace some of the rice milk with pear juice.*

YIELD: *Makes 20 waffles*

Calories (kcal): 200; **Total fat:** 7g; **Cholesterol:** 56mg; **Carbohydrate:** 29g; **Dietary fiber:** 2g; **Protein:** 6g; **Sodium:** 172mg; **Potassium:** 232mg; **Calcium:** 24mg; **Iron:** 3 3mg; **Zinc:** 1mg; **Vitamin A:** 84IU

Crispy Breakfast Bars

QUICK N EASY

gluten milk soy egg corn nuts

A versatile treat—try it for breakfast, a snack, or as an energy boost.

- 7 cups (98 g) crispy, GF puffed whole-grain cereal
- ³/₄ cup (90 g) dried cranberries
- ³/₄ cup (90 g) dried blueberries
- ¹/₂ cup (65 g) sunflower seeds (optional)
- 1 teaspoon cinnamon
- ³/₄ cup (255 g) brown rice syrup or honey
- ³/₄ cup (190 g) almond butter
- 2 tablespoons (28 g) butter substitute

Stir together cereal, dried fruits, seeds (if using), and cinnamon in large bowl. Place syrup, almond butter, and butter substitute in a large, micro-wave-safe measuring cup. Microwave 1¹/₂ minutes on high, or until the butter substitute has melted. Stir well and pour over cereal mixture. Stir to coat.

Dampen your hands with cold water. Press cereal mixture firmly into a 9-inch (22.5-cm) square baking pan, rewetting hands if necessary to keep mixture from sticking. Freeze 30 minutes. Cut into 15 bars, and store in refrigerator.

YIELD: *15 bars*

Calories (kcal): 232; **Total fat:** 12g; **Cholesterol:** 0mg; **Carbohydrate:** 31g; **Dietary fiber:** 2g; **Protein:** 4g; **Sodium:** 2mg; **Potassium:** 145mg; **Calcium:** 43mg; **Iron:** 1mg; **Zinc:** 1mg; **Vitamin A:** 3IU

Tracey Smith's Granola

gluten milk soy egg corn nuts

Never say "no" to granola again.

- ¹/₂ cup (170 g) honey
- ¹/₄ cup (60 ml) oil
- 1¹/₂ cups (150 g) quinoa flakes
- 1 cup (125 g) chopped nuts
- 1 cup (140 g) seeds (sunflower, sesame, pumpkin)

Melt honey in the oil in a double boiler. Mix dry ingredients and stir in honey mixture. Place in 9 x 13-inch (22.5 x 32.5-inch) pan and bake at 300°F (150°C, or gas mark 2) for 45 to 50 minutes. Stir granola occasionally as it cools.

YIELD: *4 cups (600 g)*

Calories (kcal): 457; **Total fat:** 28g; **Cholesterol:** 0mg; **Carbohydrate:** 47g; **Dietary fiber:** 6g; **Protein:** 10g; **Sodium:** 11mg; **Potassium:** 434mg; **Calcium:** 215mg; **Iron:** 6mg; **Zinc:** 3mg; **Vitamin A:** 5IU

Other Communion Wafer Options

- Use any GFCF unleavened (no yeast) cracker or flat bread.
- Hol-Grain Crackers brand is like a flat bread.
- Ener-G Foods, Inc. (P.O. Box 84487, Seattle, WA 98124-5787 (800) 331-5222 www.ener-g.com.

Communion Wafers

gluten milk soy egg corn nuts

This recipe, adapted to be milk-free, was originally from the Washington Celiac Support Group.

- 2 tablespoons (20 g) potato starch
- $^7/_8$ cup (114 g) cornstarch ($^7/_8$ cup is equal to 1 cup [130 g] minus 2 tablespoons [16 g])
- 3 cups (420 g) brown or (480 g) white rice flour
- 1 teaspoon baking soda
- 1 teaspoon salt
- 2 tablespoons (16 g) xanthan gum
- $^1/_2$ cup (112 g) Earth Balance Whipped Spread
- 1 cup (235 ml) GFCF buttermilk substitute (2 tablespoons [28 ml] lemon juice in 1 cup [235 ml] rice or soy milk)

Preheat oven to 350°F (180°C, gas mark 4).

Combine the dry ingredients. Cut the spread into dry ingredients. Add buttermilk substitute and mix with fingers until workable.

Roll with a rolling pin on a rice-floured surface until the dough is very thin. Cut into small circles using a bottle cap.

Bake for 6 minutes. The wafers will not brown.

YIELD: *24 to 36 wafers, depending on size*

Calories (kcal): 129; **Total fat:** 4g; **Cholesterol:** 0mg; **Carbohydrate:** 21g; **Dietary fiber:** 1g; **Protein:** 1g; **Sodium:** 186mg; **Potassium:** 19mg; **Calcium:** 5mg; **Iron:** trace; **Zinc:** trace; **Vitamin A:** 168IU

Gluten-free Communion Wafers

gluten   milk   soy   egg   corn   nuts

Adapted from Anne Evans

In addition to being gluten-free and dairy-free, these wafers are also salicylate-free, and free of pesticides, herbicides, preservatives, and artificial ingredients.

- 1¹/₂ cups (237 g) organic rice flour
- ¹/₃ cup (40 g) tapioca starch
- 2 teaspoons xanthan gum
- ¹/₂ teaspoons salt
- Dash stevia (optional)
- 3 tablespoons (42 g) ghee
- 1 organic egg, well beaten

Preheat oven to 350°F (180°C, gas mark 4). Sift all the dry ingredients together in one bowl. Add the ghee and blend using a pastry cutter, until mixture appears granular and pea-sized lumps have formed. Add the egg and mix until the dough holds together and pulls away from the sides of the bowl.

Turn dough out onto a board coated with tapioca starch and roll into a tube approximately 1¹/₂ to 2 inches (3.75 to 5 cm) in diameter. Slice into ¹/₄-inch (6 mm) thick wafers. Place on cookie sheet lined with parchment paper and bake for 10 minutes. Cool for 5 minutes, then transfer wafers to a wire cooling rack.

NOTES: *Those allergic to eggs may substitute 2 to 3 tablespoons (30 to 45 ml) of chilled water instead. After mixing, let the dough sit for 10 minutes to allow the xanthan gum to work. When shaping, the texture of the dough may necessitate the use of a rolling pin and a tiny round cookie cutter to make the wafers.*

YIELD: *3 dozen*

Calories (kcal): 45; **Total fat:** 1g; **Cholesterol:** 9mg; **Carbohydrate:** 7g; **Dietary fiber:** trace; **Protein:** 1g; **Sodium:** 32mg; **Potassium:** 7mg; **Calcium:** 2mg; **Iron:** trace; **Zinc:** trace; **Vitamin A:** 49IU.

Gluten-free Zucchini Bread

gluten   milk   soy   egg   corn   nuts

Another great way to turn veggies into a treat!

- 3 cups (420 g) GF flour blend, plus extra for dusting pans
- 1/4 teaspoon baking powder
- 1 teaspoon baking soda
- 2 1/4 teaspoons xanthan gum
- 1 teaspoon salt
- 1 tablespoon (7 g) ground cinnamon
- 2 large eggs
- 2 1/2 cups (500 g) sugar
- 1 cup (235 ml) safflower oil
- 1 tablespoon (15 ml) vanilla
- 2 cups (240 g) grated zucchini
- 1 cup (120 g) finely chopped nuts, such as walnuts or pecans

Preheat oven to 350°F (180°C, gas mark 4). Spray 2 loaf pans and lightly dust with GF flour blend, knocking out excess. Mix the dry ingredients in medium bowl and set aside.

Whisk eggs together in large mixing bowl; add sugar, oil, and vanilla, and continue whisking until light and frothy. Stir in zucchini. Add dry ingredients and stir to combine, and then fold in nuts. Divide batter evenly into pans and bake for 1 hour, or until toothpick inserted into the center comes out clean. Cool for 5 minutes, and then carefully remove loaves from pans. Cool completely on wire rack before serving.

YIELD: *2 loaves, or 24 slices*

Calories (kcal): 303; **Total fat:** 12g; **Cholesterol:** 18mg; **Carbohydrate:** 44g; **Dietary fiber:** 4g; **Protein:** 5g; **Sodium:** 163mg; **Potassium:** 84mg; **Calcium:** 15mg; **Iron:** trace; **Zinc:** trace; **Vitamin A:** 103IU.

Cornmeal Carrot Muffins

gluten milk soy egg corn nuts

The hearty dose of carrots sweetens these muffins while keeping them healthy; the cornmeal adds a nice crunch.

- 1 cup (140 g) GF flour blend
- 3/4 cup (105 g) coarsely ground cornmeal
- 1 teaspoon baking soda
- 1 teaspoon baking powder
- 1/2 teaspoon salt
- 1/2 cup (115 g) brown sugar
- 2 large eggs
- 1/2 cup (120 ml) canola oil
- 1/2 cup (120 ml) rice milk
- 1 1/2 cups (165 g) grated carrots

Preheat oven to 350°F (180°C, gas mark 4). Line a 12-cup muffin tin with paper or foil liners. Combine the flour blend, cornmeal, baking soda, baking powder, and salt in a medium bowl and set aside. Whisk the eggs and the brown sugar in a large bowl until frothy. Add the oil and milk and whisk to combine. Stir in the carrots and then the dry mixture, and mix just until no flour clumps remain. Divide the batter evenly between the muffin cups and bake 20 to 25 minutes. Cool 5 minutes, then transfer muffins to wire rack to cool completely. Serve.

YIELD: *12 muffins*

Calories (kcal): 224; **Total fat:** 10g; **Cholesterol:** 36mg; **Carbohydrate:** 30g; **Dietary fiber:** 3g; **Protein:** 4g; **Sodium:** 388mg; **Potassium:** 98mg; **Calcium:** 39mg; **Iron:** 1mg; **Zinc:** trace; **Vitamin A:** 4366IU.

Maya's Favorite Lemon Poppy Seed Muffins

gluten milk soy egg corn nuts

From Joanne Bregman (Maya's mother)

- 1 3/4 cups (245 g) GF flour blend
- 3 tablespoons (30 g) MLO Natural Brown Rice Protein Powder
- 2 teaspoons baking powder
- 1/2 teaspoon salt
- 1 tablespoon (8 g) poppy seeds
- 2 large eggs
- 2/3 cup (230 g) agave nectar
- 3/4 cup (175 ml) rice milk
- 1/4 cup (60 ml) safflower oil
- 1 tablespoon (15 ml) lemon juice
- 1 teaspoon lemon extract

Preheat oven to 375°F (190°C, gas mark 5). Grease and flour a 12-cup muffin tin. Mix all dry ingredients in a large bowl and set aside. Whisk eggs, agave nectar, rice milk, oil, lemon juice, and lemon extract together. Add to dry ingredients and mix until just combined. Divide batter evenly between the muffin cups. Bake 20 minutes, until wooden toothpick inserted into the centers comes out clean; cool on wire rack.

YIELD: *12 muffins*

Calories (kcal): 237; **Total fat:** 6g; **Cholesterol:** 37mg; **Carbohydrate:** 41g; **Dietary fiber:** 4g; **Protein:** 6g; **Sodium:** 199mg; **Potassium:** 22mg; **Calcium:** 68mg; **Iron:** 1mg; **Zinc:** tracemg; **Vitamin A:** 41IU.

Socca to Me

gluten   milk   soy   egg   corn   nuts

Socca is a flatbread made from chickpea flour hailing from Southern France. It can be found at the bustling markets in Nice, where it is cooked on giant cast iron pans in wood-fired ovens. Not only is it surprisingly easy to recreate at home, but it is naturally gluten-free, and delicious plain, or as a base for a variety of toppings.

- 1 cup (140 g) chickpea flour (or chickpea-fava flour blend)
- 1/2 teaspoon salt
- 1/4–1/2 teaspoon freshly ground black pepper (optional)
- 1 cup (235 ml) water
- 3 tablespoons (45 ml) olive oil

Whisk chickpea flour, salt, and pepper (if using) into a medium bowl. Slowly add water, whisking to eliminate lumps. Stir in 2 tablespoons olive oil. Cover and set aside for 1 hour (batter should be about the consistency of heavy cream).

Preheat oven to 475°F (240°C, gas mark 9). Heat remaining oil in 10-inch non-stick skillet over medium-high heat, swirling the pan to coat until oil is shimmering. Pour batter into the pan, swirling to coat evenly. Place pan in hot oven and cook until batter is lightly browned on top, 12 to 18 minutes. Slide pancake into cutting board, cut into quarters, and serve immediately.

NOTE: *This recipe can easily be doubled and cooked in 2 batches. If you don't have a skillet with an oven-proof handle, a cast-iron skillet can be used instead. If using toppings, they can be added halfway through the baking time or after the socca comes out of the oven.*

TIP: *If there is any socca leftover, crumble it up with your fingers, toast the crumbs, and use in any recipe that calls for breadcrumbs.*

YIELD: *4 servings*

Calories (kcal): 175; **Total fat:** 12g; **Cholesterol:** 0mg; **Carbohydrate:** 13g; **Dietary fiber:** 3g; **Protein:** 5g; **Sodium:** 283mg; **Potassium:** 198mg; **Calcium:** 14mg; **Iron:** 1mg; **Zinc:** 1mg; **Vitamin A:** 10IU.

Irish Soda Bread

gluten   milk   soy   egg   corn   nuts

Adapted from Caryn Talty (http://healthy-family.org)

Caryn credits Pamela's Wheat-Free Bread Mix for her success in replicating her Irish mother-in-law's traditional soda bread.

- 1 package (19 ounces, or 535 g) "Pamela's Wheat-Free Bread Mix"
- 1 tablespoon (14 g) baking powder
- ¹/₄ cup (50 g) sugar
- 3 large eggs, room temperature
- ¹/₄ cup (60 ml) water
- ¹/₂ cup (120 ml) rice milk
- ¹/₄ cup (60 ml) safflower oil
- ¹/₂ cup (75 g) raisins (or dried blueberries or cranberries if you are Feingold Stage 1)
- ¹/₂ cup (80 g) rice flour, for shaping

Combine the first 7 ingredients in the bowl of a standing mixer fitted with the paddle attachment. Mix on medium-high speed for 3 minutes; add raisins and mix on low speed until combined. Scrape dough onto a greased pie plate or baking sheet. Sprinkle with rice flour (it will be very sticky) and shape into a slightly flattened ball. Cover loosely with plastic wrap and let rise for 1 hour. Meanwhile, preheat oven to 400°F (200°C, gas mark 6).

After 1 hour, remove plastic and cut an "X" into the top of the loaf using a sharp knife. Bake for 40 to 50 minutes, until the crust is dark brown. Invert the loaf (carefully—it is very hot!) onto a clean, damp kitchen towel, wrap it snuggly, re-invert, and allow to cool completely. Serve with your favorite GFCF spread or fruit jam.

YIELD: *1 loaf, 12 slices*

Calories (kcal): 291; **Total fat:** 7g; **Cholesterol:** 55mg; **Carbohydrate:** 55g; **Dietary fiber:** 5g; **Protein:** 4g; **Sodium:** 519mg; **Potassium:** 64mg; **Calcium:** 78mg; **Iron:** 1mg; **Zinc:** trace; **Vitamin A:** 80IU.

Ginger-or-Not Granola

gluten   milk   soy   egg   corn   nuts

Although this recipe is for ginger lovers, this is still a great granola without the ginger. For a description of these special gluten-free oats, see the recipe for Hot Oatmeal Cereal, page oo. This granola can be eaten out of hand as a great snack, or sprinkled over baked fruit or GFCF ice cream as a special treat.

- $2^2/_3$ cups (10 ounces, or 280g) Lara's Rolled Oats (available at www.creamhillestates.com)
- $3/_4$ cup (82 g) sliced almonds
- $1/_4$ cup (55 g) melted ghee
- $1/_4$ teaspoon salt
- 6 tablespoons (125 g) honey
- 6 tablespoons (90 g) brown sugar
- 1 tablespoon (6 g) minced fresh ginger (optional)
- 2 tablespoons (30 ml) water
- $1^1/_2$ teaspoons vanilla

Preheat oven to 350°F (180°C, gas mark 4). In a large bowl, toss oats with almonds, melted ghee, and salt. Grease or line a baking sheet with parchment paper; sprinkle oat mixture evenly on top and bake for 8 to 10 minutes, until almonds are golden and oats smell toasted. Transfer mixture back to the bowl, reserving the baking sheet.

Combine honey, brown sugar, ginger (if using), and water in a small saucepan and cook over medium heat for 10 minutes, until thick and syrupy. Off heat, add vanilla, and then pour hot syrup over oat mixture. Quickly stir mixture to combine (syrup will get very thick as it cools and won't coat the oats as well). Turn mixture out onto the baking sheet once again, separating any large clusters (small clusters are good). Bake for 10 to 20 minutes, until granola is golden brown (taking care not to burn it). Let cool at room temperature until crisp. Store in an airtight container at room temperature.

YIELD: *12 servings*

Calories (kcal): 237; **Total fat:** 11g; **Cholesterol:** 12mg; **Carbohydrate:** 30g; **Dietary fiber:** 3g; **Protein:** 5g; **Sodium:** 49mg; **Potassium:** 92mg; **Calcium:** 41mg; **Iron:** 2mg; **Zinc:** trace; **Vitamin A:** 170IU.

Hot Oatmeal Cereal

gluten milk soy egg corn nuts

This recipe comes from Chateau Cream Hill Estates (www.creamhillestates.com), and is made using one of their products, Lara's Rolled Oats (Lara has celiac). The company guarantees no cross-contamination with gluten. They state that the oats are protected from cross-contamination during growth. The fields used have been free of wheat, barley and rye for at least 3 years before their oats are planted. They use only dedicated or thoroughly cleaned equipment in planting, harvesting, transport, processing and packaging. They use ELISA testing to test for gluten-free purity. They state they are in compliance with The Canadian Celiac Association Professional Advisory Board's definition of pure, uncontaminated oats. Plus . . . it tastes good!

- 1/3 cup (35 g) Lara's Rolled Oats
- 2/3 cup (160 ml) boiling water
- Pinch of salt

In a saucepan, combine the oats, water, and salt. Return to boiling, reduce heat to low and simmer for 5–6 minutes. After 4 minutes check to make sure there is enough water. For softer cereal, cook a little longer. Serve.

TIP: *Try one or more of these different flavor additions:*

- *1/4 cup (35 g) dried fruit, such as raisins, blueberries, or cranberries*
- *1/4 cup (60 g) applesauce, added at the end of cooking*
- *1/2 teaspoon GFCF vanilla*
- *1/2 teaspoon ground cinnamon*

YIELD: *1 serving*

Calories (kcal): 140; Total fat: 2g; Cholesterol: 0mg; Carbohydrate: 23g; Dietary fiber: 3g; Protein: 5g; Sodium: 5mg; Potassium: 9mg; Calcium: 23mg; Iron: 2mg; Zinc: trace; Vitamin A: 0IU.

With dried fruit: Calories (kcal): 249; Total fat: 3g; Cholesterol: 0mg; Carbohydrate: 52g; Dietary fiber: 4g; Protein: 6g; Sodium: 9mg; Potassium: 206mg; Calcium: 33mg; Iron: 3mg; Zinc: trace; Vitamin A: 632IU.

With unsweetened applesauce: Calories (kcal): 166; Total fat: 3g; Cholesterol: 0mg; Carbohydrate: 30g; Dietary fiber: 4g; Protein: 5g; Sodium: 6mg; Potassium: 46mg; Calcium: 25mg; Iron: 2mg; Zinc: trace; Vitamin A: 18IU.

With vanilla: Calories (kcal): 146; Total fat: 3g; Cholesterol: 0mg; Carbohydrate: 23g; Dietary fiber: 3g; Protein: 5g; Sodium: 5mg; Potassium: 0mg; Calcium: 23mg; Iron: 2; Zinc: trace; Vitamin A: 0IU.

With cinnamon: Calories (kcal): 143; Total fat: 3g; Cholesterol: 0mg; Carbohydrate: 24g; Dietary fiber: 4g; Protein: 5g; Sodium: 5mg; Potassium: 6mg; Calcium: 37mg; Iron: 2mg; Zinc: trace; Vitamin A: 3IU.

Quinoa Cake

gluten   milk   soy   egg   corn   nuts

Adapted from Karina's Kitchen (http://glutenfreegoddess.blogspot.com/)
This makes a great breakfast treat or afternoon snack.

- 1$^1/_2$ cups (250 g) quinoa flakes
- $^1/_2$ cup (70 g) sorghum flour
- $^1/_2$ cup (60 g) tapioca starch
- $^3/_4$ cup (90 g) almond meal flour
- 1 teaspoon baking soda
- $^1/_2$ teaspoon salt
- 1 teaspoon xanthan or guar gum
- 2 teaspoons ground cinnamon
- 2 large eggs (or the equivalent of egg replacer)
- $^1/_4$ cup (60 ml) olive oil
- $^1/_4$ cup (60 g) unsweetened applesauce
- $^1/_2$ cup (170 g) agave nectar
- $^1/_2$ cup (115 g) brown sugar
- $^1/_4$ cup (85 g) molasses
- 2 teaspoons GFCF vanilla extract
- 1 cup (110 g) grated carrots
- $^1/_2$ cup (42 g) unsweetened grated coconut

Preheat oven to 350°F (180°C, gas mark 4). Grease a 9 by 13-inch (23 by 33 cm) baking pan and then line with parchment paper.

In a medium bowl, combine the first 8 ingredients and set aside. Whisk the eggs together with the olive oil, applesauce, agave nectar, brown sugar, molasses, and vanilla. Add the dry ingredients and beat well to combine. Add carrots and coconut and stir until evenly combined. Pour batter into prepared pan and bake for 25 to 35 minutes, until cake is set in the center. Allow cake to cool on a wire rack completely before slicing.

NOTE: *Individual pieces of this cake can be wrapped in parchment or waxed paper and then stored in a zipper lock plastic bag or container and frozen for future use.*

YIELD: *16 pieces*

Calories (kcal): 251; **Total fat:** 9g; **Cholesterol:** 27mg; **Carbohydrate:** 40g; **Dietary fiber:** 3g; **Protein:** 5g; **Sodium:** 174mg; **Potassium:** 257mg; **Calcium:** 45mg; **Iron:** 2mg; **Zinc:** 1mg; **Vitamin A:** 2177IU.

Maya's Waffles

gluten

milk

soy

egg

corn

nuts

Another great high-protein waffle recipe.

- $^2/_3$ cup (95 g) GF flour blend (see note)
- $^1/_3$ cup (30 g) brown rice or soy protein powder (make sure to use a brand that stays stable when cooked)
- 2 teaspoons baking powder
- $^1/_4$ teaspoon salt
- 2 large eggs
- 1 tablespoon (20 g) agave nectar
- $^1/_4$ cup (60 ml) canola oil
- $^2/_3$ cup (160 ml) non-casein milk

Stir together all ingredients and cook in waffle maker according to manufacturer's instructions.

YIELD: *2 to 4 servings*

TIP: *You can double the recipe to make extra waffles, and then freeze the leftovers. When you are ready to eat them, simply defrost slightly and toast.*

NOTE: *You can use Bette Hagman's All-Purpose Flour Substitute or this alternative offered by Joanne Bregman:*
- *$^1/_2$ cup (70 g) brown or white rice flour*
- *$^3/_4$ cup (105 g) sorghum flour*
- *$^1/_2$ cup (60 g) buckwheat flour*
- *$^1/_4$ cup (30 g) tapioca starch*

Combine all ingredients and blend with a whisk.

YIELD: *2 cups*

Calories (kcal): 361; **Total fat:** 17g; **Cholesterol:** 106mg; **Carbohydrate:** 36g; **Dietary fiber:** 4g; **Protein:** 16g; **Sodium:** 441mg; **Potassium:** 34mg; **Calcium:** 184mg; **Iron:** 2mg; **Zinc:** trace; **Vitamin A:** 122IU.

CHAPTER 13

Main Dishes and One-Dish Meals

Breakfast Sausage

gluten   milk   soy   egg   corn   nuts

Sometimes it is difficult to come up with a varied source of protein for breakfast. This version avoids the usual additives found in commercial sausages. The recipe can also be made with turkey. Note among the ingredients is the addition of palm oil. This nonhydrogenated all-vegetable shortening is available from Spectrum Naturals.

- 1 pound (455 g) ground pork or ground turkey
- 1 egg lightly beaten (optional)
- 1 teaspoon coarse Kosher salt
- $^1/_2$ teaspoon ground sage
- $^1/_4$ teaspoon ground savory
- $^1/_8$ teaspoon ground nutmeg
- $^1/_8$ teaspoon ground ginger
- $^1/_4$ teaspoon black pepper
- 3 shakes cayenne pepper (almost $^1/_8$ teaspoon)
- 2 shakes dried thyme (about $^1/_{16}$ teaspoon)
- $1^1/_2$ tablespoons palm oil
- $^3/_4$ teaspoon honey

Place ground pork in a large bowl, add egg and mix in well. Combine salt and seasonings. Sprinkle a little of the seasonings over the meat and work in by pushing down with a closed fist, dividing the meat, stacking it, and then pushing down again. Sprinkle a little more of the seasonings and repeat. Do this until the seasonings are worked throughout. Spread the palm oil over the meat and work in. Drizzle honey over the meat and work in.

Shape into nine patties and fry at a lower temperature than normally expected for sausage. If using an electric frying pan, set the temperature to just under 250°F (120°C, or gas mark $^1/_2$), as the honey will cause the sausage to brown quickly. Cover in between turnings. Turn frequently and watch closely. Cook for approximately 10–15 minutes.

YIELD: *9 patties*

Calories (kcal): 141; **Total fat:** 11g; **Cholesterol:** 57mg; **Carbohydrate:** trace; **Dietary fiber:** trace; **Protein:** 9g; **Sodium:** 243mg; **Potassium:** 153mg; **Calcium:** 12mg; **Iron:** 1mg; **Zinc:** 1mg; **Vitamin A:** 50IU

Crustless Spinach Quiche

gluten   milk   soy   egg   corn   nuts

This is a nice adaptation of a popular recipe. It can be made with other additions, including mushrooms.

- 2 cups (500 g) silken tofu
- 2 eggs
- $1/8$ teaspoon garlic powder or minced garlic
- 1 small onion, coarsely chopped
- $1/8$ teaspoon turmeric
- $1/2$ teaspoon cumin
- $1/8$ teaspoon nutmeg
- 2 tablespoons (15 g) prepared GFCF mustard
- 1 cup (235 ml) vegetable broth
- 1 teaspoon dried parsley
- Salt and pepper to taste
- 1 pound (455 g) spinach or greens, rinsed, finely chopped, steamed, and drained, or use 1 package (16 ounces, or 455 g) frozen chopped spinach, steamed and drained
- Dash paprika

VARIATIONS

- **OPTION:** 1 jar (2.5 ounces, or 70 g) sliced mushrooms, drained, or 5 tablespoons (22 g) sliced white mushrooms
- **OPTION:** 9-inch (22.5-cm) prepared or purchased GFCF pie crust

Coat a 9-inch (22.5-cm) pie plate with vegetable cooking spray (olive oil). (If using pie crust, omit cooking spray and line pie plate with crust.) Set aside.

Preheat oven to 450°F (230°C, or gas mark 8). Place tofu, eggs, garlic, onion, spices, mustard, vegetable broth, and parsley in a blender or food processor and blend on medium speed until smooth. Season with salt and pepper to taste.

In a large bowl, combine mixture with greens. Spoon mixture into greased pie plate. Sprinkle paprika on top.

Bake at 450°F (230°C, or gas mark 8) for 1 hour or until golden brown and a knife inserted in center comes out clean.

YIELD: *8 servings*

Calories (kcal): 106; **Total fat:** 5g; **Cholesterol:** 47mg; **Carbohydrate:** 8g; **Dietary fiber:** 3g; **Protein:** 9g; **Sodium:** 314mg; **Potassium:** 486mg; **Calcium:** 139mg; **Iron:** 6 6mg; **Zinc:** 1mg; **Vitamin A:** 4494IU

Scrambled Veggie Eggs

gluten   milk   soy   egg   corn   nuts

- 8 large eggs (organic)
- 1 tablespoon (15 ml) water
- $1/4$ cup (55 g) pureed mashed cauliflower
- Salt and pepper to taste
- 1 scallion, thinly sliced
- 1 tablespoon (3 g) chopped fresh basil (optional)
- 2 tablespoons (28 g) Earth Balance Spread or ghee

In a medium bowl, lightly mix eggs with water. Stir in cauliflower, salt, pepper, scallion, and basil (optional).

In a large skillet, melt the spread or ghee. Scramble egg mixture on low heat until done.

NOTE: *To make mashed cauliflower, use the recipe in chapter 14 or puree the following in a blender:*

- *$1/2$ cup (65 g) well-steamed/cooked, drained, and dried cauliflower*
- *1 tablespoon (15 ml) or more rice or coconut milk (enough to "wet" the cauliflower)*

YIELD: *8 servings*

Calories (kcal): 97; **Total fat:** 8g; **Cholesterol:** 196mg; **Carbohydrate:** 1g; **Dietary fiber:** trace; **Protein:** 6g; **Sodium:** 58mg; **Potassium:** 70mg; **Calcium:** 24mg; **Iron:** 1mg; **Zinc:** trace; **Vitamin A:** 428IU

Ground Vegetable Omelet

gluten   milk   soy   egg   corn   nuts

Vegetables that work well in this omelet are broccoli, onions, zucchini, garlic, bell peppers, and carrots.

- 1 cup (200 g) leftover cooked, chopped vegetables
- 2 to 3 large eggs
- Sea salt
- Pinch cayenne pepper
- 2 tablespoons (30 ml) olive oil

Puree the vegetables in a food processor or blender until smooth. Beat the eggs lightly in a medium bowl and season with salt and cayenne pepper. Mix the vegetables into the eggs.

Heat the oil in a skillet over medium heat. Pour the egg-vegetable mixture into skillet, cover, and cook until egg is completely set.

YIELD: *2 servings*

Calories (kcal): 267; **Total fat:** 21g; **Cholesterol:** 323mg; **Carbohydrate:** 9g; **Dietary fiber:** 3g; **Protein:** 10g; **Sodium:** 145mg; **Potassium:** 265mg; **Calcium:** 61mg; **Iron:** 2mg; **Zinc:** 1mg; **Vitamin A:** 1930IU.

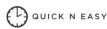 QUICK N EASY

Mexican Breakfast Pizza

gluten   milk   soy   egg   corn   nuts

Adapted from Karen Joy (http://onlysometimesclever.wordpress.com)

While she admits this is a fairly high-fat recipe, because of its redeeming qualities (it is easy to make and loved by all four of her children), Karen deems it a keeper.

For the Pizza
- 8 ounces (225 g) nitrate-free bacon, diced
- 8 large eggs
- 10 corn tortillas

Optional Garnishes
- Tofutti cheese
- Salsa
- Diced fresh tomato
- Sliced scallions
- Chopped cilantro

In a 12-inch (30 cm) non-stick skillet, cook the bacon over medium-high heat, stirring frequently, until golden and crispy. Transfer bacon with a slotted spoon to a paper towel-lined plate (leaving $^1/_4$ cup (60 ml) bacon fat in the skillet).

Whisk the eggs in a medium bowl to combine. Arrange the corn tortillas in the skillet to completely cover the bottom (they will be overlapping). Pour the eggs evenly over the tortillas and sprinkle the bacon on top. Cover and cook over medium heat until eggs are cooked through. Slide pizza from the pan onto a large cutting board, cut into six wedges and serve.

NOTE: *If you opt for tofutti cheese, try adding it to the eggs after the bacon so that it melts onto the pizza.*

YIELD: *6 servings*

Calories (kcal): 372; **Total fat:** 25g; **Cholesterol:** 308mg; **Carbohydrate:** 21g; **Dietary fiber:** 2g; **Protein:** 16g; **Sodium:** 434mg; **Potassium:** 89mg; **Calcium:** 35mg; **Iron:** 1mg; **Zinc:** 1mg; **Vitamin A:** 325IU.

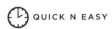 QUICK N EASY

Easy Lettuce Wraps

gluten　milk　soy　egg　corn　nuts

Tender lettuce leaves stand in for bread in these easy, quick roll-up sandwiches. This is a good way to be clever about including new kinds of vegetables (remember to start with a small amount well mixed in with vegetable favorites). If the diet is low in protein, this is a tasty way to include more.

- 8 whole Boston (or butter) or Bibb lettuce leaves, washed and dried
- 2 cups filling of choice, such as chopped vegetables, slices of chicken, chicken salad, or tuna-type salad (salmon is a healthier choice)
- 1/3 cup GFCF dressing or spread of choice (optional)

Fill each lettuce leaf with 1/4 cup filling. Sprinkle with a couple of teaspoons of dressing if using, and then roll it up like a burrito!

TIP: *Expand the variety of fillings and give more taste by adding chopped apples or cut up grapes. Offer a selection of your child's favorite fillings, and then let them fill and roll themselves!*

YIELD: *4 servings*

Calories (kcal): 319; **Total fat:** 28g; **Cholesterol:** 84mg; **Carbohydrate:** trace; **Dietary fiber:** trace; **Protein:** 15g; **Sodium:** 180mg; **Potassium:** 208mg; **Calcium:** 13mg; **Iron:** 1mg; **Zinc:** 1mg; **Vitamin A:** 873IU.

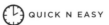 QUICK N EASY

Roll-Up Sandwiches

gluten　milk　soy　egg　corn　nuts

- 1 large GFCF tortilla (rice or corn) of choice
- 1/3 cup (77 g) GFCF cream cheese
- 2 to 3 slices GFCF luncheon meat of choice

Spread cream cheese evenly over tortilla, and then lay meat slices on top. Roll tortilla up into a tight log, and then slice into 2-inch rounds and serve.

YIELD: *1 to 2 servings*

Calories (kcal): 226; **Total fat:** 17g; **Cholesterol:** 54mg; **Carbohydrate:** 15g; **Dietary fiber:** 1g; **Protein:** 7g; **Sodium:** 459mg; **Potassium:** 48mg; **Calcium:** 26mg; **Iron:** trace; **Zinc:** 0; **Vitamin A:** 263IU.

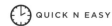 QUICK N EASY

Christina's Delicious Deviled Eggs

gluten milk soy egg corn nuts

- 6 large eggs, hard-boiled
- 1 to 1^1/$_2$ tablespoons (14 to 21 g) GFCF mayonnaise
- 1 teaspoon GFCF mustard, or to taste
- ^{1}/$_2$ teaspoon salt
- 2 tablespoons sweet pickle relish, or to taste
- Pinch of paprika

Cut each egg in half and carefully scoop out the yolk; reserve yolks in a medium bowl. Add the remaining ingredients to the yolks and mix to combine (adding additional mayonnaise to moisten if necessary). Adjust for seasoning, and then transfer mixture into a zipper lock bag. Cut one corner of the bag and squeeze the mixture evenly into the 12 egg white halves, sprinkling with additional paprika if desired. Chill and serve.

YIELD: *12 servings*

Calories (kcal): 53; **Total fat:** 4g; **Cholesterol:** 107mg; **Carbohydrate:** 1g; **Dietary fiber:** trace; **Protein:** 3g; **Sodium:** 166mg; **Potassium:** 34mg; **Calcium:** 14mg; **Iron:** trace; **Zinc:** trace; **Vitamin A:** 126IU.

Poultry Recipes

Variety is the best way to achieve good nutrition. When it comes to protein, don't focus on only poultry or just chicken within the poultry. Expand to turkey, Cornish game hens, and duck.

Avoid the commercial chicken nuggets, which are made with hydrogenated oils and are deep fried. Instead, make them at home or purchase organic GFCF chicken nuggets.

Chicken fat is not to be avoided. Almost 50 percent of the chicken fat is monounsaturated (just like the good fatty acids in olive oil). Also eat both white and dark poultry meat. The dark meat is more rich in nutrients, including fat-soluble vitamins.

Chicken Nuggets

gluten milk soy egg corn nuts

- 1¹/₂ cups (22 g) GF rice cereal
- 4 tablespoons (30 g) tapioca flour
- 1 cup (160 g) potato flour
- ¹/₂ cup (35 g) shredded coconut
- 2 tablespoons (36 g) sea salt
- 2 organic chicken breasts (deboned)
- 2 eggs
- 1¹/₂ cups (355 ml) rice milk
- ¹/₂ cup (120 ml) oil (sunflower, safflower, soy, almond, avocado, or peanut), or more as needed

Use a rolling pin to crush cereal in a resealable plastic bag. Mix dry ingredients with crushed cereal.

Cut chicken into desired sizes, wash and pat dry.

Mix eggs with rice milk, dip chicken pieces into liquid mixture, and then toss in closed resealable plastic bag and coat with mixture. Cook in oil until golden brown.

YIELD: *12 to 16 nuggets*

Calories (kcal): 401; **Total fat:** 23g; **Cholesterol:** 112mg; **Carbohydrate:** 19g; **Dietary fiber:** 1g; **Protein:** 29g; **Sodium:** 1071mg; **Potassium:** 542mg; **Calcium:** 24mg; **Iron:** 4mg; **Zinc:** 1mg; **Vitamin A:** 234IU

Roasted Apple Chicken

gluten milk soy egg corn nuts

- 1 roasting chicken (4–5 pounds, or 1.9–2.3 kg), with skin
- ¹/₂ lemon
- Salt and pepper to taste
- 1 small onion, quartered
- 1 apple, peeled and quartered
- ¹/₄ teaspoon dried rosemary
- ¹/₄ teaspoon dried thyme
- 2 sprigs fresh parsley
- ¹/₂ cup (120 ml) chicken broth
- ¹/₂ cup (120 ml) apple juice
- ¹/₄ cup (55 g) ghee, melted
- Salt and pepper

Preheat oven to 350°F (180°C, gas mark 4).

Rub inside of chicken with lemon half, sprinkle with salt and pepper.

Add the onion quarters, apple quarters, dried herbs, and parsley to chicken cavity. Pour chicken broth and apple juice in bottom of the pan. Place chicken in a shallow roasting pan and roast at 350°F (180°C, gas mark 4) for 80 to 100 minutes (20 minutes per pound). Baste with melted ghee and juices from the pan several times. Season with salt and pepper. The chicken's internal temperature should register 175°F (79°C), and the skin should be golden. Remove to a heated platter and keep warm in the oven until ready to serve. Make a sauce with pan juices, if desired.

YIELD: *6 servings*

Calories (kcal): 602; **Total fat:** 45g; **Cholesterol:** 186mg; **Carbohydrate:** 9g; **Dietary fiber:** 2g; **Protein:** 40g; **Sodium:** 230mg; **Potassium:** 655mg; **Calcium:** 61mg; **Iron:** 4 4mg; **Zinc:** 3mg; **Vitamin A:** 1690IU

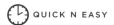 QUICK N EASY

Easy Chicken

gluten milk soy egg corn nuts

The chicken fat has the healing fatty acids. Keep the skin on the chicken.

- 4 bone-in chicken thighs or 2 breasts—with skin
- Honey

Preheat the oven to 350°F (180°C, gas mark 4).

Spread a thin layer of honey in the bottom of a casserole dish. Place chicken pieces meaty-side down on top of the honey. Squirt a little more honey on top. Cover and put in oven.

Approximately 90 minutes later, remove chicken from casserole dish with tongs.

This is great as a snack, or pull the chicken off the bone for use in salad or taco salad.

YIELD: *4 servings*

Calories (kcal): 231; **Total fat:** 14g; **Cholesterol:** 79mg; **Carbohydrate:** 9g; **Dietary fiber:** trace; **Protein:** 16g; **Sodium:** 72mg; **Potassium:** 186mg; **Calcium:** 10mg; **Iron:** 1mg; **Zinc:** 2mg; **Vitamin A:** 136IU

Stir-Fry Lemon Chicken

 gluten milk soy egg corn nuts

One of the secrets to attractive stir-fry dishes is to vary the shapes and colors of the vegetables chosen. For example, cut the carrots into ¹/₄-inch (0.6-cm) ridged diagonals; the red or green bell peppers into long, ¹/₄-inch (0.6-cm) -wide slices; and the green onions into 1-inch (2.5-cm) diagonals. Depending on taste and texture issues, this recipe can be modified.

- 1 pound (455 g) boneless, skinless chicken, cut into 1-inch (2.5-cm) pieces
- ¹/₄ cup (60 ml) GFCF tamari soy sauce
- ¹/₄ cup (60 ml) fresh lemon juice
- ¹/₄ cup (60 ml) water
- 1 tablespoon (5 g) grated lemon zest
- 1 teaspoon honey or agave nectar
- 2 teaspoons crushed red pepper flakes
- 2 garlic cloves, minced
- ¹/₂ teaspoon ground ginger
- 1 tablespoon (15 ml) olive oil
- 3 scallions, diagonally cut into 1-inch (2.5-cm) pieces
- 2 medium carrots, diagonally cut into ¹/₂-inch (1.25-cm) pieces
- ¹/₂ cup (45 g) red bell pepper, cut into ¹/₄-inch (1.25-cm) strips (optional)
- 2 teaspoons cornstarch
- 2 cups (320 g) hot cooked basmati, brown, or white rice
- Additional scallions and lemon peel strips, for garnish (optional)

Place chicken in a shallow glass dish and set aside. Combine soy sauce, lemon juice, water, lemon zest, honey, crushed red pepper, garlic, and ginger. Pour half of marinade over chicken and reserve remaining half. Marinate chicken in the refrigerator for 30 minutes.

Drain chicken and discard marinade.

In heavy skillet over medium heat, sauté chicken in olive oil until lightly browned. Transfer meat to a plate and cover with foil.

In same skillet, sauté scallions, carrots, and red bell pepper until crisp-tender. Whisk cornstarch into reserved marinade. Stir into vegetables and stir-fry until thickened. Return chicken to skillet; bring to serving temperature.

Serve immediately over cooked rice. Garnish with additional chopped scallions and lemon strips, if desired.

YIELD: *4 Servings*

Calories (kcal): 370; **Total fat:** 15g; **Cholesterol:** 70mg; **Carbohydrate:** 38g; **Dietary fiber:** 3g; **Protein:** 20g; **Sodium:** 1078mg; **Potassium:** 436mg; **Calcium:** 49mg; **Iron:** 2mg; **Zinc:** 2 2mg; **Vitamin A:** 11889IU

QUICK N EASY

Chicken Continental

gluten milk soy egg corn nuts

This recipe is easy and elegant. It makes a tasty puree for those who have texture issues.

- 1 pound (455 g) raw chicken, cut into strips
- 1 can (4 ounces, or 115 g) mushrooms, drained
- 1 garlic clove, crushed
- 2 tablespoons (28 ml) olive oil
- 2 cups (475 ml) organic chicken broth
- 1 package (9 ounces, or 255 g) frozen French-style green beans, defrosted
- 1 teaspoon salt
- $1/2$ teaspoon tarragon
- 1 teaspoon pepper
- $1^3/_4$ cups (166 g) quick-cooking rice or $1^3/_4$ cups (289 g) cooked brown, basmati, or wild rice

Sauté chicken, mushrooms, and garlic in oil until chicken is light brown.

Add broth, beans, salt, tarragon, and pepper. Bring to a boil.

Stir in rice. Remove from heat. Cover and let sit for 5 minutes.

YIELD: *4 servings*

Calories (kcal): 391; **Total fat:** 21g; **Cholesterol:** 75mg; **Carbohydrate:** 30g; **Dietary fiber:** 3g; **Protein:** 21g; **Sodium:** 1096mg; **Potassium:** 468mg; **Calcium:** 61mg; **Iron:** 3mg; **Zinc:** 2 2mg; **Vitamin A:** 1014IU

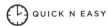 QUICK N EASY

Nut-Coated Chicken

gluten   milk   soy   egg   corn   nuts

SCD compatible.

- 1^1/$_2$ pounds (680 g) chicken breast
- 2 tablespoons (28 ml) olive oil
- Pecan Meal Coating (recipe follows)

Remove any fat from the chicken breast. Rinse with water and pat dry. Either pound meat to an even thickness or slice into each ^{1}/$_2$ breast from the thicker side to the thinner side, not cutting quite all the way through, so that it opens up like a butterfly. Then coat with olive oil.

Dip chicken breast in the pecan meal to coat completely. Cover baking sheet with kitchen parchment paper. Lay chicken, spaced apart, onto baking sheet. Bake at 425°F (220°C, or gas mark 7) for 22 to 25 minutes.

For chicken fingers, use chicken tenders or cut the chicken breast into smaller pieces. For chicken tenders, the cooking time remains the same as above, as they are still somewhat thick. However, if cutting the chicken smaller, reduce the cooking time to 18 to 20 minutes.

YIELD: *4 Servings*

Calories (kcal): 302; **Total fat:** 19g; **Cholesterol:** 87mg; **Carbohydrate:** 2g; **Dietary fiber:** trace; **Protein:** 29g; **Sodium:** 220mg; **Potassium:** 323mg; **Calcium:** 22mg; **Iron:** 1mg; **Zinc:** 1mg; **Vitamin A:** 113IU

Pecan Meal Coating

Pecan meal can be purchased seasonally from Sunnyland Farms, Inc., Albany, Georgia ([800]-999-2488). It can also be made at home by blending pecans in a blender. However, it is difficult to get the nuts ground as finely as in the purchased meal, so be aware that recipes may need adjusting, either by adding more nut meal or by reducing some of the liquid ingredients.

- 1 cup (120 g) pecan meal
- ^{1}/$_4$ teaspoon salt
- 1 tablespoon (9 g) onion powder
- ^{1}/$_2$–1 teaspoon garlic powder

Combine all ingredients.

Slow-Cooker Turkey Breast

gluten   milk   soy   egg   corn   nuts

Adapted from Angela Lowry's recipe found on Miss Roben's Web site. When not using homemade organic chicken broth, use canned or boxed organic chicken broth and add unflavored gelatin. This is much more nutritious and enhances the digestive function. See information about gelatin in chapter 8.

- Oil (safflower or light olive oil)
- 2 onions, sliced thinly
- 3–4 stalks celery, chopped
- 10–12 baby carrots
- 2 tablespoons (10 g) chopped garlic
- 4–6 pounds (1.9–2.7 kg) frozen organic, bone-in turkey breast, partially thawed
- $^1/_2$ cup (120 ml) white grape juice
- 1 can (14.5 ounces, or 411 ml) organic chicken broth mixed with 1 envelope (1 tablespoon, or 7 g) unflavored gelatin
- 3 tablespoons (6 g) chopped fresh rosemary or 1 tablespoon (3 g) dried rosemary
- Poultry seasoning (MSG-free), to taste
- Seasoned salt (MSG-free), to taste
- Pepper, to taste

Drizzle a small amount of oil onto the bottom of a slow cooker. Add the onions, celery, carrots, and garlic. Put the turkey breast halves on top of the veggies. Combine the grape juice, chicken broth–gelatin mixture, and rosemary and pour over the turkey breast. Sprinkle poultry seasoning, seasoned salt, and pepper on top. Cover and cook on low 4$^1/_2$ to 5 hours. Remove the turkey from the slow cooker. Strain veggies and store the turkey broth for use in soups and other recipes. Discard the veggies. Put turkey breast into the refrigerator until it has cooled and is easy to handle. Remove the turkey from the bones and store it in a resealable plastic bag until ready to use.

YIELD: *6–8 servings*

Calories (kcal): 500; **Total fat:** 21g; **Cholesterol:** 177mg; **Carbohydrate:** 13g; **Dietary fiber:** 2g; **Protein:** 62g; **Sodium:** 418mg; **Potassium:** 1043mg; **Calcium:** 70mg; **Iron:** 4mg; **Zinc:** 5mg; **Vitamin A:** 3081IU

Chicken Puree

 gluten
 milk
 soy
 egg
 corn
 nuts

This can be used to improve protein in many types of foods, from muffins and pancakes to tomato sauce and GFCF pizza.

- 1 ($^3/_4$–1 pound, or 340–455 g) organic boneless chicken breast
- $^1/_2$ envelope (1/2 tablespoon, or 3.5 g) unflavored gelatin
- $^1/_4$ cup (60 ml) chicken broth

POACHING METHOD: Heat $^1/_2$ inch (1.25 cm) of water in a medium skillet over medium-high heat until simmering. Add chicken breast. Water should not cover chicken, but come up about halfway. Simmer chicken until opaque and cooked through, 3 to 4 minutes per side.

OVEN METHOD: Preheat oven to 400°F (200°C, or gas mark 6). Place chicken breast on a greased baking rack over a baking pan. Bake chicken 12 minutes on each side, or until cooked through.

Add $^1/_2$ envelope unflavored gelatin to chicken broth or cooking liquid (if using poaching method) and stir well.

Coarsely chop chicken and transfer to a food processor. Process chicken for about 1 minute. While processor is running, slowly add $^1/_4$ cup (60 ml) of the liquid-gelatin mixture and continue to process until a paste forms. Add more liquid as needed to reach desired consistency.

VARIATIONS:
For a creamier texture, add tofu.
For sweetness, add $^1/_2$ cup (125 g) pureed apples.
Add $^1/_2$ cup (125 g) pureed vegetables (acorn squash or carrots work best).

Quick N Easy Version

Use organic pureed infant foods.

YIELD: *Four $^1/_2$ -cup (105 g) servings*

Calories (kcal): 140; **Total fat:** 2g; **Cholesterol:** 66mg; **Carbohydrate:** 2g; **Dietary fiber:** 0g; **Protein:** 27g; **Sodium:** 130mg; **Potassium:** 284mg; **Calcium:** 14mg; **Iron:** 1mg; **Zinc:** 1mg; **Vitamin A:** 32IU

Fruity Rice Chicken or Turkey

 gluten milk soy egg corn nuts

This recipe is a one-dish meal for children who have sensory issues and do not like "lumps and bumps" in their food.

- 1 tablespoon (15 ml) olive oil
- 1 small onion, chopped
- 3 tablespoons (45 g) applesauce or pearsauce
- 2 dried apricots
- 3 tablespoons (42 g) chicken breast or turkey breast
- 3 plum tomatoes, skinned, seeded, and chopped, or 2 tablespoons (32 g) tomato puree
- 2 tablespoons (20 g) golden raisins
- ³/₄ teaspoon finely chopped fresh rosemary
- 3 pinches each ground coriander and cinnamon
- ³/₄ teaspoon finely chopped garlic (optional)
- ³/₄ cup (175 ml) water
- ³/₄ cup (175 ml) chicken broth
- 3 tablespoons (30 g) cooked basmati rice

Heat the oil in a small pan over medium heat. Add the onion and fry until soft, about 2 minutes.

Mix in the fruits, chicken, tomatoes or tomato puree, and raisins.

Add the rosemary, spices, garlic, water, and broth. Bring to a boil, then reduce the heat, cover, and simmer for about 20 minutes, stirring occasionally to prevent sticking.

Add the cooked rice to the pan and stir.

Puree all ingredients in a blender. Add extra water if a thinner consistency is preferred, or more cooked rice if a thicker consistency is better.

YIELD: *About 2 to 3 child-sized servings*

Calories (kcal): 352; **Total fat:** 7g; **Cholesterol:** 7mg; **Carbohydrate:** 72g; **Dietary fiber:** 10g; **Protein:** 8g; **Sodium:** 217mg; **Potassium:** 1537mg; **Calcium:** 64mg; **Iron:** 5 5mg; **Zinc:** 1mg; **Vitamin A:** 6680IU

Spanish Chicken

gluten milk soy egg corn nuts

Look for the Goya seasonings in the international aisle of your supermarket.

- 3 pounds (1.35 kg) chicken pieces, such as thighs, drumsticks, or bone-in chicken breasts
- $^3/_4$ cup (150 g) sofrito (use Quick N Easy recipe on page 140, or Goya brand, found in the freezer section of most grocery stores)
- $^1/_2$ small can (8 ounces, or 225 g) tomato sauce
- 2 tablespoons (12 g) Goya Adobo all purpose seasoning w/ pepper
- 1 packet Sazón Goya w/ Coriander & Anatto
- 1 medium potato, peeled and cut into cubes
- 3 bay leaves

Put chicken into a pressure cooker, and then add just enough water to cover. Add sofrito, tomato sauce, seasonings, potatoes, and bay leaves. Cook according to your pressure cooker's instructions for cooking chicken (our pressure cooker cooks chicken for nine minutes after steady steam). Serve chicken and its juices over choice of rice.

YIELD: *4 servings*

Calories (kcal): 615; **Total fat:** 37g; **Cholesterol:** 195mg; **Carbohydrate:** 12g; **Dietary fiber:** 2g; **Protein:** 56g; **Sodium:** 1080mg; **Potassium:** 104mg; **Calcium:** 47mg; **Iron:** 3mg; **Zinc:** 5mg; **Vitamin A:** 837IU.

Thai Ginger Chicken

gluten milk soy egg corn nuts

- $^1/_4$ cup (50 ml) canola or safflower oil
- 1 tablespoon (10 g) minced garlic
- 2 tablespoons (12 g) minced ginger
- 12 ounces (340 g) ground chicken
- 2 medium red bell peppers, diced
- 2 scallions, chopped
- 1 tablespoon (15 ml) GFCF tamari
- 2 teaspoons white grape juice or apple juice
- $^1/_2$ teaspoon sugar
- $^1/_4$ teaspoons salt
- $^1/_3$ cup (20 g) basil leaves (whole, torn, or chopped)

Heat the oil in a wok or large skillet over high heat. Add the garlic and ginger and quickly fry for 30 seconds. Add the ground chicken and cook for 1 minute. Add the peppers, scallions, tamari, brandy, sugar, and salt and cook for 2 minutes. Stir in the basil and serve with rice.

YIELD: *2 to 4 servings*

Calories (kcal): 338; **Total fat:** 22g; **Cholesterol:** 80mg; **Carbohydrate:** 8g; **Dietary fiber:** 1g; **Protein:** 27g; **Sodium:** 449mg; **Potassium:** 375mg; **Calcium:** 33mg; **Iron:** 2mg; **Zinc:** 2mg; **Vitamin A:** 510IU.

Yellow Chicken and Rice

gluten milk soy egg corn nuts

This dish is named for the vibrant color given by the annatto seeds in the Goya mix, found in the International aisle of the supermarket. Goya Sofrito can be found in the freezer section, or use the Quick N Easy Sofrito recipe, page 140.

- 2 boneless, skinless chicken breasts
- 1 tablespoon (15 ml) olive oil
- $3/4$ cup (150 g) sofrito
- 1 package Goya Sazón with Coriander & Annatto
- $1^1/2$ cups (293 g) medium grain rice
- Salt to taste

In medium sauce pan, bring 3 cups (705 ml) water to a boil over high heat. Add chicken and cook for 5 minutes, or until chicken is no longer pink in the center. Remove chicken and cut into thin strips; reserve cooking water. In large pot, heat oil over medium heat. Add Goya Sofrito, Sazón Goya, and chicken and cook for 3 minutes. Add rice and stir to combine, and then add reserved chicken-water and 1 teaspoon salt. Bring to a boil, then cover, reduce heat, and simmer for 20 minutes, stirring occasionally, until rice is tender. Off heat, let mixture sit for 5 minutes, season to taste, and then serve.

YIELD: *4 servings*

Calories (kcal): 516; **Total fat:** 12g; **Cholesterol:** 68mg; **Carbohydrate:** 61g; **Dietary fiber:** 2g; **Protein:** 37g; **Sodium:** 544mg; **Potassium:** 535mg; **Calcium:** 41mg; **Iron:** 4mg; **Zinc:** 2mg; **Vitamin A:** 33IU.

Chicken Fried Rice

gluten milk soy egg corn nuts

This is a great recipe to use up leftover rice.

- 2 tablespoons (30 ml) canola or safflower oil
- $1/2$ pound (225 g) boneless, skinless chicken breast, cut into small pieces
- 1 medium onion, chopped
- 2 cloves garlic, minced
- 2 eggs, lightly beaten
- 4 cups (750 g) cooked rice
- 1 tomato, seeded and diced
- 1 tablespoon (15 ml) GFCF tamari
- 1 teaspoon sugar
- $1/2$ teaspoon ground black pepper
- 2 scallions, sliced thin

Heat the oil in large skillet over high heat. Add chicken and cook 1 minute. Add the onion and cook another 2 minutes, until chicken is lightly browned and cooked through. Add the garlic and eggs and stir constantly until eggs are cooked. Add the rice, tomato, tamari, sugar, and pepper, stir to combine and cook for 2 minutes to heat through. Sprinkle with the scallions and serve.

YIELD: *4 servings*

Calories (kcal): 431; **Total fat:** 11g; **Cholesterol:** 139mg; **Carbohydrate:** 59g; **Dietary fiber:** 2g; **Protein:** 23g; **Sodium:** 315mg; **Potassium:** 392mg; **Calcium:** 56mg; **Iron:** 2mg; **Zinc:** 2mg; **Vitamin A:** 359IU.

Easy Chicken Kebabs

gluten milk soy egg corn nuts

This very simple marinade adds flavor to and livens up a basic chicken kebab.

- 1 pound (455 g) boneless, skinless chicken breasts
- 2 tablespoons (30 ml) GFCF tamari
- 2 tablespoons (30 ml) canola or safflower oil
- 1 teaspoon ground black pepper

Cut the chicken into 1-inch cubes and place in a shallow dish. Mix the tamari, oil, and pepper with 1 tablespoon (15 ml) water and pour over the chicken; cover and refrigerate for at least 1 hour.

Thread the chicken cubes onto metal skewers and grill over medium heat for 20 minutes, turning and basting occasionally with the leftover marinade, until cooked through (be sure to discard any marinade that will not be cooked). Serve immediately.

NOTE: *Try an equal portion of flank or skirt steak in this recipe instead of chicken (cooking until desired doneness). Both are great served with Thai peanut sauce on the side for dipping.*

YIELD: *3 to 4 servings*

Calories (kcal): 195; **Total fat:** 8g; **Cholesterol:** 66mg; **Carbohydrate:** 1g; **Dietary fiber:** trace; **Protein:** 27g; **Sodium:** 551mg; **Potassium:** 297mg; **Calcium:** 15mg; **Iron:** 1mg; **Zinc:** 1mg; **Vitamin A:** 33IU.

Crispy Chicken Nuggets

gluten milk soy egg corn nuts

This recipe is adapted from Martha Holland, who says these are perfect for the child who loves crunchy things.

- $^1/_2$ cup (112 g) ghee, melted
- 2 cups (150 g) crushed GFCF potato chips or cassava chips of choice
- 1 large egg
- 2 tablespoons (30 ml) milk substitute
- 1 pound (455 g) boneless, skinless chicken breasts, cut into $1^1/_2$-inch cubes
- Salt and pepper

Preheat oven to 350°F (180°C, gas mark 4). Brush a baking sheet with 2 tablespoons (28 g) of the melted ghee. Spread the crushed chips in a shallow dish; beat the egg together with the milk substitute in a medium bowl.

Toss the chicken pieces in the egg mixture until thoroughly coated. Then drop each piece separately into the chips, cover them to coat, and then transfer to the greased baking sheet. When all the pieces are coated, drizzle the remaining ghee over the tops and lightly season with salt and pepper. Bake for 15 to 18 minutes, until golden brown. Serve with your favorite GFCF sauce or dressing.

TIP: *The chips can be quickly and easily crushed, either in the food processor, or in a zipper lock baggy with a rolling pin.*

NOTE: *These nuggets freeze well after baking.*

YIELD: *4 servings*

Calories (kcal): 533; **Total fat:** 32g; **Cholesterol:** 194mg; **Carbohydrate:** 34g; **Dietary fiber:** 2g; **Protein:** 28g; **Sodium:** 87mg; **Potassium:** 243mg; **Calcium:** 22mg; **Iron:** 2mg; **Zinc:** 1mg; **Vitamin A:** 1129IU.

Chicken Curry

gluten

milk

soy

egg

corn

nuts

The bones add a lot of flavor to this braise, but feel free to use boneless chicken instead, or sneak the bones out after the chicken is cooked.

- 3 pounds (1.4 kg) bone-in chicken pieces, skin removed (or 2 pounds boneless, skinless chicken)
- $^1/_4$ cup (55 g) ghee (or other suitable oil)
- 1 medium onion, finely chopped
- 3 cloves garlic, minced
- 2 tablespoons (16 g) grated ginger
- 1 small jalapeno pepper, seeded and diced
- Cardamom seeds from 2 pods, crushed
- 3 cloves
- 1 cinnamon stick
- 1 bay leaf
- 1 can (14 ounces, 400 g) diced tomatoes, drained
- $^1/_2$ teaspoon turmeric
- $^1/_2$ teaspoon chili powder
- 1 tablespoon (6 g) ground coriander
- 1 teaspoon salt
- $^1/_2$ teaspoon ground black pepper
- 1 pound (455 g) potatoes, peeled and diced
- Water
- $^1/_4$ cup (4 g) cilantro leaves, chopped (optional)

Heat the ghee in a large pot or Dutch oven over medium heat. Add onions and cook for 5 minutes, until golden. Add the garlic, ginger, jalapeno, cardamom, cloves, cinnamon, and bay leaf and cook for 1 minute, until fragrant. Then add the tomatoes and remaining spices and cook for 3 minutes. Add the chicken pieces and cook in the tomato mixture for 5 minutes. Add the potatoes and just enough water to cover and bring to a boil; reduce heat to low and simmer, covered, for 1 hour, until chicken and potatoes are tender. Sprinkle with cilantro if using and serve with basmati or other rice of choice.

YIELD: *4 to 6 servings*

Calories (kcal): 349; **Total fat:** 12g; **Cholesterol:** 111mg; **Carbohydrate:** 24g; **Dietary fiber:** 5g; **Protein:** 38g; **Sodium:** 572mg; **Potassium:** 1062mg; **Calcium:** 105mg; **Iron:** 4mg; **Zinc:** 2mg; **Vitamin A:** 928IU.

Orange Sesame Chicken

gluten   milk   soy   egg   corn   nuts

This stir-fry is healthier than but just as tasty as the deep-fried version.

- 1 pound (455 g) boneless, skinless, chicken breasts
- $^1/_4$ cup (60 ml) GFCF tamari, divided
- 1 tablespoon (8 g) cornstarch, divided
- $^1/_2$ cup (120 ml) orange juice
- $^1/_4$ cup (60 ml) GFCF chicken broth
- 2 teaspoons sesame oil
- 2 garlic cloves, minced
- 1 tablespoon (6 g) minced fresh ginger
- $^1/_4$ teaspoon hot pepper flakes
- 2 tablespoons (30 ml) canola or safflower oil, divided
- $^1/_2$ pound (225 g) asparagus, sliced thinly
- 1 small red bell pepper, chopped
- 2 medium carrots, grated
- 2 scallions, thinly sliced
- 2 tablespoons (16 g) toasted sesame seeds

Cut the chicken into $^1/_2$-inch pieces; combine 1 tablespoon (15 ml) tamari and 1 teaspoon cornstarch in a medium bowl and then add the chicken and toss to combine. Let sit for 5 minutes.

For the sauce, whisk the orange juice, broth, remaining tamari and cornstarch, sesame oil, garlic, ginger, and hot pepper flakes and set aside.

Heat 1 tablespoon of oil in a large skillet over high heat. Add the chicken pieces and cook 2 to 3 minutes, stirring occasionally, until lightly browned and cooked through. Transfer to a clean bowl. Heat remaining oil in skillet; add asparagus, pepper, and carrot and cook 3 minutes, until tender. Return chicken to the skillet, add the sauce ingredients and cook for 2 minutes, until thickened. Add scallions and sesame seeds and serve over rice.

YIELD: *4 servings*

Calories (kcal): 300; **Total fat:** 13g; **Cholesterol:** 66mg; **Carbohydrate:** 15g; **Dietary fiber:** 3g; **Protein:** 30g; **Sodium:** 1067mg; **Potassium:** 615mg; **Calcium:** 45mg; **Iron:** 2mg; **Zinc:** 2mg; **Vitamin A:** 105431IU.

Chicken or Steak Fajitas

gluten milk soy egg corn nuts

You can make one or the other, or do a little of both for some variety! Some good condiments to serve alongside this dish are lime wedges, diced avocados or tomatoes, minced cilantro, and plain soy yogurt.

- 1^1/$_2$ pounds (680 g) boneless, skinless chicken breasts, sliced into thin strips, or whole flank steak
- Salt and ground black pepper
- 3 tablespoons (45 ml) olive oil
- 1 green bell pepper
- 1 red bell pepper
- 1 red onion
- 2 tablespoons (30 ml) water
- 1 teaspoon chili powder
- ^{1}/$_4$ teaspoon cumin
- 1 small garlic clove, minced
- 2 tablespoons (30 ml) lime juice
- 1 tablespoon (15 ml) GFCF Worcestershire sauce
- 1 teaspoon agave nectar
- 12 small brown rice tortillas

Season the chicken or steak with salt and pepper. Heat 1 tablespoon of oil in large non-stick skillet over medium-high heat. Add meat and brown on both sides, 5 to 10 minutes total (cooking chicken thoroughly, and steak to desired doneness). Transfer meat to a plate and cover to keep warm; let steak rest for 10 minutes before slicing into thin strips.

Add another tablespoon of oil to the pan and heat over medium heat. Add peppers, onion, water, chili powder, cumin, and ^{1}/$_2$ teaspoon salt and cook for 5 minutes, until vegetables have softened. Transfer to a serving plate or bowl.

Combine remaining oil, garlic, lime juice, Worcestershire, and agave with a pinch of salt and toss with sliced meat. Warm tortillas in microwave or oven if desired, and serve with meat and vegetables.

YIELD: *4 to 6 servings*

With chicken: Calories (kcal): 484; **Total fat:** 15g; **Cholesterol:** 69mg; **Carbohydrate:** 55g; **Dietary fiber:** 5g; **Protein:** 30g; **Sodium:** 413mg; **Potassium:** 527mg; **Calcium:** 25mg; **Iron:** 1mg; **Zinc:** 1mg; **Vitamin A:** 414IU.

With steak: Calories (kcal): 550; **Total fat:**24 g; **Cholesterol:** 58mg; **Carbohydrate:** 55g; **Dietary fiber:** 5g; **Protein:** 27g; **Sodium:** 432mg; **Potassium:** 708mg; **Calcium:** 18mg; **Iron:** 3mg; **Zinc:** 4mg; **Vitamin A:** 398IU.

Herb Turkey Burgers

 gluten milk soy egg corn nuts

These are not the typical dried-out turkey burgers. The addition of mushrooms and onions gives this recipe a tender, juicy texture the family will love. It is also a good way to hide some vegetables as long as they are well minced/blended and the color does not stand out. Start with a small amount (1 tablespoon [16 g]) at first, then expand.

- 1¹/₂ pounds (680 g) ground turkey (white and dark meat)
- ¹/₂ cup (3 ounces, or 85 g) finely minced mushrooms
- ¹/₂ small onion, finely minced (about ¹/₂ cup, or 80 g)
- ¹/₈ cup (25 g) minced vegetables (squash, peas)
- 1 teaspoon prepared GFCF barbeque sauce
- 1 teaspoon chopped fresh oregano
- 1 teaspoon ground cumin
- 1 tablespoon (15 ml) balsamic vinegar
- ¹/₂ teaspoon GFCF hot sauce

To serve (optional)
- Toasted buns, pita pockets, or the child's favorite bread
- Spreads and condiments such as GFCF ketchup or mustard

In a medium bowl, combine all ingredients, using a wooden spoon or by hand. Be sure mushrooms and onion are equally distributed throughout mixture. By hand, press meat together to form 8 equal-sized patties.

Heat a grill pan or skillet over medium heat. Spray pan with cooking spray, and cook patties for 5 minutes on each side or until cooked through. For cheeseburgers, add a GFCF cheese slice to top of patty after flipping.

No bun is required. Some kids would rather dip their patties right into GFCF ketchup or mustard and don't want a bun.

YIELD: *8 servings of 1 burger each*

Calories (kcal): 132; **Total fat:** 7g; **Cholesterol:** 67mg; **Carbohydrate:** 1g; **Dietary fiber:** trace; **Protein:** 15g; **Sodium:** 88mg; **Potassium:** 234mg; **Calcium:** 16mg; **Iron:** 1mg; **Zinc:** 2mg; **Vitamin A:** 16IU

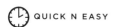 QUICK N EASY

Andrew's Turkey Tacos O' Fun

     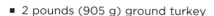

gluten   milk   soy   egg   corn   nuts

- 2 pounds (905 g) ground turkey
- 1/4 cup (60 ml) extra-virgin olive oil
- 3/4 cup (195 g) Sofrito (page 115)
- 2 cans (15 ounces, or 420 g, each) red kidney beans, drained
- 2 cans (8 ounces, or 225 g, each) tomato sauce
- 1 tablespoon (8 g) chili powder, red or green
- 1/4 teaspoon paprika
- Salt to taste

Brown turkey completely in the olive oil on high heat. Add sofrito and lower to medium heat, continuing to mix. Add beans and mix. Add tomato sauce, spices, and salt and mix well.

Serve hot with warm rice tortillas.

VARIATION: *Serve on field greens or Romaine lettuce for a taco salad. Optional condiments include onions, tomatoes, gluten-free guacamole, and chopped cilantro.*

YIELD: *6 servings*

Calories (kcal): 828; Total fat: 23g; Cholesterol: 120mg; Carbohydrate: 97g; Dietary fiber: 24g; Protein: 60g; Sodium: 631 mg; Potassium: 2672mg; Calcium: 162mg; Iron: 12mg; Zinc: 7mg; Vitamin A: 1338IU

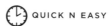 QUICK N EASY

Pureed Beef Broccoli (and Other Options)

gluten   milk   soy   egg   corn   nuts

This recipe can be modified to include a variety of meats and vegetables.

- 6 ounces (170 g) lean ground round or sirloin
- 2 cups (140 g) chopped broccoli florets
- 1/2 cup (120 ml) beef or chicken stock

Brown beef in a skillet over medium-high heat, breaking up any large pieces, about 7 minutes.

Drain off fat and return beef to skillet.

Add broccoli and stock; cover, reduce heat, and simmer until broccoli is very tender, about 15 minutes. Let cool.

Transfer to blender and puree on high speed to desired consistency.

NOTES: *To accommodate those with aversions to green foods, substitute 2 cups (260 g) chopped carrots or sweet potato for the broccoli.*

Expand this recipe to a more complete whole-dish meal by adding 1/2 cup (85 g) cooked brown, white, or basmati rice. If the consistency is too thick, add more stock to thin.

YIELD: *2 cups (430 g)*

Calories (kcal): 458; Total fat: 30g; Cholesterol: 117mg; Carbohydrate: 10g; Dietary fiber: 5g; Protein: 37g; Sodium: 1222mg; Potassium: 1097mg; Calcium: 98mg; Iron: 6mg; Zinc: 8 8mg; Vitamin A: 2715IU

Lighter Beef and Broccoli

     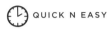

gluten   milk   soy   egg   corn   nuts

This is a simple version of a popular dish.

- 1 large bunch broccoli (about 1¹/₂ pounds, or 680 g)
- 1 pound (455 g) beef tenderloin steaks, trimmed, thinly cut into ¹/₈-inch (0.3-cm) strips
- 3 garlic cloves, crushed with garlic press
- 1 tablespoon (8 g) peeled, grated fresh ginger
- ¹/₄ teaspoon crushed red pepper
- 1 teaspoon (5 ml) olive oil, divided
- ³/₄ cup (175 ml) chicken broth
- 3 tablespoons (45 ml) GFCF soy sauce
- 1 tablespoon (8 g) cornstarch
- ¹/₂ teaspoon Asian sesame oil

Cut broccoli flowerets into 1¹/₂ -inch (3.75-cm) pieces. Peel broccoli stems and cut into ¹/₄-inch (0.6-cm) diagonal slices.

In a nonstick 12-inch (30-cm) skillet, heat ¹/₂ inch (1.25 cm) water to boiling over medium-high heat. Add broccoli and cook 3 minutes, uncovered, or until tender-crisp. Drain broccoli and set aside. Wipe skillet dry.

In a medium bowl, toss beef with garlic, ginger, and crushed red pepper. Add ¹/₂ teaspoon olive oil to skillet and heat over medium-high heat until hot but not smoking. Add half of beef mixture and cook 2 minutes or until beef just loses its pink color throughout, stirring quickly and frequently. Transfer beef to a plate. Repeat with remaining ¹/₂ teaspoon olive oil and beef mixture.

In a cup, mix broth, soy sauce, cornstarch, and sesame oil until blended. Return cooked beef to skillet. Stir in cornstarch mixture; heat to boiling. Cook 1 minute or until sauce thickens slightly, stirring. Add broccoli and toss to coat.

NOTE: *This can be pureed to suit those with texture issues or those who have difficulty chewing meats.*

YIELD: *4 main-dish servings*

Calories (kcal): 402; **Total fat:** 28g; **Cholesterol:** 80mg; **Carbohydrate:** 12g; **Dietary fiber:** 5g; **Protein:** 26g; **Sodium:** 1010mg; **Potassium:** 904mg; **Calcium:** 89mg; **Iron:** 4mg; **Zinc:** 4 4mg; **Vitamin A:** 4571IU

QUICK N EASY

Beanie Weanies

 gluten
 milk
 soy
 egg
 corn
 nuts

This is another one of Elynn DeMattia's son's favorites— he who would never eat a hot dog in its true form, devours them in this recipe. This dish also makes a great packable school lunch.

- 1 tablespoon (15 ml) safflower or canola oil
- 2 GFCF hot dogs, sliced into bite-sized pieces
- 1 can (14 ounces, or 400 g) GFCF baked beans

In a medium skillet, heat the oil over medium heat. Add the hot dog pieces and cook until golden brown on the edges. Add the beans and stir to combine, cooking until heated through, 3 to 4 minutes. Serve.

YIELD: *2 to 3 servings*

Calories (kcal): 241; **Total fat:** 10g; **Cholesterol:** 27mg; **Carbohydrate:** 31g; **Dietary fiber:** 5g; **Protein:** 10g; **Sodium:** 904mg; **Potassium:** 0mg; **Calcium:** 41mg; **Iron:** 2mg; **Zinc:** 0mg; **Vitamin A:** 0IU.

Maple-Glazed Pork Chops

 gluten
 milk
 soy
 egg
 corn
nuts

Use pure maple syrup for this dish—grade B is better for cooking because it has a stronger flavor.

- 1 cup (235 ml) GFCF chicken broth
- $^{3}/_{4}$ cup (175 ml) maple syrup
- 2 tablespoons (30 ml) cider vinegar
- $^{1}/_{2}$ teaspoon dry mustard
- Salt and ground black pepper
- 1 tablespoon (15 ml) safflower oil
- 4 boneless pork chops, 1-inch thick

Whisk together chicken broth, maple syrup, vinegar, dry mustard, and $^{1}/_{4}$ teaspoon salt in small bowl and set aside.

Heat the oil in a large skillet over medium-high heat. Season the pork chops with salt and pepper on both sides and carefully add to the hot pan. Cook for 4 minutes, or until browned on one side. Flip chops, add glaze ingredients and reduce heat to medium; cover and cook for 5 to 10 minutes, until pork registers 140°F (60°C) in the center. Remove chops and cover with foil to keep warm. Continue cooking glaze, uncovered, until thickened (adding any accumulated pork juices), 5 to 8 minutes. Pour glaze over chops and serve.

YIELD: *4 servings*

Calories (kcal): 409; **Total fat:** 18g; **Cholesterol:** 62mg; **Carbohydrate:** 40g; **Dietary fiber:** trace; **Protein:** 21g; **Sodium:** 193mg; **Potassium:** 518mg; **Calcium:** 67mg; **Iron:** 1mg; **Zinc:** 2mg; **Vitamin A:** 7IU.

Sweet and Spicy Drumsticks

gluten milk soy egg corn nuts

- 8 chicken legs, skin on
- 2 tablespoons (16 g) grated ginger
- 2 cloves garlic, minced
- 2 tablespoons (30 ml) lemon juice
- 4 tablespoons (85 g) honey
- 1 tablespoon (7 g) paprika
- 1 teaspoon chili powder
- 1 tablespoon (8 g) cornstarch
- $1/2$ teaspoon salt

Mash together the ginger, garlic, lemon juice, honey, paprika, chili powder, corn starch, and salt with a mortar and pestle or in a bowl to make a smooth paste. Wash and dry the chicken pieces, and then prick them all over with a sharp knife. Combine the paste and the chicken in a large zipper lock bag or in a shallow dish and marinate in the refrigerator for at least 20 minutes.

Preheat oven to 400°F (200°C, gas mark 6). Place the marinated chicken pieces on a wire rack set on top of a baking sheet or roasting pan (line pan with foil for easier clean up). Cook for 45 minutes, until the meat is cooked through. Serve.

YIELD: *4 to 6 servings*

Calories (kcal): 473; **Total fat:** 27g; **Cholesterol:** 185mg; **Carbohydrate:** 15g; **Dietary fiber:** 1g; **Protein:** 41g; **Sodium:** 359mg; **Potassium:** 502mg; **Calcium:** 30mg; **Iron:** 3mg; **Zinc:** 4mg; **Vitamin A:** 1117IU.

Mexican Egg "Noodles"

gluten · milk soy egg corn nuts

You'll need a good non-stick skillet to cook the thin omelets used to make the fun egg ribbons in this dish.

- $1/4$ cup (60 ml) oil
- 8 eggs, lightly beaten
- 3 cups (780 g) salsa
- 2 tablespoons (4 g) chopped cilantro

Heat 1 tablespoon (15 ml) of the oil over medium heat in a large non-stick skillet. Add one quarter of the eggs at a time, swirling the pan to coat with an even layer of egg. When the omelet is almost cooked through, flip over with a spatula and cook for an additional minute. Slide omelet onto a cutting board and repeat process to make 3 more omelets, stacking them on top of the first. Slice the stack of omelets into thin noodle-like ribbons.

Heat the salsa in the now-empty skillet until warmed through. Add the egg ribbons and toss to combine. Sprinkle with cilantro and serve.

YIELD: *4 servings*

Calories (kcal): 323; **Total fat:** 24g; **Cholesterol:** 424mg; **Carbohydrate:** 13g; **Dietary fiber:** 3g; **Protein:** 15g; **Sodium:** 983mg; **Potassium:** 550mg; **Calcium:** 111mg; **Iron:** 4mg; **Zinc:** 2mg; **Vitamin A:** 1690IU.

Singapore Noodles

gluten   milk   soy   egg   corn   nuts

This quick and simple noodle dish can pack a good amount of protein.

- ³/₄ pound (340 g) protein of choice (shrimp, chicken, pork, or firm tofu all work well), cut into bite-sized pieces
- 1 tablespoon (6.3 g) mild GFCF curry powder
- ¹/₄ cup (60 ml) GFCF tamari
- 8 ounces (225 g) rice vermicelli
- 2 tablespoons (30 ml) safflower or Canola oil, divided
- 2 eggs, lightly beaten
- 3 medium cloves garlic, minced
- 1 tablespoon (6 g) minced ginger
- 1 small onion, chopped
- 1 red bell pepper, seeded and chopped
- 1 cup (235 ml) GFCF chicken broth
- 1 tablespoon (20 g) agave nectar
- 1 cup (50 g) bean sprouts

Toss the protein with 1 teaspoon curry powder and 1 tablespoon (15 ml) tamari and let marinate at least 10 minutes. Pour enough boiling water over the noodles to cover and let stand 5 minutes; drain noodles and set aside.

In a large skillet or wok, heat 1 tablespoon (15 ml) oil over medium-high heat. Add the protein and marinade and stir fry until lightly browned and cooked through. Add the eggs and cook, stirring constantly to break up eggs, until cooked through; remove and aside. Heat remaining oil in the now empty skillet. Add the garlic, ginger, and remaining curry powder and cook until fragrant, 30 seconds. Add the onion and pepper and cook until softened, 3 minutes. Add the broth, remaining tamari, and agave nectar and stir to combine. Finally, add the reserved protein, noodles, and bean sprouts, tossing to combine ingredients and allow the noodles to absorb the sauce. Serve.

YIELD: *4 servings*

Calories (kcal): 301; **Total fat:** 15g; **Cholesterol:** 107mg; **Carbohydrate:** 29g; **Dietary fiber:** 3g; **Protein:** 14g; **Sodium:** 1130mg; **Potassium:** 288mg; **Calcium:** 123mg; **Iron:** 6mg; **Zinc:** 1mg; **Vitamin A:** 403IU.

Vietnamese Spring Rolls

gluten   milk   soy   egg   corn   nuts

There is no end to what you can stuff these fun rice paper rolls with—a great way to include hidden vegetables. These are just a few suggestions. Assembly can be a family effort, much like making your own tacos. You can also serve these with Thai Peanut Sauce, page ••.

- 2 ounces (55 g) cellophane noodles (also known as glass or bean thread noodles; rice vermicelli can also be used)
- 8 (9-inch, or 23 cm) dried rice paper wrappers
- 1 carrot, shredded
- 1 cucumber, peeled, seeded, and cut into thin strips
- 1 red bell pepper, seeded and thinly sliced
- 4 scallions, sliced into thin strips on the diagonal
- 2 cups (280 g) cooked, shredded chicken breasts
- $1/2$ cup (10 g) cilantro, basil, or mint leaves, cut into thin strips or left whole

Pour enough boiling water over the cellophane noodles to cover; let soak 5 minutes, or until tender. Drain and rinse under cold water. Cut into 7-inch lengths.

Fill a shallow dish such as a pie plate with warm water. Slide one rice paper wrapper into the water for a few seconds, until pliable. Remove and place on clean plate. Add desired fillings in a line along the center of the wrapper, leaving a 1-inch border on either end (don't overfill). Fold the bottom third of the wrapper up and over the filling, fold in the shorter sides, and then continue to roll until you reach the top (similar to making a burrito). Cut in half on the bias or leave whole.

Lime Chili Sauce

- $1/4$ cup (60 ml) fresh squeezed lime juice
- 2 tablespoons (42 g) agave nectar
- $1/4$ teaspoon hot pepper flakes
- 1 small clove garlic
- 1 teaspoon grated ginger
- $1/4$ teaspoon salt

Combine all ingredients and whisk well to dissolve salt.

NOTE: *These can be made a few hours ahead of time—simply wrap each one in waxed paper and refrigerate until needed.*

YIELD: *4 servings*

Calories (kcal): 292; **Total fat:** 9g; **Cholesterol:** 61mg; **Carbohydrate:** 31g; **Dietary fiber:** 3g; **Protein:** 22g; **Sodium:** 224mg; **Potassium:** 654mg; **Calcium:** 92mg; **Iron:** 3mg; **Zinc:** 1mg; **Vitamin A:** 625IU.

Indian Kebabs with Tomato-Onion Raita

gluten   milk   soy   egg   corn   nuts

If you can't find garam masala, you can substitute a pinch each of ground cardamom, cinnamon, cloves, and black pepper.

- 1 pound (455 g) lean ground meat of choice
- 2 tablespoons (16 g) grated ginger
- 1 small jalapeno, seeded and minced (optional)
- Salt
- $^{1}/_{2}$ teaspoon garam masala
- 1 medium onion, finely chopped
- $^{1}/_{2}$ chili powder
- $^{1}/_{2}$ teaspoon ground black pepper
- $^{1}/_{2}$ teaspoon ground cumin
- $^{1}/_{4}$ cup (4 g) cilantro leaves, chopped
- 1 large egg, lightly beaten
- 1 tablespoon (15 ml) canola or safflower oil

In the bottom of a large bowl, combine the ginger, jalapeno, $^{1}/_{2}$ teaspoon salt, and the garam masala with 1 to 2 tablespoons (15 to 30 ml) water to make a paste. Add the ground meat and the remaining ingredients and combine well. Roll the mixture into small sausage-like balls and thread onto skewers. Grill over medium heat for 20 minutes, basting with a little oil if necessary and turning frequently, until cooked through.

Tomato-Onion Raita

- $^{1}/_{2}$ cup (115 g) soy yogurt
- $^{1}/_{2}$ small onion, minced and rinsed under warm water
- 1 tablespoon (2 g) minced cilantro
- 1 tablespoon (8 g) grated ginger
- $^{1}/_{2}$ teaspoon salt
- $^{1}/_{2}$ teaspoon ground cumin, dry toasted
- $^{1}/_{2}$ cup (90 g) seeded and diced tomatoes

Combine the first six ingredients well; add tomatoes just before serving.

YIELD: *4 servings*

Kebabs Only: **Calories (kcal):** 227; **Total fat:** 13g; **Cholesterol:** 127mg; **Carbohydrate:** 4g; **Dietary fiber:** 1g; **Protein:** 25g; **Sodium:** 102mg; **Potassium:** 97mg; **Calcium:** 18mg; **Iron:** 1mg; **Zinc:** trace; **Vitamin A:** 261IU.

Tomato-Onion Raita: **Calories (kcal):** 33; **Total fat:** 1g; **Cholesterol:** 0mg; **Carbohydrate:** 6g; **Dietary fiber:** 1g; **Protein:** 1g; **Sodium:** 273mg; **Potassium:** 73mg; **Calcium:** 57mg; **Iron:** trace; **Zinc:** trace; **Vitamin A:** 151IU.

Analysis of both together: **Calories (kcal):** 260; **Total fat:** 14g; **Cholesterol:** 127mg; **Carbohydrate:** 10g; **Dietary fiber:** 1g; **Protein:** 26g; **Sodium:** 375mg; **Potassium:** 170mg; **Calcium:** 75mg; **Iron:** 1mg; **Zinc:** trace; **Vitamin A:** 412IU.

Shepherd's Pie

gluten   milk   soy   egg   corn   nuts

Traditionally this comforting dish is made with ground lamb, but lean ground beef is much more kid-friendly.

For Filling

- 1¹/₂ pounds (680 g) lean ground beef
- 1 yellow onion, minced
- 1 celery stalk, minced
- 2 teaspoons dried thyme
- ¹/₂ teaspoon salt
- 2 tablespoons (20 g) potato starch
- 1 tablespoon (16 g) tomato paste
- 2 cups (470 ml) GFCF chicken broth
- 1 tablespoon (15 ml) GFCF tamari
- Pinch cayenne pepper
- 1 cup (130 g) frozen peas
- 1 cup (130 g) diced carrots, cooked

For Mashed Potatoes

- 1¹/₂ pounds (680 g) russet potatoes, peeled, boiled, and drained
- 6 tablespoons (85 g) ghee, melted
- ¹/₃ cup (80 ml) soy milk
- ¹/₂ teaspoon salt
- ¹/₄ teaspoon pepper

FOR THE FILLING: In large non-stick skillet over medium heat, cook ground beef, stirring to break up, for 3 minutes or until no longer pink. Transfer to a plate, and drain off all but 1 tablespoon of fat. Add the onion, celery, dried thyme, and salt, and cook for 5 minutes. Add potato starch and tomato paste, stirring to combine, and cook for 1 minute. Add broth, tamari, and cayenne, and reserved meat and bring to a simmer. Cover and cook over medium-low heat 6 to 8 minutes, until sauce has thickened. Add peas and carrots and heat through, then transfer mixture to a large baking dish.

FOR THE MASHED POTATOES: Mash potatoes with potato masher or ricer. Add ¹/₄ cup melted ghee, soy milk, salt and pepper and gently mix to combine. Spread potatoes in a thin layer over beef mixture, and then brush with remaining ghee. Broil until topping is brown, 3 to 5 minutes. (If you can't keep the baking dish 6 inches away from the broiler, preheat oven to 500°F [250°C, gas mark 10] and cook on the upper-middle rack for 5 to 8 minutes.)

YIELD: *4 to 6 servings*

Calories (kcal): 363; **Total fat:** 25g; **Cholesterol:** 87mg; **Carbohydrate:** 11g; **Dietary fiber:** 3g; **Protein:** 23g; **Sodium:** 669mg; **Potassium:** 479mg; **Calcium:** 38mg; **Iron:** 3mg; **Zinc:** 5mg; **Vitamin A:** 6296IU.

Mexican Meatballs with Vegetable Chili Sauce

 gluten milk soy egg corn nuts

An interesting twist on the standard meatballs and sauce. Masa harina is the traditional flour used to make tortillas, tamales, and other Mexican dishes. Literally translated from Spanish, it means "dough flour," because the flour is made from dried masa, a dough from specially treated corn.

For the Meatballs

- 8 ounces (225g) lean ground beef
- 3 to 4 tablespoons (22.5 to 30 g) masa harina
- 1 large egg, lightly beaten
- 1 small onion, finely chopped
- 1 clove garlic, minced
- 1/2 teaspoon ground cumin
- 1 teaspoon chopped parsley
- 1 tablespoon (6 g) chopped mint
- 1 pinch dried thyme
- 1 pinch ground cloves
- Salt and pepper

For the Sauce

- 2 tablespoons (30 ml) canola oil
- 2 tablespoons (15 g) chili powder
- 1 small onion, chopped
- 2 cloves garlic, minced
- 1 can (14 ounces, or 400 g) diced or pureed tomatoes
- 1 1/2 cups (350 ml) GFCF chicken stock
- 1/8 teaspoon ground cinnamon
- 2 tablespoons (18 g) raisins or currants
- 2 teaspoons brown sugar
- 2 tablespoons (30 ml) apple cider vinegar
- 1 sweet potato, peeled and chopped
- 1 zucchini, chopped
- 2 carrots, peeled and chopped
- 2 tablespoons (4 g) chopped cilantro

FOR THE MEATBALLS: Mix the meat with the remaining ingredients and season with salt and pepper. Roll into egg-shaped meat balls and set aside in the refrigerator.

FOR THE SAUCE: Heat the oil in a large pot or Dutch oven over medium heat. Add the onion and chili powder and cook 3 minutes, until onion is soft. Add garlic and tomatoes and continue cooking 5 minutes, or until mixture has darkened and reduced slightly. Add the stock, cinnamon, raisins or currants, brown sugar, vinegar, sweet potato, zucchini and carrots, and bring to a boil. Add reserved meatballs, cover, and reduce heat to low. Simmer mixture 20 to 30 minutes, occasionally basting the meatballs with the sauce, until meatballs are cooked through. Add cilantro and serve over rice or with corn tortillas.

YIELD: *4 servings*

Meatballs: Calories (kcal): 202; Total fat: 13g; Cholesterol: 96mg; Carbohydrate: 7g; Dietary fiber: 1g; Protein: 13g; Sodium: 57mg; Potassium: 222mg; Calcium: 31mg; Iron: 2mg; Zinc: 3mg; Vitamin A: 158IU.

Sauce: Calories (kcal): 188; Total fat: 9g; Cholesterol: 2mg; Carbohydrate: 27g; Dietary fiber: 5g; Protein: 4g; Sodium: 423mg; Potassium: 672mg; Calcium: 75mg; Iron: 2mg; Zinc: 1mg; Vitamin A: 18747IU.

Combined: Calories (kcal): 391; Total fat: 22g; Cholesterol: 98mg; Carbohydrate: 34g; Dietary fiber: 6g; Protein: 17g; Sodium: 480mg; Potassium: 894mg; Calcium: 106mg; Iron: 4mg; Zinc: 3mg; Vitamin A: 18904IU.

Yummy Sloppy Joes

gluten   milk   soy   egg   corn   nuts

- 1¹/₂ pounds (680 g) lean organic ground beef
- 1 can (14 ounces, or 400 g) diced tomatoes
- 1¹/₄ cups (300 g) GFCF ketchup
- ¹/₂ cup (125 g) GFCF honey barbeque sauce
- 1 tablespoon (15 ml) GFCF Worcestershire sauce
- ¹/₂ cup (120 ml) water
- ¹/₂ teaspoon ginger
- 2 teaspoons (8 g) sugar
- Salt and pepper to taste
- 6 GFCF hamburger buns

Cook ground beef in a large skillet over medium-high heat, stirring until beef crumbles and is no longer pink. Drain well. Return cooked beef to skillet.

Stir in the rest of the ingredients. Reduce heat and simmer, stirring as the mixture heats and blends. Add more sauce for desired consistency and taste.

Spoon mixture on the buns and serve.

YIELD: *6 servings*

Calories (kcal): 564; **Total fat:** 33g; **Cholesterol:** 96mg; **Carbohydrate:** 43g; **Dietary fiber:** 3g; **Protein:** 24g; **Sodium:** 1112mg; **Potassium:** 765mg; **Calcium:** 89mg; **Iron:** 4mg; **Zinc:** 5 5mg; **Vitamin A:** 1104IU

Meatball Sauce #1—Regular Version

gluten   milk   soy   egg   corn   nuts

- 1 can (8 ounces, or 225 g) tomato sauce
- ¹/₄ cup (60 g) GFCF ketchup
- 2 tablespoons (20 g) finely chopped onion
- 1 tablespoon (15 ml) vinegar
- 1 tablespoon (15 ml) GFCF Worcestershire sauce
- ¹/₂ teaspoon salt
- ¹/₄ teaspoon black pepper
- ¹/₄ teaspoon ground allspice
- ¹/₄ cup (60 ml) water
- ¹/₃ cup (105 g) GFCF natural fruit spread—mixed berry or grape
- ¹/₄ cup (60 g) pureed vegetables (one or more of the following store-bought Stage 1 or 2 organic baby food or pureed organic fresh or frozen vegetables: carrots, squash, yam, sweet potato, peas, green beans, beets)

In a medium saucepan, combine tomato sauce, ketchup, onion, vinegar, Worcestershire sauce, salt, pepper, allspice, water, fruit spread, and pureed vegetables. Bring to a boil, lower heat, and simmer for 15 minutes. Add meatballs and simmer another 15 to 30 minutes. Spear meatballs with wooden picks.

NOTE: *When beginning to add vegetables, start with 1 tablespoon (15 g) and increase as tolerated. Expand the vegetables as each addition is tolerated.*

YIELD: *2 cups (500 g)*

Calories (kcal): 413; **Total fat:** 1g; **Cholesterol:** 0mg; **Carbohydrate:** 107g; **Dietary fiber:** 6g; **Protein:** 5g; **Sodium:** 3342mg; **Potassium:** 1390mg; **Calcium:** 99mg; **Iron:** 4mg; **Zinc:** 1mg; **Vitamin A:** 2863IU

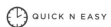

QUICK N EASY

Meatball Sauce #2—Always a Party Favorite!

gluten · milk · soy · egg · corn · nuts

- 1 jar (14 ounces, or 400 g) GFCF pasta sauce
- 1/3 cup (105 g) GFCF natural fruit spread—mixed berry or grape
- 1/4 cup (60 g) pureed vegetables (one or more of the following store-bought Stage 1 or 2 organic baby food: carrots, squash, yam, sweet potato, peas, green beans, beets)

In a medium saucepan, combine pasta/spaghetti sauce, fruit spread, and pureed vegetables. Bring to a boil, lower heat, and simmer for 15 minutes. Add meatballs and simmer another 15 to 30 minutes. Spear meatballs with wooden picks.

NOTE: *When beginning to add vegetables, start with 1 tablespoon (15 g) and increase as tolerated. Expand the vegetables as each addition is tolerated.*

YIELD: *2 cups (500 g)*

Calories (kcal): 258; **Total fat:** trace; **Cholesterol:** 0mg; **Carbohydrate:** 69g; **Dietary fiber:** 1g; **Protein:** 1g; **Sodium:** 43mg; **Potassium:** 82mg; **Calcium:** 21mg; **Iron:** trace; **Zinc:** trace; **Vitamin A:** 13IU

Meatballs with Vegetables

gluten · milk · soy · egg · corn · nuts

By Kathy Rivers. This recipe allows for any meat with your vegetable or vegetables of choice: beef, pork, turkey, or chicken. This dish is nice and moist, freezes well, and is great for adding to school lunches.

- 1 pound (455 g) beef, pork, turkey, or chicken
- 1 cup (240 g) ground vegetables
- Salt and pepper to taste
- Seasonings of choice

Mix meat, vegetables, and seasonings. Roll into 1½-inch (3.75-cm) meatballs and bake in a 350°F (180°C, gas mark 4) oven for 20 to 22 minutes (turning once) on a cookie sheet lined with parchment paper. These can also be formed into patties.

YIELD: *About 35 to 40 meatballs or 15 to 20 meat patties*

Calories (kcal): 40; **Total fat:** 3g; **Cholesterol:** 11mg; **Carbohydrate:** 0g; **Dietary fiber:** 0g; **Protein:** 2g; **Sodium:** 9mg; **Potassium:** 30mg; **Calcium:** 1mg; **Iron:** trace ; **Zinc:** trace ; **Vitamin A:** 0IU

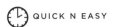

Quick N Easy Meatballs

Purchase frozen organic meatballs—check the ingredients to ensure that they are GFCF.

Nutritious, Delicious Meatballs in Sauce

 gluten   milk   soy   egg   corn   nuts

Meatballs are great for appetizers, snacks, or part of a meal. Kids love them for dipping.

The grape spread in the sauce adds a sweet and fruity taste without all the sugar found in jellies. The addition of pureed vegetables to the meatballs and the sauce makes these more nutritious and a perfect way to sneak in more vegetables.

- 1 pound (455 g) lean ground beef
- $1/2$ cup (15 g) crushed GF cornflakes or GF cracker crumbs
- $1/4$ cup (40 g) finely chopped onion
- 2 tablespoons (30 g) GFCF ketchup
- 2 tablespoons (28 ml) GFCF maple syrup
- 1 teaspoon dried thyme leaves
- 1 teaspoon salt
- $1/4$ teaspoon black pepper
- $1/4$ teaspoon chili powder
- $1/4$ cup (60 g) pureed vegetables (one or more of the following store-bought organic baby food or pureed organic fresh or frozen vegetables: carrots, squash, yam, sweet potato, peas, green beans, beets)

Preheat oven to 400°F (200°C, or gas mark 6).

Grease a baking sheet or line with parchment paper.

In a large bowl, combine beef, cornflakes, onion, ketchup, maple syrup, thyme, salt, pepper, chili powder, and pureed vegetables until well mixed. Shape into meatballs (1 tablespoon [15 g] each). Place on prepared baking sheet. Baked for 15 to 20 minutes, until nicely browned.

YIELD: *36 meatballs (1 tablespoon [15 g] each)*

Calories (kcal): 48; **Total fat:** 3g; **Cholesterol:** 11mg; **Carbohydrate:** 2g; **Dietary fiber:** trace; **Protein:** 2g; **Sodium:** 91mg; **Potassium:** 39mg; **Calcium:** 4mg; **Iron:** 1mg; **Zinc:** trace; **Vitamin A:** 47IU

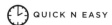

Spaghetti and Meatballs

gluten   milk   soy   egg   corn   nuts

This recipe is a good place to hide pureed or mashed vegetables.

- 1 small yellow onion
- 1 slice gluten-free rice bread
- 2 tablespoons (28 ml) water
- 1 teaspoon salt
- $^1/_2$ teaspoon oregano
- 1 pound (455 g) ground beef
- 2 jars (26 ounces, or 737 g, each) GFCF pasta sauce
- 1 pound (455 g) GF spaghetti of choice
- Extra-virgin olive oil

Put onion in a food processor and mince. Add bread, water, salt, and oregano and mix again. Pour mixture into a mixing bowl. Knead by hand together with ground beef until thoroughly mixed. Shape into desired meatball size.

Put meatballs into a slow cooker. Add spaghetti sauce and cook for 4 hours. Cook spaghetti according to package directions. Drain and sprinkle with extra-virgin olive oil and toss. Serve with meatball sauce.

OPTIONS: *Add $^1/_4$ cup (60 g) or more single or mixed vegetables (pureed or mashed) to the spaghetti sauce.*

YIELD: *4 to 6 servings*

Calories (kcal): 123 2; **Total fat:** 53g; **Cholesterol:** 97mg; **Carbohydrate:** 149g; **Dietary fiber:** 16g; **Protein:** 41g; **Sodium:** 2481 mg; **Potassium: Calcium:** 1912mg 152mg; **Iron:** 9mg; **Zinc:** 6mg; **Vitamin A:** 4535IU

Spinach Mushroom Lasagna

gluten   milk   soy   egg   corn   nuts

Adapted from Mary Frances
(www.glutenfreecookingschool.com)

Mary Frances used pureed beans as a substitute for the creamy ricotta filling in this lasagna. Not only is it gluten-free, casein-free, and soy-free, but it is also a good source of protein.

- 4 cups (946 ml) GFCF marinara sauce of choice
- ¼ cup (60 ml) olive oil, divided
- 1 pound (455 g) mushrooms, chopped
- 1 large onion, diced
- 4 cloves garlic, minced
- 2 teaspoons salt, divided
- 1 pound (455 g) frozen chopped spinach, thawed and drained
- 1 can (14 ounces, or 400g) chickpeas
- 1 can (14 ounces, or 400 g) red beans
- Water
- 2 packages GF lasagna noodles

Preheat oven to 375°F (190°C, gas mark 5). Heat 2 tablespoons (30 ml) of the oil in a large skillet over medium heat. Add mushrooms and cook until they have released their liquid. Add the onion, garlic, and 1 teaspoon salt and cook for 10 minutes, stirring occasionally. Add the spinach, reduce heat to low, and simmer until vegetables are heated through.

Drain and rinse the chickpeas and red beans. Pulse in a food processor with remaining 1 teaspoon salt 5 times, and then scrape down the side of the bowl. Add the remaining olive oil and process until smooth. Continue processing and adding 1 tablespoon (15 ml) of water at a time, until the puree is creamy and spreadable.

Spread 1 cup (235 ml) of the marinara sauce into a 9 by 13-inch baking dish. Add a layer of the dry noodles (about 4) on top. Dab one third of the bean puree on top of the noodles and spread it out with the back of a spoon or a rubber spatula. Top the bean puree with one third of the veggie mixture. Repeat 2 more times, ending with a fourth layer of noodles and sauce. Cover the lasagna with aluminum foil and bake for one hour.

YIELD: *8 servings*

Calories (kcal): 228; **Total fat:** 9g; **Cholesterol:** 0mg; **Carbohydrate:** 31g; **Dietary fiber:** 8g; **Protein:** 8g; **Sodium:** 906mg; **Potassium:** 438mg; **Calcium:** 121mg; **Iron:** 3mg; **Zinc:** 1mg; **Vitamin A:** 4223IU.

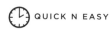

 QUICK N EASY

Quick Macaroni and Cheese

gluten   milk   soy   egg   corn   nuts

GFCF cheese doesn't melt very well and tends to lack flavor. This small tweak from Elynn DeMattia adds some salty goodness to the mix.

- 12 ounces (340 g) brown rice elbow noodles, or GFCF elbow noodles of choice
- 1¹/₂ teaspoons salt
- 1 cup GFCF chicken broth
- 1 package (8 ounces, or 225 g) GFCF cheese, grated or torn into pieces

Bring 2 quarts (2 litres) of water to a boil in a large pot. Add noodles and salt and cook according to package instructions. Drain noodles and return to pot. Over low heat, add chicken broth and cheese and stir until melted. Serve.

YIELD: *4 servings*

Calories (kcal): 485; **Total fat:** 12g; **Cholesterol:** 1mg; **Carbohydrate:** 69g; **Dietary fiber:** 10g; **Protein:** 27g; **Sodium:** 1484mg; **Potassium:** 0mg; **Calcium:** 5mg; **Iron:** 3mg; **Zinc:** 0mg; **Vitamin A:** 152IU.

Spaghetti and Marinara Sauce

gluten   milk   soy   egg   corn   nuts

Adapted from The Book of Yum *(http://www.bookofyum.com)*

- 2 tablespoons (15 ml) extra virgin olive oil
- 1 medium onion, diced
- 4 garlic cloves, minced
- ¹/₄ medium carrot, grated
- 2 cans (28-ounces, or 784 g each) peeled whole tomatoes
- ¹/₄ cup (10 g) chopped fresh basil
- Salt
- 1 pound (455 g) GFCF spaghetti of choice

In a large pot or Dutch oven, heat the oil over medium heat. Add the onion and cook until light golden brown, 8 to 10 minutes. Add the garlic and carrot and cook for 5 minutes, turning heat down if vegetables get too dark. Add tomatoes and their juices and bring mixture to a boil, stirring to break apart the tomatoes. Reduce heat and simmer on low for 30 minutes, until sauce has thickened. Add basil and salt to taste.

Meanwhile, bring a large pot of water to a boil, and cook spaghetti according to package instructions. Serve with sauce.

NOTE: *This sauce makes a great filling for vegetarian Sloppy Joes, served on GFCF hamburger buns.*

YIELD: *4 to 6 servings*

Calories (kcal): 365; **Total fat:** 6g; **Cholesterol:** 0mg; **Carbohydrate:** 76g; **Dietary fiber:** 5g; **Protein:** 5g; **Sodium:** 410mg; **Potassium:** 649mg; **Calcium:** 91mg; **Iron:** 2mg; **Zinc:** trace; **Vitamin A:** 3330IU.

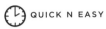 QUICK N EASY

Elynn's Quick Pizza

gluten   milk   soy   egg   corn   nuts

Adapted from Elynn Demattia

Elynn's son doesn't like any of the GFCF pizza crusts, so she came up with her own simple solution.

- 1 large (10-inch) brown rice tortilla
- ³/₄ cup (187.5 g) GFCF spaghetti sauce of choice
- ¹/₂ cup diced soy cheese
- 10 to 12 slices GFCF pepperoni

Preheat the oven to 350°F (180°C, gas mark 4). Lightly oil a baking sheet, or line with parchment paper. Place the tortilla on the baking sheet, and spread sauce on top. Sprinkle evenly with cheese, and place the pepperoni slices on top. Bake for 10 to 12 minutes, and then carefully slide the pizza from the baking sheet directly onto the rack for 2 to 3 minutes to crisp up the bottom (this is more easily done when the pizza is left on the parchment paper). Cut into wedges and serve.

YIELD: *2 to 4 servings*

Calories (kcal): 205; **Total fat:** 13g; **Cholesterol:** 21mg; **Carbohydrate:** 12g; **Dietary fiber:** 2g; **Protein:** 11g; **Sodium:** 598mg; **Potassium:** 24mg; **Calcium:** 15mg; **Iron:** 1mg; **Zinc:** 0mg; **Vitamin A:** 150IU.

Pizza with Easy Tomato Sauce

gluten milk soy egg corn nuts

Pizza sauce is an excellent way to hide pureed vegetables and meats. Add those that will be least easily detected.

- 1¹/₃ cups (185 g) garbanzo bean flour
- ¹/₂ cup (70 g) brown rice flour
- ¹/₂ cup (60 g) tapioca starch
- 1 tablespoon (8 g) and 1 teaspoon (3 g) xanthan gum
- 1 teaspoon salt
- 1 tablespoon (15 ml) oil
- 1¹/₃ cups (315 ml) water

Blend all the ingredients on low speed, then medium-high speed for 2 minutes. The dough will be sticky. Cover a pizza pan with parchment paper. Roll out dough. Bake in a 425°F (220°C, or gas mark 7) oven for 20 minutes. Add sauce (recipe to follow) and toppings and bake for another 20 minutes.

VARIATIONS: *The same recipe can be used to make pretzels or bread sticks. Cover cookie sheet with parchment paper. Place dough in cookie press. Form pretzels using nozzle with a ¹/₄- to ¹/₂-inch (0.6- to 1.25-cm) opening. Sprinkle with salt. Bake in 425°F (220°C, or gas mark 7) oven for 20 minutes. A half batch makes 1 tray of pretzels. Best eaten fresh and warm out of the oven.*

YIELD: *1 pizza (serves 6 to 8)*

Calories (kcal): 226; **Total fat:** 4g; **Cholesterol:** 0mg; **Carbohydrate:** 42g; **Dietary fiber:** 5g; **Protein:** 8g; **Sodium:** 1176mg; **Potassium:** 760mg; **Calcium:** 48mg; **Iron:** 3mg; **Zinc:** 1mg; **Vitamin A:** 1435IU

Easy Tomato Sauce

gluten milk soy egg corn nuts

- 2 cans (6 ounces, or 170 g, each) tomato paste
- 12 ounces (355 ml) water (use tomato paste cans to measure)
- 1 teaspoon salt
- 1 teaspoon onion powder
- 1 teaspoon dried basil
- 1 teaspoon dried oregano
- ¹/₈ teaspoon pepper
- ¹/₈ teaspoon garlic powder

Mix all ingredients and simmer 30 minutes.

VARIATIONS: *Add 1 tablespoon (15 g) pureed vegetables to expand nutrition. Add pureed turkey or beef to improve the protein.*

YIELD: *3 cups (750 g)*

Pizza Sauce and Crust

gluten   milk   soy   egg   corn   nuts

This recipe is tasty, even if it lacks the cheese typically associated with pizza. Having kids participate in making the recipe is not only a fun activity, it may encourage them to be more creative in their tastes. Pizza sauce is a favorite way to add hidden pureed vegetables and meats.

Pizza Sauce

- 1 can (8 ounces, or 225 g) tomato sauce
- 1 1/2 teaspoons sugar or honey
- 1 tablespoon (15 g) pureed vegetables (carrot, peas, squash)
- 1 tablespoon (15 g) pureed meat (chicken, turkey, beef)
- 1/2 teaspoon dried oregano leaves
- 1/2 teaspoon dried basil leaves
- 1/2 teaspoon crushed dried rosemary leaves
- 1/2 teaspoon fennel seed
- 1/2 teaspoon salt
- 1/4 teaspoon garlic powder

Pizza Crust

- 1 tablespoon (12 g) active dry yeast
- 2/3 cup (95 g) brown rice flour
- 1/2 cup (60 g) tapioca flour
- 2 teaspoons xanthan gum
- 1 teaspoon unflavored gelatin powder
- 1 teaspoon Italian seasoning
- 1/2 teaspoon sugar or honey
- 1/2 teaspoon salt
- 3/4 cup (175 ml) warm milk (rice or soy) (110°F [43°C])
- 1 teaspoon (5 ml) olive oil
- 1 teaspoon (5 ml) cider vinegar
- Rice flour, for sprinkling

Combine all sauce ingredients in a small saucepan. Bring to a boil over medium heat. Reduce heat to low; simmer for 15 minutes while crust is being assembled. Makes about 1 cup (250 g).

Preheat oven to 425°F (220°C, or gas mark 7). Grease a 12-inch (30-cm) pizza pan or baking sheet. In a medium mixer bowl using regular beaters (not dough hooks), blend yeast, flours, xanthan gum, gelatin powder, Italian seasoning, sugar, and salt on low speed. Add warm milk, oil, and vinegar.

Beat on high speed for 2 minutes. The dough will resemble soft bread dough. If dough is too stiff, add water 1 tablespoon (15 ml) at a time. Put mixture on a prepared pan. Liberally sprinkle rice flour onto dough, then press dough into pan, continuing to sprinkle with flour to prevent sticking to the pan. Makes edges thicker to hold the toppings.

Bake pizza crust for 10 minutes. Remove from oven. Top pizza crust with sauce and preferred toppings. Baked for another 20 to 25 minutes or until top is nicely browned.

YIELD: *Serves 6 (1 slice per serving)*

Calories (kcal): 143; **Total fat:** 2g; **Cholesterol:** 2mg; **Carbohydrate:** 30g; **Dietary fiber:** 2g; **Protein:** 3g; **Sodium:** 589mg; **Potassium:** 250mg; **Calcium:** 20mg; **Iron:** 1mg; **Zinc:** 1mg; **Vitamin A:** 409IU

🕐 QUICK N EASY

Quick N Easy Pizza Sauce & Crust

Use premade GFCF pizza sauce and pizza crust.

QUICK N EASY

Veal or Pork Scaloppini

gluten milk soy egg corn nuts

This dish tastes gourmet, yet it's incredibly easy to make.

- 4 veal or pork cutlets (1$^{1}/_{2}$ pounds, or 680 g)
- Salt and pepper to taste

Sauce

- 2 tablespoons (28 ml) olive oil
- 2 tablespoons (28 ml) fresh lemon juice
- $^{1}/_{2}$ cup (120 ml) chicken broth or white grape juice
- 2 tablespoons (28 g) ghee or $^{1}/_{2}$ teaspoon arrowroot mixed in 2 teaspoons (10 ml) water to form a paste
- 2 tablespoons (18 g) GF capers, packed in salt or salt brine, not vinegar (optional)
- 1 tablespoon dried parsley or $^{1}/_{4}$ cup (15 g) chopped fresh parsley (optional)
- $^{1}/_{8}$ teaspoon ground nutmeg (optional)

Season veal (or pork) with salt and pepper. (If using pork cutlets, pound to $^{1}/_{4}$ -inch (0.6-cm) thickness.) In a large, heavy skillet, brown meat in batches in the oil about 2 minutes on each side. Remove meat from skillet but keep warm.

To make sauce, increase skillet heat to high and add lemon juice and broth. Continue cooking until reduced by half. Add melted ghee or arrowroot paste and whisk thoroughly. Stir until liquid is reduced and thickens slightly.

To thicken the sauce, add a pinch to $^{1}/_{8}$ teaspoon arrowroot. To thin the sauce, add more broth.

VARIATIONS: *Depending on the tastes of the family, add capers, parsley, and nutmeg to the sauce and serve over rice.*

YIELD: *4 servings*

Calories (kcal): 373; **Total fat:** 25g; **Cholesterol:** 157mg; **Carbohydrate:** 1g; **Dietary fiber:** trace; **Protein:** 34g; **Sodium:** 277mg; **Potassium:** 587mg; **Calcium:** 33mg; **Iron:** 2 2mg; **Zinc:** 5mg; **Vitamin A:** 333IU

Spicy Pork Tenderloin

gluten   milk   soy   egg   corn   nuts

The ginger in this dish adds just the right flavor, moving it from ordinary to extrodinary.

- 1–3 tablespoons (3–24 g) GFCF chili powder
- 1 teaspoon salt
- $^1/_4$ teaspoon ground ginger
- $^1/_4$ teaspoon thyme
- $^1/_4$ teaspoon pepper
- 2 pork tenderloins (1 pound [455 g] each)

Combine the first five ingredients and rub over tenderloins. Cover and refrigerate 4 hours. Grill over hot heat 15 minutes per side, until juices run clear and a meat thermometer registers 155°F to 160°F (68°C–71°C).

Delicious served with a side of rice and a green salad.

YIELD: *8 servings*

Calories (kcal): 74; **Total fat:** 2g; **Cholesterol:** 37mg; **Carbohydrate:** 1g; **Dietary fiber:** 1g; **Protein:** 12g; **Sodium:** 314mg; **Potassium:** 245mg; **Calcium:** 11mg; **Iron:** 1mg; **Zinc:** 1mg; **Vitamin A:** 660IU

Seafood Dishes

 QUICK N EASY

Reddings' Really Delicious Fish

gluten   milk   soy   egg   corn   nuts

Sue and Dick Redding are experienced in the art of preparing and presenting delicious and healthy foods. They offer this easy and quick way to prepare a tasty fish dish.

- 1 pound (455 g) fish (salmon, rockfish, sea bass, white fish)
- $^1/_2$ cup (120 ml) water
- 1–2 tablespoons (8–16 g) GFCF seasoning blend for seafood

Place fish in a 9 x 13-inch (22.5 x 32.5-cm) baking dish. If desired, pan can be lined with oil-sprayed aluminum foil.

Add $^1/_2$ cup (120 ml) water to gently poach the fish. Sprinkle fish with seasoning to taste. Bake at 350°F (180°C, gas mark 4), until fish juices run clear and form a white milky curd on top of fish (approximately 30 to 45 minutes, depending on thickness of fish).

VARIATIONS: *In lieu of a seasoning blend, sprinkle salt, pepper, fresh lemon juice, herbs to taste*

YIELD: *4 servings*

Calories (kcal): 0; **Total fat:** 0g; **Cholesterol:** 0mg; **Carbohydrate:** 0g; **Dietary fiber:** 0g; **Protein:** 0g; **Sodium:** 1mg; **Potassium:** 0mg; **Calcium:** 1mg; **Iron:** trace ; **Zinc:** trace ; **Vitamin A:** 0IU

Favorite Salmon

gluten   milk   soy   egg   corn   nuts

Salmon is an excellent source of low-fat protein, plus the essential omega-3 fatty acids EPA and DHA, which are so important to those with autism spectrum issues, skin conditions, and immune problems. These good fats help with immunity and brain development and function and improve skin health. Avoid farm-raised and buy wild, ocean sockeye salmon, which has a natural orange color from eating the smaller fish that feed on algae rich in EPA and DHA.

Seasoning Rub Ingredients

- 3 tablespoons (60 g) honey or (45 ml) maple syrup
- 1 teaspoon ground cumin
- 1 teaspoon ground coriander
- 1 teaspoon (5 ml) hot water
- $3/4$ teaspoon grated fresh lime peel
- $3/4$ teaspoon salt
- $1/4$ teaspoon coarsely ground black pepper

Main Ingredients

- 4 fillets (6 ounces, or 170 g, each) salmon, skin on
- 3 tablespoons (12 g) chopped fresh cilantro

Preheat a grill pan or prepare an outdoor grill for covered, direct grilling over medium heat.

Stir together the seasoning rub until well blended. Rub mixture over fillets.

Place salmon fillets, skin-side up, on hot grill pan or rack and cook 4 minutes. Use a wide spatula to turn salmon over. Cook until opaque throughout (4 to 5 minutes longer.)

Sprinkle salmon with cilantro and serve with lime wedges.

YIELD: *4 servings*

Calories (kcal): 248; **Total fat:** 6g; **Cholesterol:** 88mg; **Carbohydrate:** 13g; **Dietary fiber:** trace; **Protein:** 34g; **Sodium:** 516mg; **Potassium:** 573mg; **Calcium:** 32mg; **Iron:** 2mg; **Zinc:** 1mg ; **Vitamin A:** 259IU

Deviled Crab

gluten   milk   soy   egg   corn   nuts

Fresh lump crabmeat is the best for this dish.

- 3 tablespoons (45 g) ghee or GFCF no-trans-fats spread
- 2 teaspoons GF flour mix
- 1 cup (235 ml) soy or rice milk, heated
- 1 teaspoon salt
- Dash cayenne pepper
- 1/4 teaspoon GFCF Old Bay seasoning
- 1 teaspoon GFCF Worcestershire sauce
- 1/4 teaspoon GFCF mustard
- 2 egg yolks, slightly beaten
- 2 cups (250 g) lump crabmeat (fresh)
- 1/2 teaspoon lemon juice

Preheat oven to 450°F (230°C, or gas mark 8).

In a medium saucepan, melt the ghee and stir in the flour mix and milk. Add the salt, pepper, Old Bay, Worcestershire sauce, and mustard. Add the egg yolks and cook over medium-high heat, stirring constantly until the mixture starts to thicken. Add the crab and cook until the sauce is thickened and the crab is hot. Remove from heat and stir in the lemon.

Spoon the mixture into 4 single-serving baking shells or ramekins. Bake about 20 to 25 minutes until brown.

YIELD: *4 servings*

Calories (kcal): 205; **Total fat:** 15g; **Cholesterol:** 185mg; **Carbohydrate:** 3g; **Dietary fiber:** 1g; **Protein:** 15g; **Sodium:** 752mg; **Potassium:** 325mg; **Calcium:** 79mg; **Iron:** 1mg; **Zinc:** 3mg; **Vitamin A:** 591IU

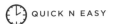 QUICK N EASY

Simple Crab Supreme

gluten   milk   soy   egg   corn   nuts

This can be served as a main dish in individual servings or in a casserole. Dana's family loves this best served as an appetizer with GFCF rice crackers or rice almond crackers.

- 2 cups (1 pound [455 g]) backfin lump crabmeat
- 1 teaspoon GFCF Old Bay seasoning
- 1 teaspoon minced garlic
- 1/2 cup (115 g) GFCF mayonnaise

Preheat oven to 350°F (180°C, gas mark 4).

Drain the crabmeat and gently sort to remove any shell pieces. Try to leave the crabmeat in lumps.

Mix the seasoning and minced garlic into the mayonnaise.

Add the mayonnaise mix just enough to moisten the crabmeat. Use less or more of the mayonnaise mix as needed.

Place in an ovenproof casserole dish and bake at 350°F (180°C, gas mark 4) for 20 to 30 minutes or until there is a touch of golden brown on top. The crab mixture can also be baked in individual ramekins (1/2 cup [145 g] each).

YIELD: *4 servings (1/2 cup [145 g] each)*

Calories (kcal): 257; **Total fat:** 24g; **Cholesterol:** 62mg; **Carbohydrate:** trace; **Dietary fiber:** trace; **Protein:** 13g; **Sodium:** 371 mg; **Potassium:** 234mg; **Calcium:** 66mg; **Iron:** 1mg; **Zinc:** 2mg; **Vitamin A:** 80IU

Fish Pockets

gluten milk soy egg corn nuts

This is a really healthy way to cook healthy fish! Essentially steaming in its own juices, the fish can be served right in the pocket—a nice sensory experience for some. You can really use any fish fillet (skin removed) for this recipe, but reduce the cooking time if they are very thin.

- 4 cod fillets, 6 ounces (170 g) each
- 8 sprigs of cilantro
- 1 piece fresh ginger, 1 1/2 inches (4 cm) long, peeled and cut into thin matchsticks
- Olive oil
- Salt and pepper to taste

Preheat oven to 425°F (220°C, gas mark 7). Cut 4 pieces of parchment paper, at least 12 by 14-inches (30 by 35 cm). Fold each piece in half to form a 12 by 7-inch (30 by 17.5 cm) piece; unfold.

Brush one side of paper with olive oil. Place one-quarter of the ginger pieces on the oiled side. Pat each piece of fish dry, season with salt and pepper, and place on top of the ginger. Place a couple of sprigs of cilantro on top of each fillet, and then fold over the parchment paper. Seal the 3 open sides well by folding them up over themselves, leaving a small amount of space inside the pocket for steam. Place the 4 pockets in a baking dish, and cook for 15 to 20 minutes (cut into 1 pocket to check doneness of fish), until fish is cooked through, opaque, and flaky. Serve in the pockets, or transfer to a plate (leaving the ginger behind).

TIP: *You can add some simple, quick-cooking vegetables to the pockets as well. Snap peas, thinly sliced carrots, zucchini, and tomatoes all work well, and lemon slices placed over the fish can add a lot of flavor too.*

YIELD: *4 servings*

Calories (kcal): 154; **Total fat:** 1g; **Cholesterol:** 73mg; **Carbohydrate:** 3g; **Dietary fiber:** trace; **Protein:** 31g; **Sodium:** 100mg; **Potassium:** 889mg; **Calcium:** 73mg; **Iron:** 2mg; **Zinc:** 1mg; **Vitamin A:** 765IU.

Vegetarian Protein Main Dishes

Lentil Loaf

gluten   milk   soy   egg   corn   nuts

From the Great Sage Restaurant. This is a staple for the vegetarian, GFCF diet. Serve with mashed potatoes and a vegetable for an updated version of a classic meal.

- 3 cups (600 g) lentils
- 4 bay leaves
- 2 tablespoons (28 ml) canola oil
- 1¹/₂ cups (240 g) diced yellow onions
- 1 cup (100 g) walnuts, toasted, cooled, and chopped
- ¹/₂ cup (60 g) finely ground rice white bread (or GF bread crumbs)
- 1 cup (165 g) cooked brown rice
- 1¹/₂ teaspoons sea salt
- ¹/₄ cup (60 ml) GF tamari
- 1¹/₂ tablespoons (15 g) minced garlic
- 2¹/₂ cups (625 g) barbeque sauce, divided
- ¹/₂ cup (120 g) GFCF ketchup
- 1 tablespoon (3 g) dried thyme
- 1 tablespoon (2 g) dried sage
- ¹/₂ teaspoon black pepper

Preheat oven to 350°F (180°C, gas mark 4). Lightly oil two 6-cup (1.4 L) loaf pans and place parchment on the bottom.

Lentils:

Wash lentils in a bowl of water, removing any broken ones that float to the top. Drain and rinse. Place lentils and bay leaves in a large pot and fill with enough water to cover lentils by 2 inches (5 cm). Place over medium heat and bring to a rolling boil.

Reduce heat to low and simmer 45 minutes, or until tender. Stir often and add water as needed, always keeping the water level 2 inches (5 cm) above lentils.

When the lentils are tender, remove from heat and drain well. Spread the lentils out on a baking sheet and chill in the refrigerator for 30 minutes to 1 hour. Remove bay leaves and transfer lentils to a mixer.

In a medium sauté pan, heat oil over medium-high heat. Add onion and sauté until tender and lightly browned, about 10 minutes. Transfer onions to the mixer with the lentils, and add the ground walnuts, bread crumbs, cooked rice, salt, tamari, garlic, ¹/₂ cup (125 g) barbeque sauce, ketchup, thyme, sage, and black pepper. Mix until all ingredients are well combined and the lentils are somewhat mashed. Turn mixer off and stir from the bottom with a rubber spatula. Combine well.

Transfer the mixture to the oiled loaf pans. Fill within ¹/₂ inch (1.25 cm) from top and smooth with a spatula. Cover the tops with parchment paper. Bake for 35 to 40 minutes or until browned around the edges and firm in the middle. Remove the parchment paper and spread 2 cups (500 g) of barbeque sauce over the loaves. Put back in oven, uncovered, for about 6 minutes or until set. Remove from oven and place on a cooling rack for about 1 hour. If not properly cooled, loaves will fall apart easily. Gently tap out of pans onto their sides. Cut each into 10 slices.

YIELD: *2 small loaves; serves 10 people (10 slices)*

Calories (kcal): 415; **Total fat:** 12g; **Cholesterol:** 0mg; **Carbohydrate:** 58g; **Dietary fiber:** 20g; **Protein:** 23g; **Sodium:** 1390mg; **Potassium:** 839mg; **Calcium:** 86mg; **Iron:** 8mg; **Zinc:** 3mg; **Vitamin A:** 755IU

Dahl (Vegetarian and with Chicken)

gluten   milk   soy   egg   corn   nuts

This traditional vegetarian dish from India is adapted from Lizzie Vann's Organic Baby & Toddler Cookbook. *The nonvegetarian version uses added chicken, which expands protein. This recipe can be served pureed.*

- 3 tablespoons (45 ml) good-quality safflower, light olive, or avocado oil
- 3 small onions, finely chopped
- $3/4$ teaspoon turmeric
- $1/2$ tablespoon ground coriander or cumin seeds
- $1^1/2$ cups (300 g) red lentils, washed and picked over
- 3 carrots, finely chopped
- $3^3/4$ cups (885 ml) water or 2 cups (475 ml) water and $1^3/4$ (410 ml) cup chicken broth (store-bought or homemade)
- $1/3$ cup (25 g) shredded cabbage
- 2 ounces (55 g) cooked chicken breast, shredded (optional)

Heat the oil in a pan over medium heat. Add the onion and fry gently until soft, about 5 minutes. Mix in the spices and cook for another 2 minutes.

Add the lentils, carrots, and water and bring to a boil. Reduce the heat and simmer for 20 minutes, until the lentils are soft and the dahl has a smooth consistency. Add the cabbage and chicken (optional) and cook for another 5 minutes, stirring from time to time.

YIELD: *4 servings ($1/2$ cup [125 g] each)*

Calories (kcal): 392; **Total fat:** 11g; **Cholesterol:** 0mg; **Carbohydrate:** 55g; **Dietary fiber:** 25g; **Protein:** 22g; **Sodium:** 37mg; **Potassium:** 989mg; **Calcium:** 80mg; **Iron:** 7mg; **Zinc:** 3mg; **Vitamin A:** 15225IU

Jonathan's Falafel

gluten milk soy egg corn nuts

Leonardo Hosh provides this tasty recipe enjoyed by his son Jonathan. This recipe is also in the Rice and Beans chapter as a side dish, but it can be a main dish as well.

- 2 pounds (905 g) dry garbanzo beans
- 1 bunch parsley (about 1 cup [60 g] finely chopped)
- 1 medium potato
- 1 medium onion
- Garlic salt to taste
- $^1/_8$ teaspoon baking soda
- $^1/_4$ teaspoon salt
- 3 cups (710 ml) canola or vegetable oil for deep-frying

Soak garbanzo beans in water for two days; drain and change water several times throughout.

Clean the parsley and potato and peel onion. Rough chop all three and place in a food processor.

Add the beans to the processor and grind until fine and homogeneous in color. Add garlic salt if desired.

Divide the mixture into serving sizes (approximately 1 cup [250 g] portions) and freeze for later use.

To cook, thaw the mixture, add to each 1-cup (250 g) batch: $^1/_8$ teaspoon baking soda and $^1/_4$ teaspoon salt and mix well.

Form into bite-size balls (may use a small ice cream scoop). Heat oil to 375° (185°C), and deep-fry the balls in hot canola or vegetable oil until they turn golden. They are best served immediately after deep-frying.

VARIATION: *Other seasonings can be added if desired:*

- *1 tablespoon (7 g) ground coriander*
- *1 tablespoon (7 g) ground cumin*
- *1 teaspoon cayenne pepper*

YIELD: *12 bite-size balls per cup*

Calories (kcal): 309; **Total fat:** 7g; **Cholesterol:** 0mg; **Carbohydrate:** 49g; **Dietary fiber:** 14g; **Protein:** 15g; **Sodium:** 79mg; **Potassium:** 759mg; **Calcium:** 89mg; **Iron:** 5mg; **Zinc:** 3mg; **Vitamin A:** 311IU

CHAPTER 14

Rice and Beans

Beans are proteins and good with spice;
They go together quite well with rice.

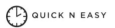

QUICK N EASY

Coconut Jasmine Rice

gluten   milk   soy   egg   corn   nuts

Both simple to make and elegant to serve, this recipe is a delicious variation from the usual rice dishes.

- 1 cup (195 g) jasmine rice
- 2 cups (475 ml) water
- $^1/_4$ cup (60 ml) coconut milk
- Sea salt to taste
- $^1/_4$ teaspoon tarragon

Cook rice in water according to package directions. Stir in coconut milk, salt, and tarragon.

YIELD: *2 servings*

Calories (kcal): 407; **Total fat:** 8g; **Cholesterol:** 0mg; **Carbohydrate:** 76g; **Dietary fiber:** 2g; **Protein:** 7g; **Sodium:** 16mg; **Potassium:** 191mg; **Calcium:** 38mg; **Iron:** 5mg; **Zinc:** 1mg; **Vitamin A:** 8IU

Brown Rice Pilaf

gluten   milk   soy   egg   corn   nuts

With the added vegetables, this provides a nice side dish.

- 1 cup (190 g) brown rice
- 1 tablespoon (15 ml) extra-virgin olive oil, divided
- $^1/_2$ cup (80 g) chopped onion
- $^1/_4$ cup (25 g) chopped celery
- $^1/_4$ cup (35 g) chopped carrots
- 1 medium garlic clove, minced
- $^1/_4$ cup (35 g) raisins
- $^1/_2$ teaspoon dried sage leaves
- $^1/_2$ teaspoon dried thyme leaves
- $^1/_4$ teaspoon black pepper
- $2^1/_2$ cups (570 ml) chicken stock (store-bought or homemade, see page 199)
- 1 bay leaf

Place rice and half of the oil in a heavy saucepan. Sauté rice over medium heat, stirring frequently, until lightly browned (about 5 minutes). Remove rice from pan. Place remaining oil in a saucepan and sauté onion, celery, and carrots over medium heat until tender, about 5 to 8 minutes.

Add remaining ingredients and bring to a boil. Cover, reduce heat, and simmer mixture for 50 minutes or until liquid is absorbed. Discard bay leaf before serving.

YIELD: *4 servings ($^1/_2$ cup [85 g] each)*

Calories (kcal): 267; **Total fat:** 6g; **Cholesterol:** 0mg; **Carbohydrate:** 47g; **Dietary fiber:** 2g; **Protein:** 7g; **Sodium:** 490mg; **Potassium:** 410mg; **Calcium:** 42mg; **Iron:** 2 2mg; **Zinc:** 1mg; **Vitamin A:** 2285IU

Colorful Celebration Rice

 gluten   milk   soy   egg   corn   nuts

This is a clever recipe children will enjoy making. The apple adds natural sweetness to the mixture.

- 1¹/₂ cups (280 g) uncooked long-grain brown rice (plain or basmati)
- 2¹/₂ cups (570 ml) chicken broth (store-bought or homemade, see page 199)
- ¹/₄ cup (35 g) peas, fresh and lightly steamed, or frozen
- ¹/₄ cup (40 g) corn, fresh and uncooked, or frozen
- ¹/₄ cup (18 g) chopped broccoli, steamed or blanched until just tender
- ¹/₄ cup (35 g) diced carrots, steamed or blanched until just tender
- 1 scallion, trimmed of roots, sliced into thin rounds (white and green parts)
- GFCF soy sauce
- Sea salt

Combine the rice and chicken broth in a saucepan and bring to a boil. Turn the heat to the lowest simmer, cover the pot, and cook undisturbed for 40 minutes, or until the rice is tender. Remove from the heat and fluff with a fork to let the steam escape, and transfer to a bowl. This can also be cooked in a rice cooker for the same amount of time.

If using frozen peas or corn, place each in a strainer or a colander and run under room-temperature tap water to thaw. Drain thoroughly and cook until tender. Combine the vegetables and rice and reheat if necessary. Let children help with this recipe and serve themselves. Place rice and all vegetables in separate bowls, letting the children create their own mixtures.

Add a few drops of soy sauce and sea salt to taste.

VARIATIONS: *Expand the vegetables to include red and green peppers if desired. Increase the amount of vegetables and decrease the rice.*

YIELD: *5 or 6 servings*

Calories (kcal): 245; **Total fat:** 2g; **Cholesterol:** 0mg; **Carbohydrate:** 48g; **Dietary fiber:** 2g; **Protein:** 8g; **Sodium:** 595mg; **Potassium:** 344mg; **Calcium:** 32mg; **Iron:** 2mg; **Zinc:** 1mg; **Vitamin A:** 1956IU

Coconut Sweet Rice

gluten   milk   soy   egg   corn   nuts

This cinnamon in this sweet rice variation makes this dish quite tasty.

- 1 cup (235 ml) water
- 1 cup (190 g) short-grain brown rice
- ½ cup (70 g) raisins or currants
- 1 cinnamon stick
- 1 cup (235 ml) coconut milk
- ¼ teaspoon turmeric

Boil water. Add rice and bring back to a boil. Reduce heat and simmer for 10 minutes. Add raisins or currants, cinnamon stick, coconut milk, and turmeric. Cook an additional 20 minutes or until water has evaporated.

YIELD: *2 servings*

Calories (kcal): 747; **Total fat:** 32g; **Cholesterol:** 0mg; **Carbohydrate:** 113g; **Dietary fiber:** 9g; **Protein:** 11g; **Sodium:** 32mg; **Potassium:** 884mg; **Calcium:** 155mg; **Iron:** 7mg; **Zinc:** 3mg; **Vitamin A:** 21IU

Rice Fruit Pudding

gluten   milk   soy   egg   corn   nuts

This is an excellent way to incorporate new fruits. It is best to start with a fruit the child already prefers, then gradually include others.

- 1 cup (235 ml) water
- ¼ cup (190 g) short-grain white or basmati rice (rinsed)
- Pinch of salt
- ¼ cup (40 g) fruit—one kind or mixed (cut up pears, peaches, apricots)
- 2 tablespoons (30 g) soy yogurt

Bring the water to a boil in a small pan. Add the rice and simmer gently for 15 minutes, stirring occasionally to prevent sticking.

Add the fruit(s) and simmer for about 5 minutes.

Puree the mixture by pushing through a sieve or by using a blender. Stir in the yogurt, and add more water if a thinner consistency is preferred.

YIELD: *About 2 to 4 servings, depending on the age and appetite of the child*

Calories (kcal): 46; **Total fat:** trace; **Cholesterol:** 0mg; **Carbohydrate:** 9g; **Dietary fiber:** trace; **Protein:** 1g; **Sodium:** 36mg; **Potassium:** 13mg; **Calcium:** 5mg; **Iron:** 1mg; **Zinc:** trace; **Vitamin A:** 0IU

Red or Black Beans and Rice

gluten   milk   soy   egg   corn   nuts

Beans

- ¹/₂ cup Sofrito (page 131)
- ¹/₄ cup (60 ml) extra-virgin olive oil
- 4 cans (15 ounces, or 420 g, each) organic beans, drained
- ¹/₂ can (3 ounces, or 85 g) tomato paste
- 3 cups (710 ml) chicken broth
- Salt to taste
- 3 bay leaves (only if using black beans)

Sauté Sofrito in oil. Add remaining ingredients. Cook on medium heat for 15 minutes. Reduce heat to low, cover, and simmer for 10 minutes.

Rice

Arborio rice is particularly tasty with this bean recipe.

- 2 cups (400 g) Arborio rice
- 2¹/₂ cups (570 ml) water or chicken broth
- Salt to taste
- 2 tablespoons (28 ml) extra-virgin olive oil

Mix rice, water or chicken broth, salt, and oil in a medium saucepan. Cook on medium-high until most of the liquid evaporates, about 5 minutes. Reduce heat to low, stir, and cover. Cook until rice is soft.

YIELD: *6 to 8 servings beans and rice*

Calories (kcal): 650; **Total fat:** 18g; **Cholesterol:** 0mg; **Carbohydrate:** 94g; **Dietary fiber:** 18g; **Protein:** 25g; **Sodium:** 1749mg; **Potassium:** 523mg; **Calcium:** 41mg; **Iron:** 4mg; **Zinc:** 1mg; **Vitamin A:** 593IU

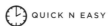 QUICK N EASY

Spicy Black Beans and Rice

gluten   milk   soy   egg   corn   nuts

This simple version of black beans and rice is ideal for busy parents trying to put dinner on the table quickly.

- ¹/₂ cup (80 g) chopped onion
- 4 cloves garlic, minced
- 2 tablespoons (28 ml) olive oil
- 1 can (15 ounces, 420 g) black beans, rinsed and drained
- 1 can (14.5 ounces, 411 g) Mexican-style stewed tomatoes
- ¹/₈–¹/₄ teaspoon ground red pepper
- 2 cups (330 g) hot cooked brown or long-grain rice

In a medium saucepan, cook onion and garlic in hot oil until tender but not brown. Carefully stir in beans, undrained tomatoes, and ground red pepper. Bring to a boil and reduce heat. Simmer uncovered for 15 minutes.

To serve, mound rice on serving plates and make a well in each mound. Spoon the black bean mixture into the wells. If desired, sprinkle with ¹/₄ cup (40 g) chopped onion.

YIELD: *4 servings*

Calories (kcal): 310; **Total fat:** 8g; **Cholesterol:** 0mg; **Carbohydrate:** 50g; **Dietary fiber:** 8g; **Protein:** 10g; **Sodium:** 357mg; **Potassium:** 324mg; **Calcium:** 54mg; **Iron:** 1mg; **Zinc:** 1mg; **Vitamin A:** 562IU

Homemade Refried Beans

gluten   milk   soy   egg   corn   nuts

Note that lard can be used and is much healthier to use than any hydrogenated oil; however, canola or olive oil can also be used.

- 2 cups (500 g) dried pinto beans
- 6 cups (1.4 L) water
- 2 cups (475 ml) chicken broth
- 1 teaspoon salt
- ¹/₄ teaspoon dried and crumbled oregano (optional)
- ¹/₈–¹/₄ cup (28–55 g) lard (bacon drippings) or (28–60 ml) canola oil or olive oil
- 1 medium onion, peeled and minced or finely chopped
- 1–2 tablespoons (10–20 g) minced garlic (optional)

Go through the beans thoroughly, removing stones or bad beans.

Place beans in a strainer and rinse well under cold water. Put beans, water, and broth into a large pot and bring to a boil. Skim any gray foam from the surface.

Lower the heat to medium and let the beans simmer rapidly for 30 minutes. Add the salt and any other seasoning.

Continue to simmer for another 1¹/₂ hours or until beans are very soft.

In a large skillet, heat lard or oil over medium heat. Add onion and garlic and sauté until almost golden.

Increase heat to medium-high and add 1 cup (100 g) of the beans and some of their cooking liquid.

Using a potato masher, mash the beans in the pan while they fry. Additional bean-cooking liquid or water may be necessary to keep the beans hydrated and not too dry. The consistency should be smooth, with some small chunks of whole beans mixed in.

Serve in a bowl or use as part of a recipe that calls for refried beans.

NOTE: *If the chunks of beans are a problem for those with texture issues, mash more thoroughly to make the mixture much more uniform in consistency.*

YIELD: *8 servings (¹/₄ cup [60 g] each)*

Calories (kcal): 240; **Total fat:** 7g; **Cholesterol:** 6mg; **Carbohydrate:** 33g; **Dietary fiber:** 12g; **Protein:** 12g; **Sodium:** 468mg; **Potassium:** 723mg; **Calcium:** 73mg; **Iron:** 3 3mg; **Zinc:** 1mg; **Vitamin A:** 6IU

White Bean Ratatouille

gluten   milk   soy   egg   corn   nuts

This recipe pleases parents and kids alike. The cooked peppers make it sweeter and kid-friendly.

- 3 tablespoons (45 ml) olive oil
- 1 onion, diced
- 6 cloves garlic, minced
- Salt to taste
- Pepper to taste
- Dried oregano to taste
- Red chili flakes (optional)
- 1 red pepper, diced
- 1 yellow or orange pepper, diced
- 1 sprig fresh rosemary, leaves stripped from stem
- 2 fresh sage leaves, chopped
- 1 zucchini, diced
- 1 small to medium eggplant, peeled and diced
- 1 cup (225 g) white beans, cooked or canned
- 15 kalamata olives (optional)
- 6 basil leaves, chopped
- 1 bag (10 ounces, or 280 g) prewashed spinach

Heat oil in a deep skillet. Add onion and garlic and sauté until soft. Add salt, pepper, oregano, chili flakes, peppers, rosemary, and sage and sauté until soft. Add zucchini and eggplant and sauté until soft. Add beans (and olives, if using) and stir. Add basil and spinach and sauté until wilted.

Serve over GFCF pasta or rice.

YIELD: *4 to 6 servings*

Calories (kcal): 276; **Total fat:** 15g; **Cholesterol:** 0mg; **Carbohydrate:** 31g; **Dietary fiber:** 10g; **Protein:** 9g; **Sodium:** 290mg; **Potassium:** 1202mg; **Calcium:** 151mg; **Iron:** 5 5mg; **Zinc:** 1mg; **Vitamin A:** 6841IU

Happy Hummus

gluten　milk　soy　egg　corn　nuts

This popular and traditional recipe was sent in by several of our parents.
It can be used for dipping or on a sandwich.

- 2 cups (480 g) chickpeas, cooked or canned
- 1/3 cup (80 ml) fresh lemon juice
- 1/4 cup (65 g) tahini
- 2 cloves garlic, minced or pressed
- 1 tablespoon (15 ml) extra-virgin olive oil
- 1 teaspoon paprika or cayenne pepper
- 1/4 cup (60 ml) or more water
- Salt to taste

Drain and rinse the chickpeas. Place in a blender or food processor with the lemon juice, tahini, minced garlic, oil, and paprika. Blend well, adding water as needed to form a smooth paste. (Add less water to make a thicker hummus for sandwich spread.) Add salt to taste.

Place hummus in a covered container. It tastes best if it is refrigerated before serving.

Spread on GFCF bread for sandwiches or serve with GFCF crackers or raw vegetables for dipping.

YIELD: *Makes about 3 cups (750 g)*

Calories (kcal): 108; **Total fat:** 52g; **Cholesterol:** 0mg; **Carbohydrate:** 132g; **Dietary fiber:** 28g; **Protein:** 35g; **Sodium:** 1509mg; **Potassium:** 1253mg; **Calcium:** 431 mg; **Iron:** 13mg; **Zinc:** 8mg; **Vitamin A:** 1566IU

Quinoa Veggie Sauté

gluten   milk   soy   egg   corn   nuts

Adapted from Lisa Barnes of Petit Appetit

Quinoa is an ancient grain with a nutty flavor and light texture, similar to couscous. Quinoa is a valuable source of protein (ounce for ounce it has as much protein as meat), which makes this not only a colorful dish side, but a viable and healthy main course as well. You can find quinoa in a box near the rice or in the bulk section of specialty and organic grocers.

- $^1/_2$ cup (85 g) quinoa
- 2 tablespoons (30 ml) olive oil, divided
- $1^1/_2$ cups (355 ml) water
- $^1/_2$ teaspoon salt
- $^1/_2$ teaspoon black pepper
- $^1/_2$ cup (80 g) chopped onion
- 1 cup (8 ounces, or 120 g) grated zucchini
- 2 tablespoons (19 g) currants
- $^1/_2$ teaspoon ground cumin
- 2 tablespoons (30 ml) fresh lemon juice
- 1 tablespoon (4 g) chopped fresh parsley
- $^1/_2$ teaspoon minced fresh basil

Preheat oven to 375°F (190°C, gas mark 5). In a small saucepan combine the quinoa in 1 tablespoon olive oil to coat. Add water, salt, and pepper and bring to a boil over medium-high heat. Cover and simmer over low heat for 20 minutes. Quinoa will be translucent when fully cooked. Remove from heat.

Pour remaining tablespoon of olive oil into a large skillet and sauté onion, zucchini, currents, and cumin over medium-high heat for 3 to 5 minutes, or until onions are translucent. Add lemon juice, parsley, basil, and mix to combine. Add quinoa to the pan and mix thoroughly until heated throughout.

YIELD: *4 servings*

Calories (kcal): 168; **Total fat:** 8g; **Cholesterol:** 0mg; **Carbohydrate:** 22g; **Dietary fiber:** 2g; **Protein:** 4g; **Sodium:** 277mg; **Potassium:** 329mg; **Calcium:** 34mg; **Iron:** 3mg; **Zinc:** 1mg; **Vitamin A:** 167IU.

Curried Quinoa Sauté

gluten   milk   soy   egg   corn   nuts

- ¹/₂ cup (85g) quinoa
- Salt
- 1 tablespoon (15 ml) safflower oil
- 1 medium yellow onion, finely diced
- 1 tablespoon (6.3 g) curry powder
- 1 cup (71 g) chopped broccoli
- 1 cup (100 g) chopped cauliflower
- 1 cup (130 g) frozen peas
- 1 medium red bell pepper, diced
- ¹/₂ cup (120 ml) GFCF chicken broth or water

To cook the quinoa: Place quinoa, 1 cup (235 ml) water, and ¹/₈ teaspoon salt in medium saucepan. Cover and bring to a boil over high heat, then reduce heat to medium-low and cook for 10 minutes, until quinoa is tender and translucent.

For the sauté: In large sauté pan, heat oil over medium-high heat. Add onion, ¹/₄ teaspoon salt, and curry powder and cook for 3 minutes, or until soft. Add remaining vegetables, and cook for another 3 minutes. Add broth, cover pan, and cook for 5 minutes. When vegetables are tender, add quinoa and stir to combine. Serve.

YIELD: *4 servings*

Calories (kcal): 178; **Total fat:** 6g; **Cholesterol:** 1mg; **Carbohydrate:** 27g; **Dietary fiber:** 6g; **Protein:** 7g; **Sodium:** 133mg; **Potassium:** 478mg; **Calcium:** 52mg; **Iron:** 3mg; **Zinc:** 1mg; **Vitamin A:** 809IU.

Edamame Succotash

gluten   milk   soy   egg   corn   nuts

This is a slight twist in the original Southern dish, but feel free to use the more traditional lima beans in place of the edamame (baby soybeans) if you are trying to avoid soy.

- 2 tablespoons (30 ml) safflower or canola oil
- 2 scallions, finely chopped
- 1 clove garlic, minced
- 2 cups (450 g) cooked corn kernels
- 2 cups (340 g) cooked, shelled edamame (soybeans)
- ¹/₂ teaspoon salt
- ¹/₄ teaspoon freshly ground black pepper
- 1 cup (150 g) grape or cherry tomatoes, halved or quartered
- ¹/₄ cup (10 g) basil leaves, torn or chopped

Heat oil in a skillet over medium heat; add scallions, garlic, corn, edamame, and salt and pepper and gently cook until heated through, about 5 minutes. Add tomatoes and basil and let cool completely. Serve chilled or at room temperature.

YIELD: *4 servings*

Calories (kcal): 326; **Total fat:** 16g; **Cholesterol:** 0mg; **Carbohydrate:** 33g; **Dietary fiber:** 8g; **Protein:** 19g; **Sodium:** 294mg; **Potassium:** 1028mg; **Calcium:** 16mg; **Iron:** 1mg; **Zinc:** trace; **Vitamin A:** 306IU.

Polenta

gluten   milk   soy   egg   corn   nuts

Polenta is simply cornmeal porridge—naturally gluten-free and a great accompaniment to saucy dishes. It is a traditional staple food throughout much of northern Italy but also popular (under other names) in Switzerland, Austria, Bosnia, Croatia, Cuba, Hungary, Romania, Corsica, Africa, Argentina, Uruguay, Brazil, Peru, Venezuela, Haiti, Mexico and Turkey.

- 1 cup (140 g) coarsely ground cornmeal
- 1 tsp salt
- 1 quart (1 litre) water

In a large pot, bring the water and salt to a boil. Reduce the heat to low and slowly add cornmeal, whisking constantly to avoid lumps. Cover and cook, stirring occasionally, for 30 minutes or until polenta is thick and creamy. Serve immediately.

TIP: *Ways to use polenta*

Polenta can be used instead of mashed potatoes or rice—with roasted chicken, sliced meat, shrimp, fish, or scallops. It can be embellished with your own mix of chopped fresh or dried herbs, garlic, chopped arugula or spinach, roasted red peppers, olives, and more. Dress it up with lots of veggies and pile them on top or mix them in and serve it casserole style.

NOTE: *For fried, sautéed, or grilled polenta, spread hot polenta into a greased 8-inch square baking dish and chill until set. Then cut into pieces and cook as desired. This can be used as the base for appetizers or snacks topped with pesto (has nuts), chopped tomatoes, olives, hummus or chicken salad.*

YIELD: *4 servings*

Calories (kcal): 126; **Total fat:** 1g; **Cholesterol:** 0mg; **Carbohydrate:** 27g; **Dietary fiber:** 3g; **Protein:** 3g; **Sodium:** 541mg; **Potassium:** 56mg; **Calcium:** 10mg; **Iron:** 1mg; **Zinc:** trace; **Vitamin A:** 142IU.

Baked Grits

gluten   milk   soy   egg   corn   nuts

Crumbled sausage can be substituted for the bacon, and feel free to vary the vegetables. Do not use the quick-cooking grits.

- 6 cups (1.4 L) water
- Salt
- 1^1/$_2$ cups (235 g) stone-ground yellow grits
- ^{1}/$_2$ pound (225 g) nitrate-free bacon, cut into ^{1}/$_2$-inch pieces
- 1 medium onion, chopped
- 2 cups (170 g) sliced mushrooms
- 1 red bell pepper, cored, seeded, and chopped
- 3 cups (90g) baby spinach
- 3 scallions, thinly sliced
- 4 large eggs, lightly beaten
- ^{1}/$_2$ teaspoon ground black pepper

In a large pot, bring water and 1 teaspoon salt to a boil; slowly pour in grits, while stirring constantly. Reduce heat and simmer 30 minutes or until thick, stirring frequently.

Preheat oven to 350°F (180°C, gas mark 4). Grease a 9 by 13-inch (23 by 33 cm) baking pan.

Meanwhile, cook bacon in a large skillet over medium heat until browned and crisp, 5 to 8 minutes. Transfer bacon with a slotted spoon to a paper towel-lined plate. Pour off all but 2 tablespoons (30 ml) fat, add onions and mushrooms and cook until onions have softened and mushroom liquid has evaporated, 5 to 8 minutes. Add peppers, spinach, and scallions and cook until tender, 2 to 4 minutes.

When the grits are done, stir in the vegetables, eggs, and pepper off heat. Pour the mixture into the prepared pan and smooth out the top. Sprinkle the top with the reserved bacon and bake 30 to 40 minutes. Cool on rack 20 minutes before serving.

YIELD: *8 servings*

Calories (kcal): 296; **Total fat:** 16g; **Cholesterol:** 127mg; **Carbohydrate:** 27g; **Dietary fiber:** 2g; **Protein:** 11g; **Sodium:** 304mg; **Potassium:** 263mg; **Calcium:** 37mg; **Iron:** 2mg; **Zinc:** 1mg; **Vitamin A:** 1159IU.

Kasha Pilaf with Mushrooms

gluten   milk   soy   egg   corn   nuts

Kasha is a traditional Slavic porridge almost always made with toasted buckwheat groats. The mushrooms can be omitted.

- ¼ cup (60 ml) olive oil, divided
- 1 pound (455 g) mushrooms, cleaned and sliced
- 1 small onion
- Salt
- 1 cup (200 g) Kasha, or buckwheat groats, rinsed well
- 2 cups (475 ml) water

Heat 2 tablespoons (30 ml) of the oil in a large skillet over medium heat. Cook mushrooms and ½ teaspoon salt until mushrooms have released their water; increase heat to medium-high and cook until mushrooms are completely dry and have turned golden brown, 10 to 12 minutes. Set aside.

Heat remaining oil in a saucepan over medium heat. Add the onion and ½ teaspoon salt and cook until softened, 3 minutes. Add the kasha and sauté until golden and fragrant, 3 minutes. Add the water, and bring to a boil. Cover, reduce heat to low, and simmer for 15 to 20 minutes, until kasha is tender. Gently stir in the mushrooms, season to taste with salt, and serve.

YIELD: *4 servings*

Calories (kcal): 294; **Total fat:** 15g; **Cholesterol:** 0mg; **Carbohydrate:** 37g; **Dietary fiber:** 6g; **Protein:** 7g; **Sodium:** 13mg; **Potassium:** 559mg; **Calcium:** 18mg; **Iron:** 2mg; **Zinc:** 2mg; **Vitamin A:** 0IU.

Vegetable Risotto

gluten   milk   soy   egg   corn   nuts

This creamy side dish is a great way to sneak in some finely chopped vegetables. The lemon juice takes the place of the more traditional wine.

- 3 cups (400 g) grated or finely chopped vegetables, such as zucchini, carrots, asparagus, or peas (which can be used whole)
- $1/4$ cup (60 ml) olive oil, divided
- 3 cups (710 ml) GFCF chicken broth
- 1 small onion, chopped fine
- $1/2$ teaspoon salt
- 1 cup (200 g) Arborio rice
- 1 tablespoon (15 ml) lemon juice
- $1/2$ cup (120 ml) water
- $1/4$ teaspoon ground black pepper
- $1/2$ teaspoon lemon zest

In a large skillet, heat 2 tablespoons (30 ml) of the olive oil over medium heat. Add the vegetables and sauté until just tender. Reserve.

Heat the chicken broth in a small pot until steaming; keep warm. In a larger pot, heat the remaining oil over medium heat. Add onion and salt and cook until softened but not browned, 3 minutes. Add the rice and cook another 3 minutes, until edges of rice are translucent. Add the lemon juice and water and cook until completely absorbed. Add the broth, $1/2$ cup (120 ml) at a time, stirring occasionally, and waiting until each addition is absorbed before adding the next. When the last bit of broth is added, add the reserved vegetables, pepper, and lemon zest, and cook until broth is absorbed. (If rice is not as tender as you'd like at this point, add $1/2$ cup [120 ml] warm water and continue cooking until absorbed.) Serve.

YIELD: *4 servings*

Calories (kcal): 382; **Total fat:** 16g; **Cholesterol:** 4mg; **Carbohydrate:** 51g; **Dietary fiber:** 4g; **Protein:** 9g; **Sodium:** 837mg; **Potassium:** 295mg; **Calcium:** 38mg; **Iron:** 1mg; **Zinc:** 1mg; **Vitamin A:** 9895IU.

Risotto Cakes

It is worth doubling this recipe so that you have enough leftover to make these cakes. The tricks to avoiding heavy breading and a lot of fat for frying is a non-stick skillet and cooking low and slow; this allows the natural starches in the rice to brown and crisp up. The risotto needs to be chilled at least overnight to be firm enough to shape into patties.

- 2 cups leftover risotto (with or without vegetables added)
- 2 tablespoons (30ml) olive oil
- Salt to taste

Shape $1/2$ cup risotto into a ball, and then flatten to form a patty (wetting your hands first helps to minimize sticking); repeat with remaining risotto, and sprinkle the cakes with salt. In a non-stick skillet, heat the oil over medium-low heat. Add the cakes and cook for 10 to 15 minutes, until crisp and light golden on the bottom. Flip and repeat for the other side. Serve plain, or topped with your favorite GFCF tomato sauce.

YIELD: *4 cakes*

Calories (kcal): 442; **Total fat:** 22g; **Cholesterol:** 4mg; **Carbohydrate:** 51g; **Dietary fiber:** 4g; **Protein:** 9g; **Sodium:** 837mg; **Potassium:** 295mg; **Calcium:** 38mg; **Iron:** 1mg; **Zinc:** 1mg; **Vitamin A:** 9895IU.

CHAPTER 15

Vegetables and Side Dishes

DON'T SKIP THIS CHAPTER!

Some of you are saying "No way! My child gags at vegetables."

Well, hang in there. One of these ideas may be your child's breakthrough.

This chapter includes creative ways to include vegetables in the diet for those who like them and those who can't stand them. From eating frozen peas to the Trojan Horse technique of hiding pureed vegetables in other foods, we hope our suggestions will be helpful.

Many parents report that their children ate a wide variety of foods when on baby food but had appetite changes once solid foods were introduced. This may be due to sensory issues, which frequently include aversions or strong dislikes to certain textures and to specific foods, especially vegetables. Most of the children who dislike vegetables are also very particular about texture and color. For this reason, it is important to carefully and slowly add anything new.

Mashed Potatoes

gluten   milk   soy   egg   corn   nuts

This simple and delicious GFCF version of mashed potatoes is destined to become a family favorite.

- 5 Yukon Gold potatoes, washed and peeled
- $^{1}/_{4}$ cup (55 g) GFCF butter substitute or ghee
- $^{1}/_{2}$ cup (120 ml) soy milk
- $^{1}/_{2}$ teaspoon sea salt
- $^{1}/_{2}$ teaspoon black peppercorns, ground

Cut potatoes into 2-inch (5-cm) cubes and place in a pot, covering with cold water by 1 inch (2.5 cm). Bring potatoes to a boil, reduce heat, and simmer 10 minutes or until tender. Drain. Place in bowl of an electric mixer. Add butter substitute, soy milk, salt, and pepper. Whip until well combined. Adjust seasoning as necessary.

YIELD: *6 or more servings*

Calories (kcal): 167; **Total fat:** 10g; **Cholesterol:** 23mg; **Carbohydrate:** 19g; **Dietary fiber:** 2g; **Protein:** 3g; **Sodium:** 189mg; **Potassium:** 586mg; **Calcium:** 11mg; **Iron:** 1mg; **Zinc:** trace; **Vitamin A:** 347IU

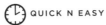

QUICK N EASY

Suzi's Guilt-Free French Fries and Sweet Fries

gluten milk soy egg corn nuts

"They taste great," says Suzi Gifford. This is a healthy version of a favorite food.

- 2 large unpeeled russet potatoes, or 2 unpeeled sweet potatoes
- 2 egg whites (large egg)
- 1 teaspoon black pepper, freshly ground
- 1–2 teaspoons salt
- Oil spray or 1 tablespoon (15 ml) light olive oil

Cut potatoes into thin strips. In a bowl, whip egg whites until foamy. Add black pepper and salt and mix.

Add potatoes and toss to coat well. Spray a cookie sheet with GFCF oil spray or wipe the surface with oil or use a nonstick cookie sheet or nonstick foil. Spread potatoes on the cookie sheet.

Bake for 30 to 35 minutes at 450°F (230°C, or gas mark 8) or until potatoes are crisp and brown.

VARIATIONS: *Sweet potatoes have excellent nutrition. Combine the two types of potatoes to expand the vegetable choices.*

Add some spice by adding the following to the egg-white foam:
- *1 tablespoon (8 g) chili powder*
- *1/2 teaspoon cayenne pepper*

Make garlic fries by adding the following to the egg-white foam:
- *1 teaspoon garlic powder*
- *1 teaspoon paprika*

YIELD: *3 to 4 servings*

Calories (kcal): 69; **Total fat:** 3g; **Cholesterol:** 0mg; **Carbohydrate:** 7g; **Dietary fiber:** 1g; **Protein:** 3g; **Sodium:** 563mg; **Potassium:** 234mg; **Calcium:** 9mg; **Iron:** trace ; **Zinc:** trace ; **Vitamin A:** 1IU

Pleasing Frozen Peas—Try this!

gluten   milk   soy   egg   corn   nuts

Frozen peas (regular or baby) are a favorite of many children and adults. They are especially well tolerated by those who favor "crunchy" textures. Many children with sensory issues and aversions to vegetables find eating the individual frozen peas a delight. Serve these as a snack or part of the meal. Of course, organic is better!

Also consider expanding to other frozen vegetables or a medley of frozen vegetables.

Calories (kcal): 55; **Total fat:** trace; **Cholesterol:** 0mg; **Carbohydrate:** 10g; **Dietary fiber:** 3g; **Protein:** 4g; **Sodium:** 81mg; **Potassium:** 107mg; **Calcium:** 16mg; **Iron:** 1mg; **Zinc:** 1mg; **Vitamin A:** 523IU

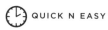 QUICK N EASY

Potato Pancakes

gluten   milk   soy   egg   corn   nuts

Not only is this recipe delicious, but also including the garbanzo bean flour in the mix means they're packed with protein.

- 3 cups (675 g) mashed potatoes
- 1¹/₄ cups (185 g) garbanzo bean flour
- ¹/₂ cup (70 g) brown rice flour
- ¹/₂ cup (60 g) tapioca starch
- ¹/₂ tablespoon xanthan gum
- ¹/₂ tablespoon (9 g) salt
- ¹/₂ tablespoon baking soda
- 3 tablespoons (45 ml) oil
- 3 tablespoons (45 ml) rice milk

Mix ingredients well in a large bowl. Roll out pancakes between two floured pieces of wax paper. Cook on high heat on a griddle until brown, turning once.

YIELD: *Makes 20 pancakes*

Calories (kcal): 68; **Total fat:** 3g; **Cholesterol:** 1mg; **Carbohydrate:** 10g; **Dietary fiber:** 1g; **Protein:** 1g; **Sodium:** 265mg; **Potassium:** 109mg; **Calcium:** 11mg; **Iron:** trace; **Zinc:** trace; **Vitamin A:** 28IU

Sweet Potato Pancakes

gluten   milk   soy   egg   corn   nuts

A sweet and savory version of an old standby.

- 1 pound (455 g) sweet potatoes, peeled
- 1/2 cup (70 g) brown rice flour, or GF flour blend of choice
- 2 teaspoons (8 g) sugar or Sucanat
- 1 teaspoon brown sugar
- 1 teaspoon baking powder
- 1 teaspoon cinnamon
- 1/8 teaspoon cayenne (optional)
- 1 teaspoon curry powder
- 1/2 teaspoon cumin
- Salt and pepper to taste
- 2 large eggs, beaten
- 1/2 cup (120 ml) milk substitute
- 1 large onion, diced
- Oil for frying

Grate sweet potatoes coarsely. In a separate bowl, mix flour, sugars, baking powder, cinnamon, cayenne, curry powder, cumin, salt, and pepper. Add eggs and just enough milk substitute to make a stiff batter. Add potatoes and diced onion and mix. The batter should be moist but not runny. If too stiff, add milk substitute. Heat 1/4 inch (0.6 cm) of oil in a frying pan until smoking. Drop batter by tablespoon and flatten. Fry over medium-high heat on each side until golden. Drain on paper towels.

YIELD: *16 pancakes*

Calories (kcal): 52; **Total fat:** trace; **Cholesterol:** 0mg; **Carbohydrate:** 12g; **Dietary fiber:** 1g; **Protein:** 1g; **Sodium:** 34mg; **Potassium:** 72mg; **Calcium:** 27mg; **Iron:** trace; **Zinc:** trace; **Vitamin A:** 4107IU

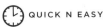 QUICK N EASY

Sautéed Cinnamon Carrots

gluten   milk   soy   egg   corn   nuts

Sally Fallon notes in her book, Nourishing Traditions, *that peeling carrots does not affect the nutrient content because nutrients are well distributed, unlike potatoes, which have the nutrients concentrated under the skin.*

- 1 pound (455 g) carrots
- 1/4 cup (55 g) ghee or (60 ml) olive oil
- 1/4–1/2 teaspoon cinnamon (optional)
- 1/4 teaspoon sea salt (optional)

Peel carrots and slice into rounds or cut into sticks about 3 inches (7.5 cm) long and 1/4 inch (0.6 cm) wide. They may also be cut julienne-style (using a food processor).

Sauté in ghee or olive oil about 20 minutes, until golden but still slightly firm.

Add cinnamon and sea salt.

YIELD: *4 to 6 servings*

Calories (kcal): 109; **Total fat:** 9g; **Cholesterol:** 23mg; **Carbohydrate:** 7g; **Dietary fiber:** 2g; **Protein:** 1g; **Sodium:** 105mg; **Potassium:** 221 mg; **Calcium:** 21mg; **Iron:** 1mg; **Zinc:** trace; **Vitamin A:** 19284IU

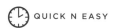

QUICK N EASY

Simple Steamed Veggies

gluten   milk   soy   egg   corn   nuts

This easy recipe lends itself to any variety of greens, depending on the likes and dislikes of your children.

- 2 cups (120 g) green vegetable (spinach, swiss chard, broccoli, kale, asparagus)
- 1 tablespoon (15 ml) olive oil
- $1/4$ teaspoon sea salt
- $1/8$ teaspoon white pepper
- $1/8$ teaspoon dried oregano
- $1/8$ teaspoon garlic powder
- $1/8$ teaspoon red chili flakes (optional)

Steam the green vegetable.

While steaming, combine the rest of the ingredients to taste in a large bowl. Add steamed vegetables. Stir and coat thoroughly and serve.

YIELD: *4 servings ($1/2$ cup [30 g] each)*

Calories (kcal): 40; **Total fat:** 4g; **Cholesterol:** 0mg; **Carbohydrate:** 2g; **Dietary fiber:** 1g; **Protein:** 1g; **Sodium:** 127mg; **Potassium:** 117mg; **Calcium:** 18mg; **Iron:** trace; **Zinc:** trace; **Vitamin A:** 1072IU

Roasted Veggies

gluten   milk   soy   egg   corn   nuts

A colorful crowd pleaser.

- 2-3 sweet potatoes, cubed
- 1 butternut squash, cubed
- 1 red pepper, chopped
- 1 yellow pepper, chopped
- 1 zucchini, cubed
- 1 red onion, chopped
- $1/2$ cup (120 ml) balsamic vinegar
- 6 tablespoons (90 ml) olive oil
- 2 teaspoons (8 g) sugar or Sucanat
- 2 teaspoons fennel seed, crushed or whole, or dried rosemary
- 1 teaspoon salt
- $1/2$ teaspoon pepper

Lightly grease a roasting pan. Combine veggies. Mix remaining ingredients to make a sauce. Combine sauce with veggies. Bake uncovered for 45 minutes in a 450°F (230°C, or gas mark 8) oven, stirring twice during baking.

VARIATIONS: *Include turnips, parsnips, fennel bulbs, and/or new potatoes.*

YIELD: *10 to 12 servings*

Calories (kcal): 211; **Total fat:** 9g; **Cholesterol:** 0mg; **Carbohydrate:** 35g; **Dietary fiber:** 5g; **Protein:** 3g; **Sodium:** 227mg; **Potassium:** 820mg; **Calcium:** 106mg; **Iron:** 2 2mg; **Zinc:** trace; **Vitamin A:** 21878IU

Mashed Cauliflower—
The New Comfort Food

(Oven and Microwave Versions)

gluten   milk   soy   egg   corn   nuts

Many children on the spectrum have strong aversions to vegetables, especially greens. They tend to focus on "the white diet." By substituting mashed cauliflower for mashed potato, the result is a healthy, high-fiber, nutrient-dense white food. To make the transition from mashed potatoes to cauliflower, combine both at the start. Depending on the type of milk substitute used, the recipe may or may not include soy or nut (almond) milks.

- 1 head cauliflower, or 1 pound (455 g) frozen cauliflower florets
- $1/8$–$1/4$ cup (28–60 ml) rice milk (or soy milk, coconut milk, almond milk)
- Salt and pepper to taste
- 1 tablespoon (15 g) ghee
- Optional seasoning: paprika, garlic

Boil, steam, or microwave (8–10 minutes) cauliflower until fork-tender. Drain thoroughly (squeeze excess water out, or it will be like soup).

Place cauliflower pieces in the blender, then add milk (rice, soy, coconut, or almond), ghee, salt, and pepper. Whip until smooth.

Pour cauliflower into a small baking dish. If desired, sprinkle with paprika and seasonings. Bake in a hot oven until bubbly or heat quickly in the microwave.

VARIATION: *For those children who eat only white foods, white rice can be added as well as potato.*

YIELD: *4 servings*

Calories (kcal): 40; **Total fat:** 3g; **Cholesterol:** 9mg; **Carbohydrate:** 2g; **Dietary fiber:** 1g; **Protein:** 1g; **Sodium:** 9mg; **Potassium:** 78mg; **Calcium:** 6mg; **Iron:** trace; **Zinc:** trace; **Vitamin A:** 132IU

Broccoli or "Little Tree" Puree

gluten   milk   soy   egg   corn   nuts

According to Lisa Barnes in The Petit Appetit Cookbook, *no matter how old you are, everyone has referred to broccoli as "little trees." Look for compact heads that are dark green, sage green, or a purple-green color. The floret clusters should be firm, compact, and tightly closed. Avoid bunches that are wilted or shriveled and those with a pungent odor.*

- 2 medium heads organic broccoli, stems removed, separated into equal-size florets, or 16 ounces (455 g) frozen broccoli florets
- Water
- Ghee, melted, if desired

Steamer Method:

Place broccoli in a steamer basket set in a pot filled with about 2 inches (5 cm) of lightly boiling water. Do not let water touch broccoli. Cover tightly for best nutrient retention and steam for 10 to 12 minutes or until broccoli is tender. Florets should pierce easily with a toothpick. Immediately transfer steamer basket to sink and run cold water over florets until completely cool, 2 to 3 minutes.

Puree broccoli in a food processor with a steel blade. Additional liquid is not usually needed.

Microwave Method:

Place broccoli florets in a microwave-safe dish. Add 1/2 cup (120 ml) water and cover tightly, lifting a corner to vent. Microwave on high for 4 minutes and stir broccoli. Re-cover and cook for 4 to 6 minutes or until tender. Check for doneness, cook, and proceed with directions above.

Top with melted ghee.

If the child has an aversion to green, mix the broccoli puree into spaghetti sauce or other food source in which the color will not be obvious.

NOTE: *The recipe is even more Quick N Easy when using the frozen organic broccoli florets.*

YIELD: *4 servings (1/2 cup [120 g] each)*

Calories (kcal): 79; **Total fat:** 7g; **Cholesterol:** 17mg; **Carbohydrate:** 4g; **Dietary fiber:** 2g; **Protein:** 2g; **Sodium:** 21mg; **Potassium:** 227mg; **Calcium:** 34mg; **Iron:** 1mg; **Zinc:** trace; **Vitamin A:** 2333IU

Butternut Squash "Fries"

gluten   milk   soy   egg   corn   nuts

Elaine Gotschall is the inspiration for this recipe. It is also good for those on the SCD eating plan.

- 1 butternut squash
- 2 tablespoons (28 g) GFCF butter substitute or ghee, melted
- Salt to taste

Preheat oven to 450°F (230°C, or gas mark 8).

Using only the neck of the squash, slice thinly (1/4 inch, or 0.6 cm)

Place the squash on a cookie sheet or pizza pan, dot with butter or melted ghee, and sprinkle with salt. Bake until one side is brown. Turn over and brown the other side.

YIELD: *2 to 3 servings*

Calories (kcal): 335; **Total fat:** 10g; **Cholesterol:** 23mg; **Carbohydrate:** 66g; **Dietary fiber:** 10g; **Protein:** 6g; **Sodium:** 25mg; **Potassium:** 2000mg; **Calcium:** 273mg; **Iron:** 4mg; **Zinc:** 1mg; **Vitamin A:** 44606IU

Barb's Vegetable Combo

gluten   milk   soy   egg   corn   nuts

- 3 tablespoons (45 g) ghee
- 3/4 cup (175 ml) chicken broth
- 1 tablespoon (15 g) Dijon mustard
- 1 tablespoon (8 g) cornstarch
- Dash pepper
- 1/2 teaspoon dried basil leaves, crushed
- 1/4 teaspoon garlic powder
- 1 package (16 ounces, or 455 g) frozen Italian green beans
- 1 cup (50 g) cooked GFCF shell pasta or (165 g) cooked brown rice
- 1 can (3 ounces, 85 g) button mushrooms, drained
- 1 small tomato, chopped
- 1/4 cup (25 g) sliced black olives (optional)

Melt ghee in a large saucepan. Stir in broth, mustard, cornstarch, pepper, basil, and garlic. Cook until bubbling, stirring constantly. Add green beans, pasta shells or rice, and mushrooms. Stir until heated. The Italian green beans should be cooked to tender-crisp. Just before serving, stir in tomato and olives (optional). Heat to serving temperature.

YIELD: *4 servings*

Calories (kcal): 222; **Total fat:** 12g; **Cholesterol:** 26mg; **Carbohydrate:** 26g; **Dietary fiber:** 5g; **Protein:** 5g; **Sodium:** 275mg; **Potassium:** 435mg; **Calcium:** 73mg; **Iron:** 5 5mg; **Zinc:** 1mg; **Vitamin A:** 1171IU

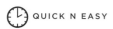 **QUICK N EASY**

Fried Summer Squash

gluten   milk   soy   egg   corn   nuts

SCD compatible.

This delicious summer squash recipe is good in any season.

- 1 egg
- 1 teaspoon (5 ml) water
- 2 medium summer squash
- Pecan meal or GFCF bread crumbs
- Olive oil

Beat egg and add 1 teaspoon (5 ml) water. Peel the squash and slice it about ¼ inch (0.6 cm) thick. Drop squash slices into egg mixture to coat, then drop them into pecan meal or crushed bread crumbs, turning to coat evenly. Place on a plate until pan is ready.

A regular frying pan can be used, but be careful that it doesn't get too hot. Nut meal will brown quickly, so remember to cook below medium temperature. If using an electric frying pan, set the temperature to 250°F (120°C). Add a little oil to the pan (watch the amount of oil—just a little under each slice is sufficient) and add the squash slices. Cover the pan and cook 5 to 7 minutes on the first side. Flip the squash, add oil as necessary, and cover and cook for 3 to 4 minutes. Remove the cover and cook 2 to 3 minutes longer.

YIELD: *3 to 4 servings*

Calories (kcal): 147; **Total fat:** 8g; **Cholesterol:** 47mg; **Carbohydrate:** 12g; **Dietary fiber:** 3g; **Protein:** 8g; **Sodium:** 16mg; **Potassium:** 257mg; **Calcium:** 30mg; **Iron:** 1mg; **Zinc:** 1mg; **Vitamin A:** 281IU

Pecan Meal

Pecan meal is sold in health food stores and online. Pecan "meal" refers to the flakes that occur as the result of chopping pecans. The meal is used in pie crusts, sprinkled on salads, and substituted as a breading for pan-fried foods.

Fall Harvest Veggies

gluten   milk   soy   egg   corn   nuts

Colorful, sweet, nutritious, and kid-friendly, this dish has it all.

- 2 jewel yams (or 1 jewel and 1 Japanese yam)
- 4 carrots
- 3 parsnips
- 2 tablespoons (28 ml) olive oil
- Fresh rosemary, to taste
- Dried oregano, to taste
- Salt
- Pepper

Preheat oven to 350°F (180°C, gas mark 4). Peel the vegetables and cut into small, thin pieces. Combine in a bowl. Add the remaining ingredients. Bake uncovered for 1 hour or until soft but not too mushy.

For those with sensory issues, this can be pureed.

VARIATION: *To sweeten the flavor, add 1 tablespoon (20 g) honey.*

YIELD: *4 to 6 servings*

Calories (kcal): 205; **Total fat:** 5g; **Cholesterol:** 0mg; **Carbohydrate:** 39g; **Dietary fiber:** 9g; **Protein:** 3g; **Sodium:** 33mg; **Potassium:** 989mg; **Calcium:** 62mg; **Iron:** 1mg; **Zinc:** 1mg; **Vitamin A:** 1350IU

Glenda's Oven-Roasted Vegetables

gluten   milk   soy   egg   corn   nuts

This is an Ingham Family favorite. Vegetable choices can be changed to accommodate the people being served.

- 2–3 zucchini, sliced (medium thickness)
- 2 yellow squash, sliced (medium thickness)
- 3 peppers—one each of red, yellow, and green—sliced (medium thickness)
- 1 large onion, sliced (medium thickness)
- 3–4 cloves garlic, chopped
- 1 can (13.5 ounces, or 378 g) chopped tomatoes
- 1–2 tablespoons GFCF herbs de Provence (basil, oregano, rosemary, parsley, thyme)
- $1/8$ cup (8 g) fresh chopped cilantro (optional)
- $1/2$ cup (120 ml) olive oil

Place all vegetables in a 9 x 13-inch (22.5 x 32.5-cm) or other large pan. Sprinkle with herbs. Pour olive oil over top and mix well.

Cover with tin foil and roast in very hot (450°F [230°C, or gas mark 8]) oven for 7 to 10 minutes. Remove tin foil and roast for an additional 7 to 10 minutes.

VARIATIONS: *The vegetables can also be marinated in a GFCF marinade and then roasted in a grill pan. Leftovers can be served over brown rice for a quick, nutritious meal addition.*

With the addition of chicken broth or stock, this recipe also makes a good soup.

YIELD: *6 servings*

Calories (kcal): 223; **Total fat:** 19g; **Cholesterol:** 0mg; **Carbohydrate:** 14g; **Dietary fiber:** 4g; **Protein:** 3g; **Sodium:** 12mg; **Potassium:** 612mg; **Calcium:** 40mg; **Iron:** 1mg; **Zinc:** 1mg; **Vitamin A:** 1252IU

Joyce's Versatile Vegetable Medley

 gluten milk soy egg corn nuts

Joyce Mulcahy's recipe is a family favorite and her standby when asked to bring a side dish to a party. Whether using the basic recipe or adding the optional vegetables, the dish is consistently delicious. Joyce provides two popular versions—Italian and Mexican—which depend on the herb combination used.

Basic Recipe

- $1/2$ onion, sliced or chopped
- 1 garlic clove, minced
- 1 red (or green) pepper
- 1 tablespoon (15 ml) olive oil

Basic vegetables

- 1 can (14.5 ounces, or 411 g) diced tomatoes with juice, or 1–2 fresh chopped tomatoes
- 2–3 sliced zucchini
- Salt and pepper to taste

Optional additions (one or more of the following):

- $1/2$ fennel bulb, chopped
- $2/3$ cup (100 g) white corn (frozen or fresh)
- 1 small eggplant, peeled and sliced

Herb Options:

Italian Herbs:

- 4–5 fresh basil leaves, minced, or $1/2$ –1 tablespoon (15 g) pesto
- $1/2$ teaspoon oregano

Mexican Herbs:

- 1 teaspoon cumin
- 1–2 tablespoons (4–8 g) chopped fresh cilantro

Sauté onion, garlic, and peppers in olive oil until the onions are translucent.

Add basic (and optional) vegetables and herbs and simmer on medium-low heat for 15 minutes, stirring occasionally.

VARIATIONS: *Puree the vegetable medley and serve it over GFCF pasta or rice. Add organic chicken broth and puree to make a delicious soup.*

YIELD: *4 to 6 servings*

Calories (kcal): 89; **Total fat:** 3g; **Cholesterol:** 0mg; **Carbohydrate:** 15g; **Dietary fiber:** 5g; **Protein:** 3g; **Sodium:** 24mg; **Potassium:** 662mg; **Calcium:** 35mg; **Iron:** 1mg; **Zinc:** trace; **Vitamin A:** 1006IU

Sweet Potato Enchilada

gluten milk soy egg corn nuts

This hearty Mexican dish is easy to make and its combination of sweet and spicy is something your whole family will love.

- 1 large onion, diced
- 1 teaspoon garlic, minced
- $^1/_4$ teaspoon cumin
- $^1/_4$ teaspoon coriander
- $^1/_8$ teaspoon chili powder
- Dash cayenne pepper
- $^1/_8$ teaspoon chipotle chili powder
- $^1/_8$ teaspoon garlic powder
- Approximately 3–4 cups (360–480 g) sweet potatoes, boiled and mashed
- $^1/_4$ cup (55 g) salsa
- 8 corn tortillas (cut in quarters)
- CF cheese (optional)

Sauté onion and garlic. Add spices to onion mixture and sauté until translucent. Add to mashed sweet potatoes. Adjust seasonings. Spray a baking pan with oil. Layer with half of the salsa, half of the tortillas, sweet potatoes, remaining salsa, and remaining corn tortillas. Top with CF cheese, if using. Bake at 350°F (180°C, gas mark 4) for 20 to 30 minutes, until done.

YIELD: *8 servings*

Calories (kcal): 193; **Total fat:** 1g; **Cholesterol:** 0mg; **Carbohydrate:** 43g; **Dietary fiber:** 4g; **Protein:** 4g; **Sodium:** 172mg; **Potassium:** 349mg; **Calcium:** 89mg; **Iron:** 2 2mg; **Zinc:** 1mg; **Vitamin A:** 19361IU

Grandma Lillie's Sweet Potato Tzimmes Kugel

gluten milk soy egg corn nuts

Jody Cutler finds this unusual and delicious version of tzimmes perfect for any Jewish holiday.

- 1 cup (120 g) grated sweet potato
- 1 cup (120 g) grated carrots
- 1 cup (120 g) grated apples
- $^1/_2$ cup (70 g) chopped raisins
- $^1/_2$ cup (85 g) chopped prunes
- $^1/_2$ cup (100 g) sugar (may use honey, Sucanat, or agave nectar)
- $^1/_2$ cup (70 g) brown rice flour
- 2 tablespoons (28 ml) lemon juice
- $^1/_2$ teaspoon cinnamon
- $^1/_2$ teaspoon salt
- $^1/_2$ cup (112 g) butter substitute

In a large mixing bowl, mix all the ingredients together with a spoon. Pour into a greased 8 x 4-inch (20 x 10-cm) loaf pan and bake in a preheated 350°F (180°C, gas mark 4) oven for about 60 minutes or until brown.

YIELD: *6 to 8 servings*

Calories (kcal): 273; **Total fat:** 12g; **Cholesterol:** 0mg; **Carbohydrate:** 42g; **Dietary fiber:** 3g; **Protein:** 2g; **Sodium:** 276mg; **Potassium:** 288mg; **Calcium:** 27mg; **Iron:** 1mg; **Zinc:** trace; **Vitamin A:** 8340IU

Purees

Purees are a great way to include vegetables in the diet. This approach is most helpful to those with sensory issues involving food choices, tastes, smells, and textures. One of the markers is a good appetite that becomes limited with the introduction of solids.

Please refer to detailed information in chapter 8. Purees are helpful for hiding vegetables within sauces, especially spaghetti sauce, and in muffins, cakes, brownies, pancakes, peanut butter, meatballs, smoothies, and anything chocolate. See also the main-dish recipes for adding meat purees to sauces to expand the protein content.

Reminders:

- The secret is to add a very small amount (1 tablespoon [15 g] or less) blended well with a usual and well-liked food.

- Expand as tolerated to larger amounts, depending on the food in which it is mixed (e.g., ¼ cup [60 g] or more in a recipe for spaghetti sauce or baked goods, less in a smoothie).

- Mix pureed/blended fruits with pureed/blended vegetables for flavor.

- Use lighter-colored vegetables in baked goods or smoothies:

Sweet potato	Cauliflower
Yellow squash	Turnips
Butternut squash	

- Darker colors work well in meatballs, spaghetti sauce, and chocolate items:

Baby peas	Broccoli
Green beans	Beets
Asparagus	

Use 1 tablespoon to ¼ cup (15–60 g) organic baby-food vegetables or pureed vegetables, as suitable for the child.

Select single vegetables or combinations and use the amount appropriate for the recipes.

NOTE: This works well as long as the first introduction is a very small amount that is gradually increased according to tolerance. Eventually the child may begin to eat the new vegetables alone and may expand beyond the purees and hidden vegetables. The purees are listed first and are followed by more diverse family-friendly vegetable recipes.

Potato-Carrot Mash

gluten   milk   soy   egg   corn   nuts

This recipe improves upon the standard mashed-potato recipe and is easy to make anytime. This can be made with leftover baked potatoes or leftover carrot puree for children. Russet potatoes work best in this recipe, as they have a high starch content and will become fluffy.

- 4 medium organic carrots, peeled and cut into chunks (about 2 cups, or 260 g)
- 3 medium organic baking potatoes, peeled and cut into chunks (about 3 cups, or 330 g)
- $1/2$ teaspoon sea salt
- $1/4$ cup (60 g) GMO soy yogurt
- 1 tablespoon (15 g) ghee, melted
- $1^1/2$ teaspoons sweet GFCF mustard
- Sea salt and white pepper, to taste

Put carrots and potatoes in a large stockpot, cover with cold water, and sprinkle with the salt. Bring to a boil over medium-high heat, and boil until tender, about 10 minutes. Transfer potatoes and carrots to a food processor and puree. Stir in yogurt, ghee, and mustard. Season with salt and pepper.

VARIATION: *There are many colored and healthy mashed-potato variations that can be created by adding vegetables. How about asparagus for a green potato puree for St. Patrick's Day? Or maybe beets for red potato puree for Valentine's Day? Or make both, green and red, for the Christmas table.*

YIELD: *4 servings of 6 ounces (170 g) each*

Calories (kcal): 179; **Total fat:** 4g; **Cholesterol:** 9mg; **Carbohydrate:** 33g; **Dietary fiber:** 4g; **Protein:** 4g; **Sodium:** 293mg; **Potassium:** 985mg; **Calcium:** 31mg; **Iron:** 2 2mg; **Zinc:** 1mg; **Vitamin A:** 20381IU

Yummy Mashed Carrots

gluten   milk   soy   egg   corn   nuts

Children who dislike vegetables have difficulty tasting the natural flavors. Here is a way to bring more flavor to the food. Adding salt is not a problem. Most of the children have higher needs for salt (sodium chloride).

- 1 pound (455 g) carrots
- 3 cups (710 ml) chicken stock (see page 199 or use chicken broth from the store)
- $1/4$ teaspoon sea salt

Optional ingredients
- 1 tablespoon (20 g) honey
- 2 tablespoons (30 g) applesauce (unsweetened)
- $1/4$ to $1/2$ teaspoon cinnamon

Peel carrots and slice into rounds or cut into sticks about 3 inches (7.5 cm) long and $1/4$ inch (0.6 cm) in width. They may also be cut julienne-style (using a food processor).

Combine carrots with chicken stock and cook in the microwave or simmer until soft enough to mash in a processor (medium speed) or in a mixer. Add salt.

Add one or more of the optional ingredients (honey, applesauce, cinnamon) to suit the child's taste.

YIELD: *4 servings*

Calories (kcal): 381; **Total fat:** 22g; **Cholesterol:** 127mg; **Carbohydrate:** 20g; **Dietary fiber:** 4g; **Protein:** 26g; **Sodium:** 295mg; **Potassium:** 737mg; **Calcium:** 72mg; **Iron:** 3 3mg; **Zinc:** 2mg; **Vitamin A:** 33714IU

Aidan's Favorite Meat/Vegetable Mix

gluten   milk   soy   egg   corn   nuts

Carla reports that Aidan loves this recipe and takes it with her on the school bus as her snack/meal. It is excellent for children who resist chunky textures. It can be served plain or on cucumbers or rice crackers as an appetizer. Portable and ready, this recipe can be made in large batches and frozen.

- 8 slices ($^1/_2$ inch, or 1.25 cm, each) roast turkey breast
- 1–2 bunches (total 5–6 leaves) chard without the stems, or a 1-quart (9464-ml) bag stuffed generously with watercress
- 3 acorn squash, cut in half and baked in oven at 350°F (180°C, gas mark 4) for 45 minutes to 1 hour
- $^1/_4$ cup (60 ml) high-oleic safflower oil
- $^1/_4$ cup (20 g) dried tarragon leaves
- $^1/_4$–$^1/_2$ teaspoon salt, or to taste
- White pepper to taste

Grind turkey in a grinder or food processor until almost a paste.

Steam the green leafy vegetable until slightly soft. Add steamed vegetable to the food processor with the turkey.

Scoop out the meat of the squash and add to the food processor to mix with the turkey and chard/watercress.

Add oil and tarragon, and salt and pepper to taste, to the mixture in the food processor and blend on medium speed. Serve by placing a small amount (1 tablespoon [15 g]) on cucumber slices or GFCF rice crackers.

FOR TAKEOUT: Spoon $^1/_2$ cup (125 g) of mixture into a resealable plastic bag and push to the bottom of the bag (about $1^1/_2$ inch [3.75 cm] deep). Roll up bag and freeze. To serve, thaw (it thaws well in a lunch cooler with freezer pack by lunch time) and cut small hole in one corner of the bag. Use like a frosting piping bag to extrude onto sliced cucumbers.

VARIATIONS: *Use chicken instead of turkey. Substitute wild rice or turnips for squash.*

YIELD: *14 servings ($^1/_2$ cup [125 g] each)*

Calories (kcal): 111; **Total fat:** 5g; **Cholesterol:** 27mg; **Carbohydrate:** 1g; **Dietary fiber:** trace; **Protein:** 15g; **Sodium:** 976mg; **Potassium:** 250mg; **Calcium:** 23mg; **Iron:** 1mg; **Zinc:** 1mg; **Vitamin A:** 227IU

Veggie Platter

gluten   milk   soy   egg   corn   nuts

Adapted from Lisa Barnes of Petit Appétit

Show your child how exciting and beautiful a vegetable platter can be with a rainbow of colors and flavors. You can make this a simple snack with two or three veggies, or dress it up with some Happy or Spinach Hummus alongside.

- 1 large organic carrot, peeled, or 12 baby organic carrots
- 4 ounces (115 g) organic green beans, trimmed
- ¹/₂ small jicama, peeled
- ¹/₂ small cucumber, peeled
- 10 organic cherry tomatoes

Bring a medium pot of water to a boil. Cut carrot (if whole) into 2-inch (5 cm) sticks. Add beans and carrots to boiling water and blanch about 1 minute. Remove vegetables from water with a slotted spoon and place in a bowl of cold water to stop cooking.

Cut jicama and cucumber into similarly-shaped 2-inch (5 cm) sticks; pat vegetables dry. Arrange all vegetables in various glasses, ramekins, and bowls for vegetables to stand up. Create small arrangements of color and sizes for little hands to grab and dip.

TIP: *Blanching hard and fibrous vegetables such as beans and carrots make them easier for small children to eat and enjoy and reduce choking hazard. You can also partially steam vegetables in a microwave rather than turning on the stove. Raw is of course quicker, easier, and crunchier if you're serving older children.*

YIELD: *Makes about 4 cups vegetables, or 8 servings*

Calories (kcal): 23; **Total fat:** trace; **Cholesterol:** 0mg; **Carbohydrate:** 5g; **Dietary fiber:** 2g; **Protein:** 1g; **Sodium:** 7mg; **Potassium:** 164mg; **Calcium:** 13mg; **Iron:** trace; **Zinc:** trace; **Vitamin A:** 2793IU.

Carrot Soufflé

gluten   milk   soy   egg   corn   nuts

This is Welby Griffin's family's Thanksgiving favorite!

For Soufflé

- 1 pound (455 g) carrots, peeled and cut into 2-inch pieces
- 3 large eggs
- ¹/₄ cup (50 g) sugar
- 1 teaspoon baking powder
- ¹/₄ teaspoon salt
- 1 teaspoon GF vanilla extract
- ¹/₃ cup (80 ml) oil
- 3 tablespoons (26 g) GF flour blend or white rice flour

For Topping

- ¹/₄ cup (7.5 g) GF corn flakes (or other similar cereal), crushed
- 1 tablespoon (14 g) melted ghee or GFCF spread
- 2 tablespoons (28 g) brown sugar

Preheat oven to 350°F (180°C, gas mark 4). Grease a 9-inch round casserole or soufflé dish. Boil carrots until tender, drain, and then mash them (they don't have to be perfectly smooth). Add remaining soufflé ingredients and beat well to combine. Pour mixture into the prepared dish. Blend topping ingredients together and sprinkle on top. Bake for 30 minutes or until lightly browned and bubbly.

NOTE: *This soufflé can be baked in small, individual ramekins or soufflé dishes, but be sure to reduce the baking time by 10 to 15 minutes.*

YIELD: *6 servings*

Calories (kcal): 270; **Total fat:** 17g; **Cholesterol:** 114mg; **Carbohydrate:** 25g; **Dietary fiber:** 3g; **Protein:** 5g; **Sodium:** 239mg; **Potassium:** 260mg; **Calcium:** 79mg; **Iron:** 1mg; **Zinc:** trace; **Vitamin A:** 19192IU.

Carrot Soufflé II

gluten   milk   soy   egg   corn   nuts

Adapted from Shelly L. Sheetz

- 1 pound (455 g) carrots, peeled and roughly chopped
- 3 large eggs
- ¹/₄ cup (55 g) GFCF spread or ghee, plus extra for greasing pan
- 3 tablespoons (26 g) GFCF flour
- ¹/₂ cup (100 g) sugar or ¹/₂ cup (170 g) honey or a combination of both
- 1 teaspoon baking powder
- 1 teaspoon GFCF vanilla extract

Preheat oven to 350°F (180°C, gas mark 4). Grease an 8-inch square baking pan. Boil or steam the carrots until tender and drain. Place carrots and remaining ingredients into the food processor and blend until smooth. Pour into the baking dish and bake for 30 to 35 minutes, until cooked through. Serve warm or at room temperature.

NOTE: *This recipe can be easily doubled and baked in a 9 by 13-inch baking pan.*

YIELD: *6 servings*

Calories (kcal): 237; **Total fat:** 12g; **Cholesterol:** 131mg; **Carbohydrate:** 30g; **Dietary fiber:** 3g; **Protein:** 5g; **Sodium:** 142mg; **Potassium:** 252mg; **Calcium:** 77mg; **Iron:** 1mg; **Zinc:** trace; **Vitamin A:** 19442IU.

Apple Butternut Squash Casserole

gluten milk soy egg corn nuts

The apples add a nice twist to this vegetable casserole. For a nut-free version, simply omit the pecans and increase the cereal to 2 cups (80 g).

- 1¹/₂ cups (60 g) GF flaked cereal, crushed
- ¹/₂ cup (55 g) chopped pecans
- ¹/₂ cup (115 g) brown sugar, plus 1 tablespoon (15 g)
- ¹/₂ cup (112 g) ghee, melted and divided
- 1 small butternut squash, cooked and mashed (to yield 3 cups)
- ¹/₄ teaspoon salt
- 6 large or 8 small tart apples, peeled, cored, and sliced (to yield 6 cups)
- ¹/₄ cup (50 g) granulated sugar

Preheat oven to 350°F (180°C, gas mark 4). Combine the rice cereal, pecans, ¹/₂ cup brown sugar, and 2 tablespoons (28 g) of the melted ghee in a medium bowl and set aside. In a separate bowl, mix the squash with ¹/₄ cup (56 g) ghee, 1 tablespoon brown sugar, and salt.

Heat 2 tablespoons (28 g) of ghee in a large skillet over medium-low heat. Add apples and granulated sugar, cover, and simmer for 5 to 8 minutes, until just tender. Spread apples in the bottom of a 3-quart (3-litre) casserole dish. Top with squash mixture, and then sprinkle with cereal-nut topping. Bake for 15 to 20 minutes, until just beginning to bubble at the edges. Cool on wire rack 10 minutes and serve.

YIELD: *8 to 10 servings*

Calories (kcal): 359; **Total fat:** 16g; **Cholesterol:** 28mg; **Carbohydrate:** 58g; **Dietary fiber:** 7g; **Protein:** 3g; **Sodium:** 100mg; **Potassium:** 800mg; **Calcium:** 101mg; **Iron:** 2mg; **Zinc:** 1mg; **Vitamin A:** 13783IU.

Maple Mashed Sweet Potatoes

gluten milk soy egg corn nuts

A sweet alternative to mashed potatoes.

- 2 pounds (910 g) sweet potatoes
- ¹/₄ cup (60 ml) maple syrup (preferably grade B)
- 2 tablespoons (28 g) ghee
- ¹/₂ teaspoon ground nutmeg (optional)
- Salt and pepper

Peel and cut the sweet potatoes into large chunks. Place in a large pot with 1 teaspoon salt, cover with cold water, and bring to a boil. Reduce heat and simmer for 15 to 20 minutes, until tender. Drain and return to the pot. Add remaining ingredients, season with salt and pepper, and mash with a potato masher or fork. Serve.

YIELD: *6 servings*

Calories (kcal): 190; **Total fat:** 5g; **Cholesterol:** 12mg; **Carbohydrate:** 35g; **Dietary fiber:** 3g; **Protein:** 2g; **Sodium:** 17mg; **Potassium:** 251mg; **Calcium:** 38mg; **Iron:** 1mg; **Zinc:** trace; **Vitamin A:** 22031IU.

Grilled Zucchini "Parmesan"

gluten   milk   soy   egg   corn   nuts

Adapted from The Book of Yum
(http://www.bookofyum.com)

If your child likes eggplant, try it in place of the zucchini.

- ¹/₂ cup (120 ml) extra virgin olive oil
- ¹/₄ cup (60 ml) GFCF balsamic vinegar
- Salt and pepper, to taste
- 2 pounds (910 g) zucchini, washed and cut into ¹/₂-inch slices lengthwise
- 2 cups (475 ml) GFCF marinara sauce of choice
- 4 ounces (115 g) Tofutti mozzarella cheese, cut into pieces
- 2 medium garlic cloves, minced

Preheat oven to 375°F (190°C, gas mark 5). Prepare grill for medium heat. Whisk oil, vinegar, salt, and pepper in a large shallow dish. Quickly dip each zucchini slice into the mixture and then place onto the grill. Cook until golden brown on both sides (flipping as necessary) but not mushy.

Grease a baking sheet. Arrange zucchini slices in an even layer on top. Spoon an equal portion of marinara sauce on top of each slice, and then sprinkle with cheese and a small pinch of fresh garlic. Bake until cheese is melted and lightly browned. Serve as is, or over your favorite GFCF pasta or polenta.

YIELD: *4 servings*

Calories (kcal): 384; **Total fat:** 32g; **Cholesterol:** 0mg; **Carbohydrate:** 21g; **Dietary fiber:** 4g; **Protein:** 7g; **Sodium:** 221mg; **Potassium:** 686mg; **Calcium:** 249mg; **Iron:** 2mg; **Zinc:** 1mg; **Vitamin A:** 1546IU.

Indian-Spiced Cauliflower and Potatoes

gluten   milk   soy   egg   corn   nuts

- 4 tablespoons (60 ml) olive oil
- 2 medium onions, chopped
- 1 pound Russet potatoes, peeled and cut into bite-sized pieces
- 1 small head of cauliflower, cut into bite-sized pieces
- 2 tomatoes, chopped
- ¹/₂ teaspoon ground turmeric
- ¹/₂ teaspoon chili powder
- 1 teaspoon cumin
- 1 teaspoon salt
- 1¹/₂ cups (200 g) frozen peas

Heat the oil in a large stock pot or Dutch oven over medium-high heat. Cook the onions for 3 to 4 minutes, until light brown. Add the potatoes, cauliflower, tomatoes, spices, and salt, and cook for another 3 minutes. Add the peas, cover, and reduce heat to medium low and cook for 20 minutes, stirring occasionally to keep vegetables from sticking, until potatoes and cauliflower are tender. Serve.

NOTE: *For a smooth puree version, add 1 cup (235 ml) of water along with the peas, cook 20 minutes, and then mash everything together with a potato masher or food mill.*

YIELD: *6 servings*

Calories (kcal): 196; **Total fat:** 10g; **Cholesterol:** 0mg; **Carbohydrate:** 25g; **Dietary fiber:** 5g; **Protein:** 5g; **Sodium:** 413mg; **Potassium:** 678mg; **Calcium:** 33mg; **Iron:** 2mg; **Zinc:** 1mg; **Vitamin A:** 597IU.

Stuffed Vegetables

gluten   milk   soy   egg   corn   nuts

This recipe can be a lot of fun with a variety of vegetables, but feel free to stick to just one or two that you know your child will like.

- 4 to 5 firm vegetables, such as tomatoes, bell peppers, zucchini, or small eggplants
- 3 tablespoons (45 ml) olive oil, divided
- 1 small onion, chopped
- $^2/_3$ cup (124 g) long grain rice
- 1 clove garlic, minced
- $^1/_2$ teaspoon ground cinnamon
- $^1/_4$ cup (35 g) raisins
- $^1/_2$ teaspoon salt
- $^1/_4$ teaspoon ground black pepper
- $^1/_2$ cup (70 g) pine nuts (optional)
- 2 tablespoons (12 g) chopped mint

Cut the tops off each vegetable and reserve. Scoop out and reserve seeds from the tomato. Remove and discard seeds from the zucchini and eggplant, and then scoop out and reserve enough flesh so that the walls are $^1/_4$-inch thick. Remove and discard the pepper seeds. Preheat oven to 350°F (180°C, gas mark 4).

Heat 2 tablespoons (30 ml) of oil in a large skillet over medium-high heat. Cook the onion for 3 minutes, than add the rice, garlic, cinnamon, raisins, salt, pepper, and the reserved vegetable seeds and flesh. Add enough water to cover the rice and simmer, covered, for 7 to 10 minutes, until rice is tender and most of the liquid has been absorbed. Add the pine nuts and mint and stir to combine.

Stuff each vegetable with the rice filling and replace reserved tops. Arrange vegetables to fit snuggly in a baking dish and add enough water to cover the base of the pan. Drizzle with remaining olive oil and cook for 45 to 50 minutes, until vegetables are tender, basting several times during cooking. Serve warm or cold.

YIELD: *4 to 5 servings*

Calories (kcal): 332; **Total fat:** 16g; **Cholesterol:** 0mg; **Carbohydrate:** 44g; **Dietary fiber:** 7g; **Protein:** 8g; **Sodium:** 226mg; **Potassium:** 789mg; **Calcium:** 48mg; **Iron:** 4mg; **Zinc:** 1mg; **Vitamin A:** 689IU.

Salads

Incredible, Edible Gelatin

GELATIN IS NOT JUST A FUN FOOD FOR KIDS, IT IS A healthy food. Gelatin in meat broths, desserts, and gelatin salads improves digestion by attracting digestive juices to the surface of cooked food particles. According to Sally Fallon in *Nourishing Traditions,* gelatin has been used throughout history in the treatment of many digestive and intestinal disorders. It is one of the "healing" ingredients in meat broths in chapter 16. Note that the vegetarian gelatin source, carrageenan, does not have the same healthy effect and can hinder the actions of digestive enzymes. The recipes here use only unflavored gelatin.

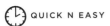

QUICK N EASY

Fruit Knox Blocks

gluten   milk   soy   egg   corn   nuts

This simple recipe is from the makers of Knox gelatin.

- 4 envelopes (1 tablespoon, or 7 g, each) unflavored gelatin
- 1 cup (235 ml) cold fruit juice (orange, grape, cranberry-apple, raspberry/cranberry)
- 3 cups (710 ml) fruit juice, heated to boiling
- 2 tablespoons (25 g) sugar or (40 g) honey (optional)

Sprinkle gelatin over cold juice in a large bowl and let stand 1 minute.

Add hot juice and stir with a metal spoon until gelatin completely dissolves (about 5 minutes). Stir in sugar or honey, if desired. Pour into 13 x 9 x 2-inch (32.5 x 22.5 x 5-cm) pan.

Refrigerate until firm, about 3 hours. To serve, cut into 1-inch (2.5-cm) squares.

YIELD: *9 dozen 1-inch (2.5-cm) squares*

Calories (kcal): 3; **Total fat:** 0g; **Cholesterol:** 0mg; **Carbohydrate:** 1g; **Dietary fiber:** 0g; **Protein:** trace; **Sodium:** 1mg; **Potassium:** trace; **Calcium:** trace; **Iron:** trace; **Zinc:** trace; **Vitamin A:** 0IU

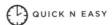

QUICK N EASY

Gelatin Fruit Puree

gluten   milk   soy   egg   corn   nuts

This is a great way for children to enjoy gelatin as part of a meal or dessert without the added sugars and preservatives of the boxed versions. The nutritional content of this real fruit version is far superior and more tasty. This recipe is also a way to sneak in a few vegetables. Pureed carrots or sweet potato will mix nicely with the fruit. For a sick child, this is an easy way to increase liquids via the healing and soothing qualities of gelatin.

- 1 envelope (1 tablespoon, or 7 g) gelatin
- 1/3 cup (80 ml) hot juice (apple, pear, white grape, or grape)
- 1 cup (245 g) pureed fruit (apple, pear, peach) or applesauce or pearsauce.
- If adding vegetables, reduce fruit to 3/4 cup (185 g) and add 1/4 cup (60 g) pureed carrots or sweet potato. Baby food may also be used.

In a medium bowl, dissolve gelatin in hot juice, stirring continuously. Add puree and stir with a rubber spatula to combine. Pour mixture into an 8-inch (20-cm) square or round shallow glass dish, and chill in the refrigerator until firm, about 2 hours.

YIELD: *8 to 10 child-size servings*

Calories (kcal): 7; **Total fat:** 0g; **Cholesterol:** 0mg; **Carbohydrate:** 2g; **Dietary fiber:** 0g; **Protein:** trace; **Sodium:** 5mg; **Potassium:** trace; **Calcium:** trace; **Iron:** trace ; **Zinc:** 0mg ; **Vitamin A:** 0IU

Great Gelatin Fruit Salad

gluten   milk   soy   egg   corn   nuts

This fruit gelatin salad recipe can be adapted many ways, using a variety of fruits. Do not use fresh or frozen pineapple, guava, figs, kiwifruit, or gingerroot in molded salads. They contain bromelin, a protein-dissolving enzyme, which will break up the gelatin's protein bonds. The canned versions are fine because the heat used in canning denatures the bromelin enzymes. For those with sensitive digestive tracts, the fruits in this recipe may be partially cooked and pureed.

- 2 envelopes (1 tablespoon, or 7 g, each) unflavored gelatin
- 3 cups (710 ml) fruit juice (orange, grape, cranberry-apple, raspberry/cranberry, mixed fruit juices), divided as follows:
    - 1 cup (235 ml) cold
    - 2 cups (475 ml) heated to boiling
- 2 tablespoons (25 g) sugar or (40 g) honey (optional)
- 2 cups (300 g) assorted fresh fruits (sliced bananas or strawberries, chopped apples or melon, grapes or blueberries, cut-up peaches or pears)

Sprinkle gelatin over cold juice in a large bowl and let stand 1 minute.

Add hot juice and stir with a metal spoon until gelatin completely dissolves (about 5 minutes). Stir in sugar or honey, if desired.

Refrigerate gelatin mixture until partially chilled (about 1 hour). The gelatin will look like thick, unbeaten egg whites. This allows the added fruits to be evenly distributed. Fold in fruits.

Coat the inside of a 5-cup mold or individual dessert dishes with light oil (safflower) to prevent sticking, and turn the mixture into a mold or dishes. Refrigerate until completely set.

VARIATIONS: *Fruits can also be pureed to avoid lumps for those with oral sensory issues.*

This is another way to hide vegetables. If the pureed fruits work, then hide a few pureed vegetables with the fruits in the gelatin.

TIP: *Mix supplements into the gelatin solution once cooled and pour into ice-cube trays for full chilling so that 1 cube = 1 dose.*

YIELD: *8 servings*

Calories (kcal): 26; **Total fat:** 0g; **Cholesterol:** 0mg; **Carbohydrate:** 6g; **Dietary fiber:** 0g; **Protein:** trace; **Sodium:** 9mg; **Potassium:** trace; **Calcium:** trace; **Iron:** trace; **Zinc:** trace; **Vitamin A:** 0IU

Dotty Lucey's Tangy Tomato Aspic

gluten   milk   soy   egg   corn   nuts

Dana adapted this recipe from her mother's signature party dish. It is another way to sneak vegetables into children's diets. For those who have sensory issues with textures, try adding the vegetables as a puree.

- 3 envelopes (1 tablespoon, or 7 g, each) unflavored gelatin
- 3 cups (710 g) cold tomato juice, divided
- 2 cups (475 ml) tomato juice, heated to boiling
- 1/4 cup (60 ml) lemon juice
- 1/2 teaspoon vinegar
- 1 1/2 teaspoons GFCF Worcestershire sauce
- 1/2 teaspoon salt
- 2 tablespoons (25 g) sugar

Optional for spicier version:

- 1/2 teaspoon onion juice
- 1/8 teaspoon red pepper sauce
- Dash of cloves

Optional addition:

- 1 cup (120 g) finely chopped celery
- 1 cup (180 g) cooked and cut-up asparagus

Spinkle gelatin over 1 cup (235 ml) cold tomato juice in a large bowl; let stand 1 minute to soften gelatin. Add 2 cups (475 ml) hot tomato juice; stir 5 minutes or until gelatin is completely dissolved.

Add remaining 2 cups (475 ml) cold tomato juice, lemon juice, vinegar, Worcestershire sauce, salt, and sugar. For spicier version, add onion juice, red pepper sauce, and dash of cloves.

If adding celery and asparagus, chill for 1 hour until slightly thickened but not set.

Fold in finely chopped or pureed celery and asparagus and spoon into a lightly oiled ring gelatin mold.

Refrigerate for 3 to 4 hours or until firm. Unmold onto a serving platter. Place a dish of GFCF mayonnaise in the center of the ring.

YIELD: *Serves 8 to 12*

Calories (kcal): 49; **Total fat:** trace; **Cholesterol:** 0mg; **Carbohydrate:** 12g; **Dietary fiber:** 1g; **Protein:** 1g; **Sodium:** 566mg; **Potassium:** 283mg; **Calcium:** 13mg; **Iron:** 1mg; **Zinc:** trace; **Vitamin A:** 680IU

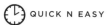

QUICK N EASY

Quick Pasta Salad

gluten   milk   soy   egg   corn   nuts

- 1 package (10–12 ounces, or 280–340 g) rice pasta
- 1 head garlic, baked in a 350°F (180°C, or gas mark 4) oven for 20 minutes or until soft
- 1/8 cup (28 ml) olive oil
- Salt
- Pepper
- Red chili flakes (optional)
- 1 jar (12–15 ounces, or 340–420 g) artichoke hearts, in water or oil, drained and diced
- 15 sundried tomatoes, diced
- 30 kalamata olives, sliced
- 1/4 cup (35 g) pine nuts

Cook pasta according to package directions. After garlic cools, push out the soft garlic from the out-side casing. Combine garlic, oil, and spices and stir with a spoon. Combine all remaining ingredients.

YIELD: *4 to 6 servings*

Calories (kcal): 382; **Total fat:** 13g; **Cholesterol:** 0mg; **Carbohydrate:** 57g; **Dietary fiber:** 7g; **Protein:** 10g; **Sodium:** 471 mg; **Potassium:** 473mg; **Calcium:** 46mg; **Iron:** 2 2mg; **Zinc:** 1mg; **Vitamin A:** 171IU

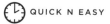

QUICK N EASY

Wild Rice Fruit Salad

gluten   milk   soy   egg   corn   nuts

- 2 cups (330 g) cooked wild rice, cooled
- 1 cup (100 g) chopped celery
- 1/4 cup (35 g) golden raisins
- 1 cup (180 g) pineapple chunks, drained
- 1 cup (190 g) mandarin oranges, drained
- 1 cup (160 g) green seedless grapes
- 1 bunch scallions, sliced
- 1/2 cup (54 g) slivered almonds

Salad Dressing Options

- 1/2–3/4 cup (115–175 g) GFCF mayonnaise
- 1/2 cup (120 ml) Really Quick N Easy Raspberry Vinaigrette (page 107)

Combine all the ingredients. Add enough dressing to moisten the salad.

VARIATION: *Add 2 cups (280 g) chopped cooked chicken for a one-dish meal.*

YIELD: *6 servings*

Calories (kcal): 401; **Total fat:** 30g; **Cholesterol:** 10mg; **Carbohydrate:** 34g; **Dietary fiber:** 4g; **Protein:** 6g; **Sodium:** 181mg; **Potassium:** 410mg; **Calcium:** 64mg; **Iron:** 2mg; **Zinc:** 1mg; **Vitamin A:** 456IU

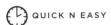 QUICK N EASY

Apple Salad

gluten   milk   soy   egg   corn   nuts

- 2 large Red Delicious apples, unpeeled, cored and cut into 1-inch (2.5-cm) chunks
- ²/₃ cup (135 g) crushed pineapple, drained, or fresh pineapple, minced—reserve juice
- ¹/₃ cup (40 g) celery, diced
- 2 tablespoons (18 g) raisins

Dressing

- 3 tablespoons (45 g) soy yogurt
- 2 teaspoons GFCF mayonnaise
- 1 tablespoon (15 ml) pineapple juice
- ¹/₈ teaspoon cinnamon

In a medium bowl, combine the salad ingredients.

In a small bowl, combine the dressing ingredients. Pour the dressing over the fruit mixture and blend.

YIELD: *4 servings (1 cup [140 g] each)*

Calories (kcal): 105; **Total fat:** 3g; **Cholesterol:** 1mg; **Carbohydrate:** 22g; **Dietary fiber:** 3g; **Protein:** 1g; **Sodium:** 23mg; **Potassium:** 199mg; **Calcium:** 19mg; **Iron:** trace; **Zinc:** trace; **Vitamin A:** 73IU

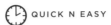 QUICK N EASY

Apple Cole Slaw

gluten   milk   soy   egg   corn   nuts

This great combination of fruit and vegetables in a sweet dressing is a definite favorite.

- 3 cups (270 g) chopped cabbage
- 1 unpeeled red Fuji or Gala apple, cored and chopped
- 1 unpeeled Granny Smith apple, cored and chopped
- 1 medium to large carrot, grated
- 1 scallion, finely chopped (optional)
- 1 cup (75 g) GFCF mayonnaise
- ¹/₃ cup (75 g) GFCF brown sugar
- 1 teaspoon (5 ml) lemon juice
- Salt and pepper to taste

In a large bowl, combine cabbage, apples, carrot, and scallion. In a small bowl, mix together mayonnaise, brown sugar, and lemon juice. Whisk well and add more mayonnaise as needed. Season with salt and pepper to taste. Pour over salad.

YIELD: *6 to 8 servings*

Calories (kcal): 251; **Total fat:** 24g; **Cholesterol:** 10mg; **Carbohydrate:** 14g; **Dietary fiber:** 2g; **Protein:** 1g; **Sodium:** 167mg; **Potassium:** 170mg; **Calcium:** 29mg; **Iron:** 1mg; **Zinc:** trace; **Vitamin A:** 2669IU

260 The Kid-Friendly ADHD and Autism Cookbook

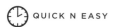 QUICK N EASY

Pasta Salad Supreme

gluten   milk   soy   egg   corn   nuts

This dish can made for all tastes in the family. The basic recipe should be acceptable to even the most picky tastes. If only white foods are preferred, then adding the mashed cauliflower should be a good way to sneak in a vegetable. For a heartier dish, simply add the family's favorite protein, such as cooked shrimp or diced cooked chicken.

- 2 cups (210 g) GFCF pasta of choice, uncooked

Basic Version

- ¹⁄₄ cup (60 ml) red wine vinegar
- 2 tablespoons (28 ml) fresh lemon juice
- 1 teaspoon GFCF mustard
- ¹⁄₄ teaspoon salt
- ¹⁄₄ teaspoon white pepper
- ¹⁄₄ cup (60 ml) olive oil
- ¹⁄₂ cup (120 g) mashed cauliflower (page 176) (optional)

Expanded Version (add these ingredients as suitable to the family members)

- 1 tablespoon dried basil leaves
- 1 small garlic clove, minced
- 1 cup (63 g) snow peas, blanched
- 1 cup (70 g) broccoli florets, blanched
- 1 small red bell pepper
- ¹⁄₄ cup (25 g) black olives, halved
- ¹⁄₄ cup (35 g) pine nuts, toasted

Cook pasta in boiling, salted water to desired degree of doneness. Drain, chill.

For the basic version, whisk together vinegar, lemon juice, mustard, salt, pepper, olive oil, and optional mashed cauliflower. Add to pasta, toss, and chill.

For the expanded version, whisk together all of the dressing ingredients in a large bowl, then add desired optional ingredients. Toss with cooked pasta. Chill.

If making both versions of this salad to accommodate differing tastes, mix the pasta with the first set of ingredients and divide into 2 portions. Reserve the first portion as is (with or without the mashed cauliflower), and to the other portion add half of the listed rest of the ingredients: basil leaves, minced garlic, snow peas, broccoli flowerets, bell pepper, black olives, and pine nuts.

YIELD: *4 servings; 6 if child-size servings*

Calories (kcal): 85; **Total fat:** 9g; **Cholesterol:** 0mg; **Carbohydrate:** 2g; **Dietary fiber:** trace; **Protein:** trace; **Sodium:** 102mg; **Potassium:** 43mg; **Calcium:** 4mg; **Iron:** trace; **Zinc:** trace; **Vitamin A:** 3IU

Cilantro Sweet Slaw

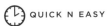

⏱ QUICK N EASY

gluten　　milk　　soy　　egg　　corn　　nuts

- 3 tablespoons (45 ml) canola or avocado oil
- 1 tablespoon (20 g) honey or white grape juice syrup (concentrate from frozen 100% juice)
- 3 tablespoons (45 ml) fresh lime juice
- ½ teaspoon coarse kosher salt
- ½ teaspoon ground black pepper
- 7 cups (12 ounces, or 340 g) purchased shredded three-color coleslaw mix
- 1 cup (60 g) coarsely chopped fresh cilantro

In a medium bowl, whisk and blend oil, honey/juice syrup, lime juice, salt, and pepper.

In a large bowl, add the dressing to the coleslaw mix and cilantro. Toss to coat.

YIELD: *5 cups (600 g)*

Calories (kcal): 567; **Total fat:** 42g; **Cholesterol:** 0mg; **Carbohydrate:** 50g; **Dietary fiber:** 12g; **Protein:** 8g; **Sodium:** 1039mg; **Potassium:** 1367mg; **Calcium:** 252mg; **Iron:** 3mg; **Zinc:** 1mg; **Vitamin A:** 1698IU

⏱ QUICK N EASY

Cabbage Coleslaw

gluten　　milk　　soy　　egg　　corn　　nuts

The mother of one of our patients passed this recipe on as a household favorite.

- 1 small cabbage, shredded
- 1 medium carrot, coarsely grated
- 2 celery stalks (cut into ¼-inch, or 0.6-cm, diagonals)
- 1 bunch scallions (cut into ¼-inch, or 0.6-cm, diagonals)

Dressing Ingredients

- 2 tablespoons (28 ml) apple cider vinegar
- 3 tablespoons (45 ml) fresh lemon juice
- 1 teaspoon honey
- ½ tablespoon (8 g) GFCF mustard
- ⅓ cup (80 ml) cooking oil (high oleic safflower, avocado, almond, extra-virgin olive oil)
- ½ teaspoon celery seed
- ½ teaspoon salt
- ¼ teaspoon ground white pepper
- ¼ teaspoon paprika

In a large bowl, toss together cabbage, carrot, celery, and scallions. In a blender or food processor, blend the dressing ingredients, except paprika. Toss vegetables with dressing. Garnish with paprika. Serve chilled.

YIELD: *4 servings*

Calories (kcal): 190; **Total fat:** 18g; **Cholesterol:** 0mg; **Carbohydrate:** 7g; **Dietary fiber:** 2g; **Protein:** 1g; **Sodium:** 319mg; **Potassium:** 205mg; **Calcium:** 36mg; **Iron:** 1mg; **Zinc:** trace; **Vitamin A:** 5224IU

Wonderful Waldorf Salad

gluten   milk   soy   egg   corn   nuts

There are numerous popular versions of this ageless salad. Contents can be adjusted according to individual tastes.

- 1 cup (155 g) pineapple chunks, fresh or unsweetened canned
- 3 cups (450 g) apples, cut in chunks or ¹/₂-inch (1.25-cm) cubes, peeled or unpeeled
- ¹/₃ cup (50 g) raisins
- 1 stalk celery, chopped
- 1 cup (120 g) carrots, thinly sliced
- ¹/₃-¹/₂ cup (40–60 g) walnut pieces
- 1 cup (225 g) GFCF mayonnaise
- ¹/₄-¹/₂ cup (20–45 g) green pepper, thinly sliced (optional)

Combine all ingredients except mayonnaise. Blend with the mayonnaise.

Serve plain or on lettuce leaves.

YIELD: *4 to 6 servings*

Calories (kcal): 413; **Total fat:** 37g; **Cholesterol:** 13mg; **Carbohydrate:** 24g; **Dietary fiber:** 4g; **Protein:** 4g; **Sodium:** 223mg; **Potassium:** 358mg; **Calcium:** 36mg; **Iron:** 1mg; **Zinc:** 1mg; **Vitamin A:** 5980IU

Colleen's Fresh Salad Topped with Chicken and Pine Nuts

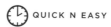

gluten   milk   soy   egg   corn   nuts

Colleen Godbout offers this quick, healthy, and delicious salad, perfect for family and company.

- 1–2 tablespoons (15–30 ml) olive oil
- ¹/₂ cup (70 g) pine nuts
- 10 ounces (280 g) chicken breast strips (packaged or cut from baked or roasted chicken)
- 4 cups (120 g) organic baby spinach (well washed and dried)
- 4 cups (80 g) organic mixed greens (well washed and dried)
- 1 teaspoon sea salt, to taste

Splash the olive oil in a small frying pan on medium heat and toast the pine nuts until golden brown. Put the pine nuts/olive oil mixture in a dish and let cool.

Heat the chicken strips in the pan used for toasting the pine nuts.

Combine and mix spinach, mixed greens, and chicken or beef or shrimp. Top with pine nuts. Season with sea salt to taste.

VARIATIONS: *Add cranberries, raisins, or sliced strawberries. Substitute chicken with grilled steak tips or shrimp.*

YIELD: *4 servings*

Calories (kcal): 269; **Total fat:** 21g; **Cholesterol:** 36mg; **Carbohydrate:** 5g; **Dietary fiber:** 3g; **Protein:** 17g; **Sodium:** 583mg; **Potassium:** 426mg; **Calcium:** 72mg; **Iron:** 3mg; **Zinc:** 1mg Vitamin A (i.u.): 3020IU

Simple Egg Salad

gluten   milk   soy   egg   corn   nuts

This recipe is easy and a favorite among kids. They enjoy helping with boiling the eggs, peeling them, and "smashing" them.

- 6 large eggs
- $^3/_8$ cup (85 g) GFCF mayonnaise
- Salt to taste
- Pepper to taste

Hard-boil eggs at least 15 minutes. Run under cold water and peel.

Place eggs in a bowl and smash with a fork until chopped up, or use an egg slicer to slice them one way first and then again at a 90-degree angle.

Add the mayonnaise and mix well. Add salt and pepper to taste.

Serve on GFCF bread as a sandwich, or simply on lettuce, or a sliced tomato, or garnish with a thin slice of avocado.

YIELD: *4 servings*

Calories (kcal): 246; **Total fat:** 24g; **Cholesterol:** 288mg; **Carbohydrate:** 1g; **Dietary fiber:** 0g; **Protein:** 8g; **Sodium:** 200mg; **Potassium:** 87mg; **Calcium:** 36mg; **Iron:** 1mg; **Zinc:** 1mg; **Vitamin A:** 477IU

Egg Salad with Zest

gluten   milk   soy   egg   corn   nuts

This recipe is nice for sandwiches or for snacks and appetizers. Children enjoy helping, especially with peeling and slicing the eggs.

- 4 hard-boiled eggs
- 2 tablespoons (30 g) GFCF mayonnaise
- 1$^1/_2$ teaspoons mustard
- 2 teaspoons (10 ml) rice vinegar, cider vinegar, or pickle juice
- 1 teaspoon honey or real maple syrup
- $^1/_4$ teaspoon salt, or to taste
- 1 stalk celery, minced
- 2 teaspoons pickle relish
- Paprika, for garnish

Options

- GFCF bread or crackers, lettuce leaves, sliced tomato

Place eggs in a bowl and smash with a fork until chopped up, or use an egg slicer to slice them one way first and then again at a 90-degree angle. Add all ingredients, except paprika, including salt to taste. Mix well, chill for at least 5 minutes, and spoon on bread, crackers, lettuce leaves, or tomato slices.

Sprinkle with paprika.

YIELD: *3 servings*

Calories (kcal): 185; **Total fat:** 15g; **Cholesterol:** 286mg; **Carbohydrate:** 5g; **Dietary fiber:** trace; **Protein:** 9g; **Sodium:** 383mg; **Potassium:** 134mg; **Calcium:** 44mg; **Iron:** 1mg; **Zinc:** 1mg; **Vitamin A:** 422IU

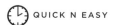

QUICK N EASY

Egg Salad

gluten   milk   soy   egg   corn   nuts

Each version of egg salad has its own special flavor.

- 4 hard-boiled eggs
- 2 tablespoons (30 g) GFCF mayonnaise
- 1¹/₂ teaspoons GFCF mustard
- 2 teaspoons (10 ml) rice vinegar
- 1¹/₂ teaspoons granulated sugar
- ¹/₄ teaspoon salt, or to taste
- 1 stalk celery, minced
- 2 teaspoons pickle relish
- Paprika, for garnish

Place eggs in a bowl and smash with a fork until chopped up.

Add all ingredients, except paprika, including salt to taste.

Mix well, chill for at least 5 minutes, and spoon onto lettuce leaves or tomato slices.

Sprinkle with paprika.

YIELD: *3 servings*

Calories (kcal): 186; **Total fat:** 15g; **Cholesterol:** 286mg; **Carbohydrate:** 5g; **Dietary fiber:** trace; **Protein:** 9g; **Sodium:** 383mg; **Potassium:** 133mg; **Calcium:** 44mg; **Iron:** 1mg; **Zinc:** 1mg; **Vitamin A:** 422IU

Popular Potato Salad

gluten   milk   soy   egg   corn   nuts

This is a popular recipe for an old standard.

- 3 cups (675 g) peeled and diced cooked potatoes
- 4 hard-boiled eggs, peeled and chopped
- ¹/₂ cup (60 g) celery, finely chopped
- ¹/₄ cup (25 g) scallions, finely chopped
- 2 tablespoons (30 g) sweet pickle relish
- ¹/₂ cup (115 g) GFCF mayonnaise
- 1 tablespoon (15 ml) vinegar
- 1 teaspoon sugar or honey
- ¹/₂ teaspoon celery salt
- ¹/₂ teaspoon celery seeds
- ¹/₄ teaspoon white pepper
- ¹/₂ teaspoon dry mustard
- Paprika, for garnish

Combine potatoes, eggs, celery, scallions, and relish in a large bowl. In a small bowl, whisk all remaining ingredients, except paprika, until smooth. Pour over potato mixture and toss until thoroughly coated. Turn into a serving bowl and sprinkle with paprika. Refrigerate until serving time.

YIELD: *6 servings*

Calories (kcal): 264; **Total fat:** 19g; **Cholesterol:** 148mg; **Carbohydrate:** 19g; **Dietary fiber:** 3g; **Protein:** 6g; **Sodium:** 659mg; **Potassium:** 403mg; **Calcium:** 90mg; **Iron:** 2 2mg; **Zinc:** 1mg; **Vitamin A:** 275IU

Lady Di's Summertime Chicken Salad

gluten   milk   soy   egg   corn   nuts

Diana Haan's family and friends love this recipe. This is a real child-pleaser.

- 4 organic chicken breasts, roasted and diced
- 2 celery stalks, diced
- 1 tablespoon (10 g) chopped red onion
- 1 cup (160 g) red grapes
- 1 cup (145 g) blueberries
- 1 can (10.5 ounces, or 294 g) mandarin oranges
- 1¹/₂ cups (340 g) GFCF mayonnaise
- 2 tablespoons (40 g) honey
- 1 tablespoon (15 ml) lemon juice
- 1 teaspoon sugar
- Salt to taste
- Pepper to taste
- 2 tomatoes, cut into wedges

Mix all ingredients except tomato wedges and stir. Add more mayonnaise for desired dressing consistency. Serve on mixed greens with tomato wedges.

YIELD: *4 to 6 servings*

Calories (kcal): 811; **Total fat:** 65g; **Cholesterol:** 143mg; **Carbohydrate:** 22g; **Dietary fiber:** 2g; **Protein:** 42g; **Sodium:** 454mg; **Potassium:** 718mg; **Calcium:** 50mg; **Iron:** 2 2mg; **Zinc:** 2mg; **Vitamin A:** 1042IU

 QUICK N EASY

Bonnie's Easy Chicken Salad

gluten   milk   soy   egg   corn   nuts

Bonnie Gutman's version is without mayonnaise. It is perfect for summer meals.

- 5 cups (700 g) cubed cooked chicken
- 2 tablespoons (28 ml) oil (avocado, almond, safflower, light olive)
- 2 tablespoons (28 ml) orange juice
- 2 tablespoons (28 ml) vinegar
- 2 teaspoons salt
- 3 cups (495 g) cooked white rice, cooled
- 1¹/₂ cups (150 g) celery, sliced
- 1 can (15.75 ounces, or 440 g) pineapple chunks in juice, drained
- 1 can (10.5 ounces, or 294 g) mandarin oranges
- 1 cup (92 g) toasted sliced almonds (optional)

Combine chicken, oil, orange juice, vinegar, and salt. Let stand 30 minutes.

Add the remaining ingredients except the almonds and mix together well.

Sprinkle almonds over the top and serve.

YIELD: *12 servings*

Calories (kcal): 286; **Total fat:** 11g; **Cholesterol:** 50mg; **Carbohydrate:** 24g; **Dietary fiber:** 2g; **Protein:** 22g; **Sodium:** 416mg; **Potassium:** 376mg; **Calcium:** 60mg; **Iron:** 1mg; **Zinc:** 1mg; **Vitamin A:** 213IU

Asian Cucumber Salad

gluten   milk   soy   egg   corn   nuts

If you can't find English cucumbers (sometimes sold as seedless cucumbers), substitute 2 medium regular cucumbers instead. Also, feel free to peel and seed the cucumbers if your child prefers them this way.

- 2 tablespoons (30 ml) rice vinegar
- 2 tablespoons (26 g) sugar
- 1 English cucumber
- 2 teaspoons minced fresh ginger
- 1 teaspoon sesame oil

In a small saucepan, bring the sugar and vinegar to a boil; cook for 1 minute, until mixture has thickened slightly. Remove from heat and cool completely.

Cut cucumber in half lengthwise, and then cut each half into very thin slices. Toss with ginger and sesame oil and allow to marinate for 10 to 15 minutes.

Just before serving, pour the vinegar-sugar dressing over the cucumbers and toss to combine.

YIELD: *4 servings*

Calories (kcal): 46; **Total fat:** 1g; **Cholesterol:** 0mg; **Carbohydrate:** 9g; **Dietary fiber:** 1g; **Protein:** 1g; **Sodium:** trace; **Potassium:** 305mg; **Calcium:** 1mg; **Iron:** trace; **Zinc:** trace; **Vitamin A:** 200IU.

Sesame Green Bean Salad

gluten   milk   soy   egg   corn   nuts

- $^1/_2$ pound (225 g) green beans, trimmed and cut into 2-inch (5 cm) pieces
- 1 medium red bell pepper, cored, seeded, and cut into thin 2-inch (5 cm) strips
- 1 tablespoon (6 g) minced fresh ginger
- 1$^1/_2$ teaspoon salt
- $^1/_2$ teaspoon maple syrup
- 1 tablespoon (15 ml) sesame oil
- 1 tablespoon (8 g) toasted sesame seeds

Bring a pot of water to a boil; set up a bowl of ice water nearby. Boil the green beans until just tender, and then transfer them to the ice water until completely cool. Drain and transfer to a medium bowl. Add the remaining ingredients and toss well to combine and serve.

YIELD: *2 to 4 servings*

Calories (kcal): 68; **Total fat:** 4g; **Cholesterol:** 0mg; **Carbohydrate:** 7g; **Dietary fiber:** 3g; **Protein:** 2g; **Sodium:** 804mg; **Potassium:** 173mg; **Calcium:** 30mg; **Iron:** 1mg; **Zinc:** trace; **Vitamin A:** 512IU.

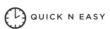

Chickpea Chicken Salad

gluten   milk   soy   egg   corn   nuts

This salad can be served as is with some GFCF crackers, or on top of a bed of salad greens.

- 1 can (14 ounces or 400 g) chickpeas, drained and rinsed
- 2 cups (280 g) cooked, shredded chicken
- 4 scallions, thinly sliced
- 1 stick of celery, finely chopped
- $1/2$ cup (120 ml) olive oil
- $1/4$ cup (60 ml) lemon juice
- 1 teaspoon lemon zest
- 2 cloves garlic, minced
- 3 tablespoons (12 g) chopped parsley
- 1 tablespoon (4 g) chopped fresh dill
- $1/4$ teaspoon mustard powder
- Salt and freshly ground black pepper

In a large bowl, combine the chickpeas, chicken, scallions, and celery. In a separate bowl, whisk together the oil, lemon juice, zest, garlic, parsley, dill, mustard powder, and salt and pepper to taste. Pour over the chickpea mixture, toss to combine, and then cover and chill for 2 hours to allow flavors to meld.

YIELD: *4 to 6 servings*

Calories (kcal): 328; **Total fat:** 21g; **Cholesterol:** 40mg; **Carbohydrate:** 17g; **Dietary fiber:** 3g; **Protein:** 18g; **Sodium:** 243mg; **Potassium:** 305mg; **Calcium:** 44mg; **Iron:** 2mg; **Zinc:** 1mg; **Vitamin A:** 184IU.

QUICK N EASY

Corn and Black Bean Salad

gluten   milk   soy   egg   corn   nuts

This is great with sweet, summertime corn, but frozen corn can be substituted.

- 3 tablespoons (45 ml) fresh lime juice
- $1/4$ teaspoon cumin
- $1/4$ teaspoon chili powder
- $1/4$ teaspoon salt
- 1 teaspoon agave nectar
- 3 tablespoons (45 ml) safflower oil
- 2 cups (450 g) cooked corn kernels
- 1 medium red bell pepper, seeded and chopped fine
- 1 can (15.5 ounces) black beans, rinsed
- 2 tablespoons (8 g) minced cilantro leaves

In a large bowl, whisk the lime juice, spices, and agave nectar together. Slowly add the oil while whisking vigorously, until the dressing is emulsified. Add the corn, pepper, beans, and cilantro and toss to combine. Serve.

YIELD: *4 servings*

Calories (kcal): 267; **Total fat:** 12g; **Cholesterol:** 0mg; **Carbohydrate:** 33g; **Dietary fiber:** 9g; **Protein:** 9g; **Sodium:** 486mg; **Potassium:** 283mg; **Calcium:** 8mg; **Iron:** 1; **Zinc:** trace; **Vitamin A:** 478IU.

CHAPTER 17

Soups and Stews

Stocks and Broths

THE PERFECT BEGINNING FOR THIS SECTION IS WITH the stocks that become the basis for many of the great soups. Whether homemade or purchased, these are an important part of healthy eating. The homemade versions of meat stocks contain natural gelatin, so important to digestion and healing. Unflavored gelatin can be added to store-bought versions to boost the healthy qualities of these broths. We have also included a vegetable broth; however, without the gelatin, the vegetable stocks are not as beneficial to digestion. Read the information on gelatin in chapter 9.

Chicken Stock

gluten   milk   soy   egg   corn   nuts

For those who prefer to make their own nutritious chicken stock, this recipe from Nourishing Traditions, *by Sally Fallon, is the best. It is nutritious and has healthy fatty acids and gelatin, which give chicken soup its healing reputation. See page 186 for a discussion of the health benefits of animal-source gelatin.*

- 1 whole organic chicken or 2–3 pounds (0.9–1.4 kg) bony chicken parts such as necks, backs, breastbones, and wings
- Gizzards from one chicken (optional)
- Chicken feet (optional)
- 4 quarts (3.8 L) cold filtered water
- 1 tablespoon (15 ml) vinegar
- 1 large onion, coarsely chopped
- 2 carrots, peeled and coarsely chopped
- 3 celery stalks, coarsely chopped
- 1 bunch parsley

If using a whole chicken, remove the fat glands and the gizzards from the cavity. Chicken feet provide healthy, healing gelatin. Place chicken or chicken pieces, and gizzards and feet if using them, in a large stainless steel pot with the water, vinegar, onion, carrots, and celery. Bring to a boil and remove any scum that rises to the top. Cover and simmer for 12 to 24 hours. The longer the stock is cooked, the richer and more flavorful it will be. Add parsley 5 minutes before finishing the stock. (Parsley is a good source of minerals.)

Remove from heat and take out the chicken with a slotted spoon. Let it cool and remove chicken meat from the bones. Reserve the chicken meat for other uses such as chicken salads, enchiladas, sandwiches, or curries.

Strain the stock into a large bowl and reserve in your refrigerator until the fat rises to the top and congeals. Skim off this fat and reserve the stock in covered containers in your refrigerator or freezer.

VARIATIONS: Turkey Stock and Duck Stock

Prepare as chicken stock, using turkey wings and drumsticks or duck carcasses from which the breasts, legs, and thighs have been removed. These stocks will have a stronger flavor than chicken stock and will profit from the addition during cooking of several sprigs of fresh thyme tied together. The reserved duck fat is highly prized for cooking purposes.

YIELD: *2 quarts (1.9 L)*

Calories (kcal): 3361; **Total fat:** 234g; **Cholesterol:** 1358mg ; **Carbohydrate:** 34g; **Dietary fiber:** 10g; **Protein:** 263g; **Sodium:** 1347mg; **Potassium:** 4287mg; **Calcium:** 419mg; **Iron:** 26mg; **Zinc:** 22mg; **Vitamin A:** 56507IU

Clarified Stock

gluten milk soy egg corn nuts

If a perfectly clear stock is needed, the following will give the desired result.

- 2 egg whites, lightly beaten
- 2 quarts (1.9 L) defatted stock

Add egg whites to stock and bring to a boil, whisking with a wire whisk. When the stock begins to boil, stop whisking. Let it boil for 3 to 5 minutes. On the surface, a white foam will gradually form and become a spongy crust. Remove the pot from the heat, lift off the crust, and strain the stock through a strainer lined with several layers of cheese cloth.

YIELD: *2 quarts (1.9 L)*

Calories (kcal): 209; **Total fat:** 2g; **Cholesterol:** 0mg; **Carbohydrate:** 8g; **Dietary fiber:** 0g; **Protein:** 14g; **Sodium:** 17287mg; **Potassium:** 779mg; **Calcium:** 24mg; **Iron:** 12mg; **Zinc:** 0mg; **Vitamin A:** 0IU

 QUICK N EASY

Quick N Easy Chicken Stock

     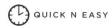

gluten milk soy egg corn nuts

This lacks the flavor and nutritive properties of home-made stock, but it will do for a quick solution.

- 1 can (14 ounces, or 425 ml) chicken stock
- 1 tablespoon (7 g) unflavored gelatin

Mix stock with gelatin, bring to a boil.

YIELD: *Approximately 2 cups (475 ml) stock*

Calories (kcal): 92; **Total fat:** trace; **Cholesterol:** 0mg; **Carbohydrate:** 15g; **Dietary fiber:** 0g; **Protein:** 3g; **Sodium:** 3530mg; **Potassium:** 140mg; **Calcium:** 4mg; **Iron:** 2mg; **Zinc:** 0mg; **Vitamin A:** 0IU

 QUICK N EASY

Quick Beef Stock

gluten milk soy egg corn nuts

This lacks the flavor and nutritive properties of home-made stock, but will do for a quick solution.

- 1 can (14 ounces, or 425 ml) beef stock
- 1 tablespoon (7 g) unflavored gelatin

Mix stock with gelatin, bring to a boil.

YIELD: *Approximately 2 cups (475 ml) stock*

Calories (kcal): 92; **Total fat:** trace; **Cholesterol:** 0mg; **Carbohydrate:** 15g; **Dietary fiber:** 0g; **Protein:** 3g; **Sodium:** 3530mg; **Potassium:** 140mg; **Calcium:** 4mg; **Iron:** 2mg; **Zinc:** 0mg; **Vitamin A:** 4IU

Beef Stock

gluten   milk   soy   egg   corn   nuts

Good beef stock must be made with several kinds of beef bones: knuckle bones and feet impart large quantities of gelatin to the broth, marrow bones impart flavor and the particular nutrients of the bone marrow, and meaty rib or neck bones add color and flavor. In moving away from animal-source foods, we have lost many of the nutrients so common in human diets throughout the ages. Organic sources are important. See page 186 for a discussion of the health benefits of gelatin.

- 6 pounds (2.7 kg) beef marrow and knuckle bones
- 1 calf's foot, cut into pieces (optional)
- 4 quarts (3.8 L) or more cold filtered water, divided
- 5 pounds (2.3 kg) meaty rib or neck bones
- ¼ cup (60 ml) vinegar
- 3 onions, coarsely chopped
- 3 carrots, coarsely chopped
- 3 celery stalks, coarsely chopped
- 2 sprigs fresh thyme, tied together
- 1 teaspoon dried green peppercorns, crushed
- 1 bunch parsley

Place the beef marrow and knuckle bones and optional calf's foot in a very large pot and cover with water.

Let stand for 1 hour.

Meanwhile, place the meaty bones in a roasting pan and brown at 350°F (180°C, gas mark 4) in the oven. When well browned, add to the pot along with vinegar and vegetables.

Pour fat out of the roasting pan, add cold water, set over a high flame and bring to a boil, stirring with a wooden spoon to deglaze. Add this liquid to the pot. Add additional water if needed to cover the bones. The liquid should not be higher than within 1 inch (2.5 cm) of the rim of the pot since the volume expands during cooking. Bring to a boil.

Using a spoon, remove the scum that comes to the top. Reduce the heat and add thyme and crushed peppercorns.

Simmer stock for at least 12 and as long as 72 hours.

Before finishing, add parsley. Let it wilt, then remove from the stock.

At this point, the brown liquid with gelatinous fatty material is unattractive and smelly. But you are not finished yet! Clear, delicious broth is just ahead.

Remove bones with tongs or a slotted spoon. Strain the stock into a large bowl.

Let cool in the refrigerator and remove the congealed fat that rises to the top.

Reheat and transfer to storage containers.

This is now a wonderful stock for soups.

YIELD: *2 quarts (1.9 L)*

Calories (kcal): 306; **Total fat:** 2g; **Cholesterol:** 0mg; **Carbohydrate:** 71 g; **Dietary fiber:** 21 g; **Protein:** 10g; **Sodium:** 345mg; **Potassium:** 2097mg; **Calcium:** 523mg; **Iron:** 19mg; **Zinc:** 4mg; **Vitamin A:** 64377IU

Anne Evans Bone Marrow Stock

gluten   milk   soy   egg   corn   nuts

Anne's daughter Sarah, who has recovered from autism, wants to share this recipe because it made a huge difference in Sarah's health.

Beef marrow bones are a completely natural, easily digestible, and easy-to-assimilate source of all the amino acids. Amino acids improve immunity and are sources for the brain neurotransmitters. Stocks made the traditional way improve digestion and have a healing effect on the digestive tract.

- 8–10 pounds (3.6–4.5 kg) stew bones from (sliced 1–2 inches, or 2.5–5 cm, thick)
- Filtered water
- $^1/_2$ teaspoon salt

In a large stockpot or Dutch oven, brown the bones and drain off the fat. Add enough filtered water to the pot to cover the bones. Add salt and bring to a boil.

Boil until the marrow falls out of the bones (approximately 45 minutes). Be sure to push all the marrow from all the bones back into the pot (this is essential).

Remove the bones from the pot. Let cool. Puree the stock plus marrow in small quantities in the blender. Store in the fridge—it keeps for a week.

Use this stock for sauces, gravies, soups, boiling rice pasta, moistening mashed potatoes, cooking vegetables, etc.

Calories (kcal): 0; **Total fat:** 0g; **Cholesterol:** 0mg; **Carbohydrate:** 0g; **Dietary fiber:** 0g; **Protein:** 0g; **Sodium:** 1066mg; **Potassium:** 0mg; **Calcium:** 7mg; **Iron:** 0mg; **Zinc:** 0 0mg; **Vitamin A:** 0IU

Vegetable Broth for the Whole Family

gluten   milk   soy   egg   corn   nuts

This recipe is perfect for use in a baby bottle or sippy cup. It is very nutritious and an easy way to hide nutritional supplements.

- 4 cups (945 ml) cold water, or 3 cups (710 ml) cold water and 1 cup (235 ml) chicken broth
- 1 cup (150 g) cauliflower florets
- 1 cup (170 g) broccoli florets
- 1 cup (55 g) collard or dandelion greens, rinsed and roughly chopped
- 1 cup (130 g) carrots, cut into rounds

Place water (and chicken broth) in a medium pot with a lid. Add vegetables and bring to a boil over high heat. Reduce heat to a simmer and cover pot. Cook for 1 hour. Strain broth and reserve vegetables. These can be pureed or mashed. This broth freezes well in ice-cube trays for later use.

YIELD: *Makes about 3 cups (serving size $^1/_2$ cup [120 ml])*

Calories (kcal): 85; **Total fat:** 1g; **Cholesterol:** 0mg; **Carbohydrate:** 18g; **Dietary fiber:** 7g; **Protein:** 4g; **Sodium:** 98mg; **Potassium:** 693mg; **Calcium:** 139mg; **Iron:** 1mg; **Zinc:** 1 1mg; **Vitamin A:** 37894IU

Soups and Stews

All soups and stews can be pureed to achieve a texture that is best suited to your child's sensory development.

Chicken Noodle Soup

gluten   milk   soy   egg   corn   nuts

Here's another tasty alternative to a childhood favorite. This GF version really satisfies a hungry tummy.

- 2 cups (475 ml) chicken broth
- 10 cups (2.4 L) water
- 2 medium onions, diced
- 3 large carrots, diced
- 2 medium potatoes, diced
- 1$^1/_2$ tablespoons parsley flakes
- 1 tablespoon (18 g) salt
- 1 teaspoon pepper
- $^1/_2$ teaspoon garlic
- 16–20 ounces (455–560 g) brown rice spaghetti
- 1 cooked chicken, diced

Put all ingredients except spaghetti and chicken in a stockpot. Simmer 1 hour. Break spaghetti into 1-inch (2.5-cm) lengths and boil in a separate pot (rice pasta is very starchy). Add chicken to stock pot and simmer 15 additional minutes. Add noodles and serve.

YIELD: *12 servings*

Calories (kcal): 443; **Total fat:** 20g; **Cholesterol:** 113mg; **Carbohydrate:** 36g; **Dietary fiber:** 3g; **Protein:** 27g; **Sodium:** 761 mg; **Potassium:** 481 mg; **Calcium:** 33mg; **Iron:** 2 2mg; **Zinc:** 2mg; **Vitamin A:** 6125IU

Jane's Lentil Vegetable Soup

gluten   milk   soy   egg   corn   nuts

This recipe is quick to put together and can be a meal in itself.

- 2 cups (400 g) lentils
- 6 cups (1.4 L) water
- 2 cups (475 ml) beef broth
- 2 slices bacon, diced (optional)
- $^1/_2$ cup (80 g) chopped onion
- $^1/_2$ cup (50 g) chopped celery
- $^1/_4$ cup (35 g) chopped carrot
- 3 tablespoons (12 g) parsley
- 1 clove garlic, minced
- 2 teaspoons salt
- $^1/_4$ teaspoon pepper
- $^1/_2$ teaspoon oregano
- 1 tablespoon (15 ml) GFCF Worcestershire sauce
- 1 can (14.5 ounces, or 411 g) diced tomatoes
- 2 tablespoons (28 ml) apple cider vinegar

Rinse lentils and place in a large soup kettle. Add water and beef broth and the remaining ingredients except tomatoes and vinegar. Cover and simmer for 1$^1/_2$ hours.

Add tomatoes and vinegar and simmer for $^1/_2$ hour more.

YIELD: *8 servings*

Calories (kcal): 207; **Total fat:** 1g; **Cholesterol:** 1mg; **Carbohydrate:** 33g; **Dietary fiber:** 16g; **Protein:** 17g; **Sodium:** 920mg; **Potassium:** 714mg; **Calcium:** 51mg; **Iron:** 5 5mg; **Zinc:** 2mg; **Vitamin A:** 1561IU

Joyce's Versatile Vegetable Medley Soup

gluten   milk   soy   egg   corn   nuts

Joyce Mulcahy uses her vegetable medley as the basis for a delicious pureed soup with the addition of organic chicken broth.

- $1/2$ onion, sliced or chopped
- 1 garlic clove, minced
- 1 red or green pepper, chopped
- 1 tablespoon (15 ml) olive oil

Basic vegetables

- 1 can (14.5 ounces, or 411 g) diced tomatoes with juice, or 1–2 fresh chopped tomatoes
- 2–3 sliced zucchini
- Salt and pepper to taste

Optional additions (one or more of the following):

- $1/2$ fennel bulb, chopped
- $2/3$ cup (105 g) white corn, frozen or fresh
- 1 small eggplant, peeled and sliced

Herb Options:

Italian Herbs:

- 4–5 minced basil leaves or $1/2$–1 tablespoon (15 g) pesto
- $1/2$ teaspoon oregano

Mexican Herbs:

- 1 teaspoon cumin
- 1–2 tablespoons (8 g) chopped cilantro (fresh)

- 1–2 cups (235–475 ml) chicken broth, depending on desired consistency of soup

Sauté onion, garlic, and pepper in olive oil until the onions are translucent.

Add basic (and optional) vegetables and herbs and simmer on medium-low heat for 15 minutes, stirring occasionally.

Place the ingredients in a blender. Add $1/2$ cup (120 ml) chicken broth and begin blending. Continue to add chicken broth and blend until the desired consistency is reached.

YIELD: *5 to 6 servings*

Calories (kcal): 667; **Total fat:** 21g; **Cholesterol:** 0mg; **Carbohydrate:** 107g; **Dietary fiber:** 33g; **Protein:** 31g; **Sodium:** 1676mg; **Potassium:** 4850mg; **Calcium:** 247mg; **Iron:** 9mg; **Zinc:** 4 4mg; **Vitamin A:** 6144IU

Turkey Noodle Soup

 gluten milk soy egg corn nuts

Turkey is not just for Thanksgiving, although turkey soup is one of the most popular ways to serve leftovers from Thanksgiving. Perfect as a meal or part of a meal, like chicken noodle soup, it is soothing to digestion and healing. If using ready-to-eat chicken broth, add gelatin to enhance the quality.

- 4 cups (940 ml) homemade Chicken Stock (see page 198) or ready-to-eat chicken broth with 1 envelope (1 tablespoon, or 7 g) plain gelatin added
- 1/2 cup (80 g) yellow onion, chopped
- 1/2 cup (65 g) carrot, chopped
- 1 tablespoon (4 g) minced fresh parsley
- 1/2 teaspoon minced fresh thyme
- 1 bay leaf
- 1/2 teaspoon black pepper
- 4 ounces (115 g) uncooked GF macaroni or small pasta shells
- 2 cups (about 3/4 pound, or 340 g) cubed cooked turkey
- 1 cup (180 g) chopped tomatoes

In a large sauce pot over medium heat, combine broth, onion, carrot, parsley, thyme, bay leaf, and pepper. Bring to a boil. Stir in macaroni, cover, and reduce heat. Simmer for about 6 minutes. Stir in turkey and tomatoes. Cook until heated through and macaroni is tender. Discard bay leaf before serving.

YIELD: *Makes 8 servings of 1 cup (215 ml) each*

Calories (kcal): 336; **Total fat:** 17g; **Cholesterol:** 111mg; **Carbohydrate:** 16g; **Dietary fiber:** 2g; **Protein:** 28g; **Sodium:** 115mg; **Potassium:** 478mg; **Calcium:** 43mg; **Iron:** 3 3mg; **Zinc:** 3mg; **Vitamin A:** 6232IU

Greek Lemon Chicken Soup

 gluten milk soy egg corn nuts

- 2 chicken breasts
- 6 cups (1.4 L) broth or water
- 3 celery ribs
- 1 onion
- 5 garlic cloves
- Salt to taste
- 1/2 cup (90 g) long-grain rice
- 3 eggs, room temperature
- 1/4 cup (60 ml) lemon juice
- 1/2 teaspoon xanthan gum
- 1 teaspoon dill
- Salt to taste

Boil chicken in broth with celery ribs, onion, garlic, and salt for 30 minutes or longer. Pour mixture through a sieve. Put broth back into pot. Add rice.

Beat eggs in a blender. Add lemon juice. Add xanthan gum.

When rice is cooked, add lemon juice/egg mixture slowly, stirring constantly. Add dill and cut-up chicken. Adjust seasonings and salt to taste.

YIELD: *6 to 8 servings*

Calories (kcal): 311; **Total fat:** 13g; **Cholesterol:** 155mg; **Carbohydrate:** 18g; **Dietary fiber:** 1g; **Protein:** 29g; **Sodium:** 871 mg; **Potassium:** 578mg; **Calcium:** 55mg; **Iron:** 2 2mg; **Zinc:** 2mg; **Vitamin A:** 259IU

Peter's Beef Stew

gluten   milk   soy   egg   corn   nuts

- 2 pounds (905 g) cubed beef
- 1 bag (1 pound, or 455 g) baby carrots
- 1/2 celery head, cubed
- 1 teaspoon oregano
- 2 teaspoons salt
- 3 tablespoons Sofrito (45 g) (page 115)
- 1/2 cup (130 g) tomato paste
- 1 1/2 cups (355 ml) water
- 1 teaspoon (5 ml) apple cider vinegar
- 4 medium potatoes, cubed
- 1 teaspoon xanthan gum

Put all ingredients in a slow cooker except potatoes and xanthan gum. Cook on low for 6 hours. One hour before it's finished cooking, add potatoes. When fully cooked, take out 1 cup (235 ml) of liquid and blend it with xanthan gum in the blender. Pour into slow cooker and mix gently.

Serve with rice or quinoa.

YIELD: *8 servings*

Calories (kcal): 373; **Total fat:** 22g; **Cholesterol:** 76mg; **Carbohydrate:** 20g; **Dietary fiber:** 3g; **Protein:** 23g; **Sodium:** 753mg; **Potassium:** 1007mg; **Calcium:** 41mg; **Iron:** 3 3mg; **Zinc:** 5mg; **Vitamin A:** 8951IU

> "The diet has changed my life in many ways. I am able to do things now that I was not capable of doing before."
>
> —**Peter,** *14 years old*

Best Beef Soup Ever

gluten   milk   soy   egg   corn   nuts

This hearty and yummy winter soup is good any time of the year.

- 8–10 cups (1.9–2.4 L) water
- 2 large onions, quartered
- 5 pounds (2.3 kg) short ribs with bone cut into 1-inch (2.5-cm) chunks (results in 2 1/2 pounds, or 1.1 kg, beef chunks)
- 1 tablespoon (18 g) kosher salt
- 1 tablespoon (6 g) ground black pepper
- 4 medium potatoes, quartered
- 1 small head cabbage, cut into bite-size pieces
- 1 large carrot, sliced into thick coins
- 1–2 tablespoons (15–30 ml) GFCF soy-free fish sauce

Combine the first 5 ingredients in a large saucepan or stockpot. Cooked (uncovered) on medium-high heat until beef is tender.

Simmer (covered) for about 3 hours. Add potatoes for the last 30 minutes. Add cabbage and carrot for the last 15 to 20 minutes. Add fish sauce to taste. (This is quite salty but does add to the taste.)

NOTE: *When buying fish sauce, check the ingredient list. Some have hydrolyzed wheat protein added. Thai Kitchen fish sauce is GFCF and soy-free (www.thaikitchen.com).*

YIELD: *8 to 10 servings*

Calories (kcal): 117; **Total fat:** 104g; **Cholesterol:** 216mg; **Carbohydrate:** 16g; **Dietary fiber:** 2g; **Protein:** 43g; **Sodium:** 861 mg; **Potassium:** 1095mg; **Calcium:** 50mg; **Iron:** 5mg; **Zinc:** 9mg; **Vitamin A:** 2545IU

Mary Lou's North African Vegetable Stew

gluten · milk · soy · egg · corn · nuts

This tasty stew is perfect for a cold winter day. It warms you from the inside.

- 2 teaspoons vegetable oil
- 1 medium onion, sliced
- 1/2 teaspoon ground coriander
- 1/4 teaspoon turmeric
- 1/2 teaspoon cinnamon
- 1/2 teaspoon ground ginger
- 1/4 teaspoon ground cumin
- 2 medium tomatoes, chopped
- 1 medium sweet potato, peeled and cut
- 1/4 cup (60 ml) water
- 2 tablespoons (28 ml) lemon juice
- 1 can (15 ounces, or 420 g) garbanzo beans, drained and rinsed
- 1 small zucchini, cut into 1-inch (2.5 cm) chunks
- 1/2 cup (30 g) chopped fresh parsley
- 1/4 cup (35 g) raisins
- Hot pepper sauce to taste (optional)

Heat oil. Add onion and spices, cooking until onion is limp, about 10 minutes, stirring frequently. Add tomatoes, sweet potato, water, and lemon juice. Bring to a boil, reduce heat, cover, and simmer approximately 30 minutes. Add beans, zucchini, parsley, and raisins. Cover and simmer another 10 minutes, until zucchini is tender. Season with hot pepper sauce to taste, if desired.

VARIATION: *Add sautéed boneless chicken to stew.*

YIELD: *4 to 6 servings*

Calories (kcal): 506; **Total fat:** 9g; **Cholesterol:** 0mg; **Carbohydrate:** 88g; **Dietary fiber:** 22g; **Protein:** 23g; **Sodium:** 44mg; **Potassium:** 1430mg; **Calcium:** 157mg; **Iron:** 8mg; **Zinc:** 4mg; **Vitamin A:** 7536IU

QUICK N EASY

Doug's Potato Leek Soup

gluten   milk   soy   egg   corn   nuts

Doug and Jeannette DeLawter enjoy sharing this recipe. It is a delicious light soup that is also easy on the digestive system and a good addition to any meal. As with all soups, this soup can be pureed as needed for those children with sensory food-texture issues.

- 3 medium leeks
- 1 medium onion
- 4 carrots, peeled or scrubbed
- 2 stalks celery
- 3 medium white potatoes, peeled
- Salt and pepper to taste
- $1/4$ teaspoon garlic powder
- 2 bay leaves
- 3 cans (14.5 ounces, or 411 g, each) chicken broth
- 3 chicken broth cans water

Under cool running water, clean dirt from leeks. Split leeks lengthwise into 4 sections, and chop into small pieces up to and including part of the green stalk.

Chop onion, carrots, and celery into small pieces. Cut potatoes into $1/4$-inch (0.6-cm) cubes.

Place leeks, onion, carrots, and celery into a large dry pot and simmer until ingredients soften.

Wash potato cubes in colander to rinse off starch and dry with paper towel before adding to vegetables. Add seasonings. Stir all ingredients frequently, not allowing them to stick to bottom of pot. When vegetables are softened, add broth and water. Bring the soup to a boil and then simmer until potatoes are cooked. Remove bay leaves before serving.

YIELD: *8 to 10 servings*

Calories (kcal): 105; **Total fat:** 1g; **Cholesterol:** 0mg; **Carbohydrate:** 19g; **Dietary fiber:** 3g; **Protein:** 5g; **Sodium:** 543mg; **Potassium:** 613mg; **Calcium:** 49mg; **Iron:** 2 2mg; **Zinc:** 1mg; **Vitamin A:** 10173IU

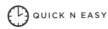 QUICK N EASY

Carrot Veggie Stew

gluten   milk   soy   egg   corn   nuts

From The Lambert Hill Farm, originally from Marilyn Lammers, with quite a bit of revising along the way, as it has been passed down through generations! This nutrient-rich stew has a good amount of beta-carotene. This is a good stew for adding more vegetables into the diet, easily mixed in with the others. It can also be pureed in a blender for those who do not tolerate "lumps and bumps" in foods.

- 1 large onion, chopped (Vidalia recommended)
- 2 cloves garlic, diced
- 1 tablespoon (15 ml) olive oil
- 2 cans (12 ounces, or 355 ml, each) carrot juice
- 1/2 cup (120 ml) chicken broth
- 1 tablespoon (8 g) chili powder (this is very conservative; use more or use cayenne for a spicier stew)
- 1 tablespoon (15 ml) vinegar
- 20 ounces (570 ml) water
- 3 cups (360 g) chopped fresh vegetables (carrots or cook's choice of vegetables)
- 1 can (19 ounces, or 530 g) red kidney beans

Sauté onion and garlic in olive oil until transparent, about 5 minutes. Add juice (reserve empty cans), broth, chili powder, and vinegar. Bring to a boil. Pour water into empty carrot-juice cans and swish around; add to soup. Add veggies. Cover and simmer slowly (so the veggies keep their texture) until veggies are tender, about 15 minutes. Add beans and simmer for another couple of minutes to heat through.

YIELD: *12 servings*

Calories (kcal): 192; **Total fat:** 2g; **Cholesterol:** 0mg; **Carbohydrate:** 34g; **Dietary fiber:** 8g; **Protein:** 11g; **Sodium:** 62mg; **Potassium:** 814mg; **Calcium:** 57mg; **Iron:** 3 3mg; **Zinc:** 1mg; **Vitamin A:** 14823IU

Vegetable Puree Soup

gluten   milk   soy   egg   corn   nuts

This is a tasty way to expand on vegetables in a way that is acceptable with most who have sensory issues.

- 12 cups (2.8 L) water
- 1/4 cup (35 g) yellow split peas
- 1/4 cup (35 g) green split peas
- 4-6 medium carrots
- 2 sweet potatoes
- 2 medium zucchini
- 2 medium parsnips
- 1 large onion
- 1 teaspoon salt
- 1 teaspoon dried dill

Bring water to a boil. Lower heat and add yellow and green peas. Cover and simmer for 1 hour. Peel and cut remaining vegetables into large chunks. Add vegetables, salt, and dill. Bring to a boil, then lower heat and simmer, covered, for 1 more hour. Puree with an immersion blender in the pot or in batches in a blender (at low/medium speed) or a food processor.

YIELD: *8 to 12 servings*

Calories (kcal): 120; Total fat: trace; Cholesterol: 0mg; Carbohydrate: 26g; Dietary fiber: 7g; Protein: 4g; Sodium: 245mg; Potassium: 554mg; Calcium: 54mg; Iron: 1mg; Zinc: 1mg; Vitamin A: 15497IU

Super Carrot Soup

gluten   milk   soy   egg   corn   nuts

- 1 small onion, chopped
- 2 tablespoons (30 g) ghee, divided
- 5-6 medium carrots, peeled and chopped
- 1 large potato, peeled and cubed
- 1 can (14.5 ounces, or 406 ml) chicken broth
- 1 1/2 cups (105 g) chopped fresh mushrooms
- 1 stalk celery, chopped
- 1 clove garlic, minced
- 1/2 teaspoon sugar
- 1/2 teaspoon salt
- 1/2 teaspoon dried thyme
- 1/4 teaspoon GFCF hot pepper sauce
- 1/2 cup (120 ml) milk substitute (rice, soy, coconut)
- Salt and pepper to taste

In a large saucepan, sauté onion in 1 tablespoon (15 g) ghee until tender. Add carrots and potato and cook for 2 minutes. Add broth, mushrooms, celery, garlic, sugar, salt, thyme, and pepper sauce. Bring to a boil and reduce heat. Cover and simmer for 50 minutes.

Let mixture cool slightly, then transfer to a blender and blend on medium until smooth.

Return to saucepan. Stir in milk substitute and remaining ghee and heat.

Season with salt and pepper.

YIELD: *6 to 8 servings*

Calories (kcal): 88; Total fat: 4g; Cholesterol: 9mg; Carbohydrate: 12g; Dietary fiber: 2g; Protein: 2g; Sodium: 327mg; Potassium: 390mg; Calcium: 27mg; Iron: 1mg; Zinc: trace; Vitamin A: 15328IU

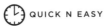 QUICK N EASY

Dana's Really Quick N Easy Vegetable Soup or Puree

gluten milk soy egg corn nuts

This soup can be made as a soup or pureed for those with sensory issues who do not tolerate the "lumps and bumps" in soups or stews. Adding an envelope of gelatin provides a better food that helps digestion. The addition of apple juice adds natural sweetness and enhances the flavor.

- 1 tablespoon (15 ml) olive oil
- 3 tablespoons (30 g) frozen minced onion
- 1/4 teaspoon minced garlic (optional)
- 4 cups (945 ml) store-bought GFCF chicken broth
- 1 cup (235 ml) apple juice (or apple cider)
- 1 envelope (1 tablespoon, or 7 g) unflavored gelatin
- 1 bag (16 ounces, or 455 g) frozen mixed vegetables (peas, corn, carrots)
- Pepper to taste
- Salt, or GFCF fish sauce, to taste

Heat oil over medium-high heat in a 3- to 4-quart (2.8- to 3.8-L) pot or stockpot. Sauté onion (and optional garlic) until translucent and soft. Add chicken broth and apple juice (or cider). Add in gelatin and stir until it dissolves. Add in vegetables. Cook (covered) on medium heat for 15 to 20 minutes.

Add pepper to taste and salt or fish sauce to taste.

Serve as a soup, or puree in blender (medium/high speed) until smooth. Add more liquid if needed.

VARIATION: *Add chicken, turkey, or beef to this for a hearty soup/stew or puree.*

YIELD: *Serves 6 to 8*

Calories (kcal): 94; **Total fat:** 3g; **Cholesterol:** 0mg; **Carbohydrate:** 14g; **Dietary fiber:** 2g; **Protein:** 5g; **Sodium:** 414mg; **Potassium:** 267mg; **Calcium:** 22mg; **Iron:** 1mg; **Zinc:** trace; **Vitamin A:** 2880IU

Asparagus Vichyssoise

gluten   milk   soy   egg   corn   nuts

- 1 tablespoon (15 ml) canola oil
- 1 leek, white part only, cleaned and chopped
- 1 large russet potato, chopped
- 1 pound (455 g) asparagus, trimmed and cut into 1-inch (2.5-cm) pieces
- 4 cups (945 ml) water
- 2 sprigs fresh thyme
- 2 sprigs fresh parsley
- $^3/_4$ teaspoon salt
- $^1/_2$ teaspoon freshly ground pepper
- $^1/_4$ cup (12 g) fresh chives, chopped, for garnish

Heat oil over medium heat in a large saucepan. Add leek, cover, and cook 5 to 7 minutes, stirring occasionally, until softened.

Add chopped potato, asparagus, water, thyme and parsley sprigs, salt, and pepper. Bring to a boil and cook 30 minutes over medium-low heat or until potatoes are tender. Remove thyme and parsley sprigs; pour soup in batches into a food processor (or use an immersion blender) and puree on medium/high to a creamy consistency. Chill well. Garnish with chives before serving.

YIELD: *8 servings*

Calories (kcal): 43; **Total fat:** 2g; **Cholesterol:** 0mg; **Carbohydrate:** 6g; **Dietary fiber:** 2g; **Protein:** 2g; **Sodium:** 215mg; **Potassium:** 243mg; **Calcium:** 41mg; **Iron:** 2mg; **Zinc:** trace; **Vitamin A:** 1041IU

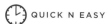 QUICK N EASY

Corn Chowder

      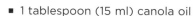

gluten   milk   soy   egg   corn   nuts

This is a good way to add in a few more vegetables in order to expand variety.

- 2 tablespoons (28 ml) oil
- 1 large yellow onion, diced
- 5 medium Yukon Gold potatoes, peeled and chopped
- Salt to taste
- Pepper to taste
- 3 cups (710 ml) water
- 1 bag (16 ounces, or 455 g) frozen corn, defrosted and drained
- 1 cup (235 ml) rice milk

Heat oil over medium-high heat in a large pot or stockpot. Sauté onion until translucent and soft. Add potatoes and mix to coat with oil; sauté 1 to 2 minutes. Add salt and pepper. Add water and corn. Cook until potatoes are soft. Add rice milk and puree until smooth.

VARIATIONS: *Add some squash, carrots, or yams in place of some of the potatoes.*

YIELD: *8 servings*

Calories (kcal): 153; **Total fat:** 4g; **Cholesterol:** 0mg; **Carbohydrate:** 28g; **Dietary fiber:** 3g; **Protein:** 4g; **Sodium:** 10mg; **Potassium:** 557mg; **Calcium:** 13mg; **Iron:** 1mg; **Zinc:** 1mg; **Vitamin A:** 74IU

Thai-Style Pumpkin Soup

gluten   milk   soy   egg   corn   nuts

Here is another excellent recipe by Jody Cutler. This is wonderful blend of colors and flavors. Guaranteed to warm you!

- 1 quart (945 ml) vegetable or chicken broth
- 1 can (15 ounces, or 420 g) pumpkin puree
- 1 can (12 ounces, or 355 ml) mango nectar
- 1/4 cup (65 g) chunky GFCF peanut butter
- 2 tablespoons (28 ml) rice vinegar
- 1 1/2 tablespoons (9 g) minced scallion
- 1 teaspoon grated peeled fresh ginger
- 1/2 teaspoon grated orange rind
- 1/4 teaspoon crushed red pepper
- 1 clove garlic, crushed
- Chopped fresh cilantro (optional)

Combine first 3 ingredients in a large Dutch oven and bring to a boil. Cover, reduce heat, and simmer 10 minutes. Combine 1 cup (235 ml) pumpkin mixture and peanut butter in a blender or food processor; process until smooth. Return mixture to pan. Stir in vinegar and next 5 ingredients (through garlic); cook 3 minutes or until thoroughly heated. Ladle into soup bowls. Sprinkle with cilantro, if using.

YIELD: *6 servings (1 cup [235 ml] each)*

Calories (kcal): 121; Total fat: 6g; Cholesterol: 0mg; Carbohydrate: 11g; Dietary fiber: 2g; Protein: 6g; Sodium: 567mg; Potassium: 322mg; Calcium: 25mg; Iron: 2 2mg; Zinc: 1mg; Vitamin A: 9017IU

Mulligatawny Soup

gluten   milk   soy   egg   corn   nuts

Adapted from The Quick Recipe, by the editors of Cook's Illustrated Magazine. *This is a wonderfully aromatic soup, which is made extra rich (and exotic) with the addition of coconut and banana.*

- 3 tablespoons (42 g) ghee
- 2 medium onions, chopped
- 1 teaspoon tomato paste
- 1/2 cup (42.5 g) unsweetened shredded coconut
- 3 medium cloves garlic, minced
- 1 piece ginger (about 11/2 inches or 3.75 cm), peeled and grated
- 11/2 tablespoons (9.5 g) curry powder
- 1 teaspoon ground cumin
- 1/4 teaspoon cayenne pepper
- 6 tablespoons (45 g) tapioca flour
- 7 cups (1.6 L) GFCF chicken broth
- 2 medium carrots, peeled and chopped
- 1 medium rib celery, chopped
- 1 medium banana, very ripe, peeled
- Table salt and ground black pepper

Optional Garnish

- 2 tablespoons (2 g) minced fresh cilantro leaves
- 3/4 cup (180 g) soy yogurt

Heat the ghee in a large pot over medium heat. Add the onions and tomato paste and cook for 3 minutes, stirring frequently, until the onions have softened. Stir in the coconut, garlic, ginger, curry powder, cumin, cayenne, and tapioca flour, and cook for 1 minute. Gradually whisk in the chicken broth. Add the carrots, celery, and banana; increase heat to medium-high and bring to a boil. Reduce the heat to low, cover, and cook for 20 minutes, or until the vegetables are tender.

Puree the soup in batches in the blender, and then season to taste with salt and pepper. (Return the soup to the pot to reheat if necessary.) Serve and garnish with cilantro and soy yogurt, if desired.

TIP: *Turn this soup into a meal by adding 2 bone-less, skinless chicken breasts once the soup has reached a boil. After the soup has simmered for 20 minutes, remove the chicken and shred with 2 forks; return to the soup after it is has been pureed.*

YIELD: *6 to 8 servings*

Calories (kcal): 169; **Total fat:** 11g; **Cholesterol:** 17mg; **Carbohydrate:** 16g; **Dietary fiber:** 3g; **Protein:** 3g; **Sodium:** 529mg; **Potassium:** 246mg; **Calcium:** 26mg; **Iron:** 1mg; **Zinc:** trace; **Vitamin A:** 5329IU.

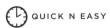

Black Bean Soup

gluten   milk   soy   egg   corn   nuts

- 1 tablespoon (15 ml) extra-virgin olive oil
- 1 medium onion, diced
- 1 tablespoon (7.5 g) chili powder
- 1 teaspoon ground cumin
- 1 teaspoon dried oregano
- 1/2 teaspoon salt
- 3 cups (705 ml) GFCF chicken broth
- 2 cans (15 ounces, or 420 g, each) black beans, drained and rinsed
- 2 garlic cloves, minced
- 1 can (15 ounces, or 420 g) pumpkin puree
- 1/4 cup (15 g) minced fresh cilantro
- 1 tablespoon (15 ml) lime juice

Heat olive oil in large pot over medium-high heat and cook onion, chili powder, cumin, oregano, and salt for 2 minutes, stirring frequently. Add the garlic and cook for 30 seconds. Add the broth and black beans and bring to a boil over high heat; reduce heat and simmer for 3 minutes. Off heat, stir in the cilantro and lime juice and serve.

YIELD: *4 to 6 servings*

Calories (kcal): 197; **Total fat:** 5g; **Cholesterol:** 3mg; **Carbohydrate:** 27g; **Dietary fiber:** 11g; **Protein:** 10g; **Sodium:** 921mg; **Potassium:** 216mg; **Calcium:** 36mg; **Iron:** 2mg; **Zinc:** trace; **Vitamin A:** 16093IU.

QUICK N EASY

Special Ingredient Noodles

gluten   milk   soy   egg   corn   nuts

Inspired by a certain blockbuster Panda, Ellen Demattia came up with this tasty dinner for her family. Their favorite part about this dish is using a special noodle spoon—the flat, ceramic kind they offer in Chinese restaurants.

- 1 quart (.95 L) GFCF chicken broth
- 8 ounces (225 g) dried Pad Thai style Rice Noodles
- 2 cups (280 g) chopped precooked chicken
- 2 cups (about 400 g) chopped cooked mixed vegetables of your choice

Bring the broth to a boil in a large pot. Off heat, add noodles and let sit for 10 to 15 minutes, until noodles are tender. Add chicken and vegetables and cook over medium heat, about 3 minutes. Serve.

YIELD: *4 servings*

Calories (kcal): 462; **Total fat:** 16g; **Cholesterol:** 83mg; **Carbohydrate:** 58g; **Dietary fiber:** 5g; **Protein:** 19g; **Sodium:** 920mg; **Potassium:** 344mg; **Calcium:** 49mg; **Iron:** 3mg; **Zinc:** 2mg; **Vitamin A:** 6952IU.

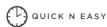
 QUICK N EASY

Simple Egg Drop Soup

gluten   milk   soy   egg   corn   nuts

- 1 large egg
- Salt and ground black pepper
- 1 clove garlic, minced
- 1 tablespoon (8 g) chopped fresh ginger
- 3 scallions, chopped fine
- 4 cups (940 ml) GFCF chicken broth
- 1 teaspoon sesame oil

In a small bowl, lightly beat the egg with a pinch of salt and pepper.

In a large saucepan, bring the chicken broth, garlic, ginger, and 1 teaspoon salt to a boil over high heat; reduce heat and simmer for 3 minutes. Pour the egg in a very thin stream along the prongs of a fork over the surface of the soup. When the egg has set, add the scallions and sesame oil and serve.

YIELD: *4 servings*

Calories (kcal): 69; **Total fat:** 5g; **Cholesterol:** 59mg; **Carbohydrate:** 1g; **Dietary fiber:** trace; **Protein:** 4g; **Sodium:** 598mg; **Potassium:** 55mg; **Calcium:** 16mg; **Iron:** trace; **Zinc:** trace; **Vitamin A:** 123IU.

Tomato Rice Soup

gluten   milk   soy   egg   corn   nuts

- 2 tablespoons (30 ml) olive oil
- 1 small onion, chopped
- 1 clove garlic, minced
- 2 teaspoons tomato paste
- 1 large can (28 ounces, or 800 g) whole tomatoes
- 2 teaspoons agave syrup
- $1/2$ teaspoon salt
- $1/4$ teaspoon coarsely ground pepper
- $1^1/2$ cups (355 ml) GFCF chicken broth
- 1 cup (165 g) cooked rice

Heat oil in large pot over medium heat; cook onion, garlic, and tomato paste 5 minutes, or until onion is soft. Add the tomatoes and their juices, agave syrup, salt and pepper and cook another 5 minutes. Carefully puree mixture in a blender or a food processor until smooth, and then return to the pot. Add the broth and cooked rice and return soup to a boil. Serve.

NOTE: *If you are using white rice, the rice can be pureed along with the tomato mixture for a completely smooth and creamy soup.*

YIELD: *4 servings*

Calories (kcal): 188; **Total fat:** 8g; **Cholesterol:** 2mg; **Carbohydrate:** 26g; **Dietary fiber:** 3g; **Protein:** 4g; **Sodium:** 801mg; **Potassium:** 508mg; **Calcium:** 72mg; **Iron:** 1mg; **Zinc:** 1mg; **Vitamin A:** 1248IU.

Cream of Cauliflower Soup

gluten milk soy egg corn nuts

Coconut milk is the secret to this "creamy" soup, and is healthy for the GI tract. See the discussion about the health benefits of this fabulous food on page 60.

- 1 medium head (about 2 pounds, or 910 g) cauliflower
- 4 tablespoons (60 ml) olive oil, divided
- 2 to 3 teaspoons mild GFCF curry powder
- Salt and ground black pepper
- 1 medium onion, chopped fine
- 2 cups (475 ml) GFCF chicken broth
- 1 can (14 ounces, or 425 ml) unsweetened coconut milk

Preheat oven to 450°F (230°C, gas mark 8). Cut the cauliflower into 1-inch florets, and toss with 3 tablespoons (45 ml) of the oil, curry powder, and 1/2 teaspoon salt in a large bowl. Transfer to a baking sheet and roast for 15 to 20 minutes, until cauliflower is golden brown on the edges, stirring once halfway through.

In a large pot, heat remaining oil over medium heat. Add onion and cook until softened, 5 minutes. Add roasted cauliflower and stock and bring to a boil; reduce heat and simmer, covered, until cauliflower is very soft. Carefully puree soup in a blender with the coconut milk until smooth; season to taste with salt and pepper. Serve, or return to pot to gently reheat if necessary, but do not boil.

YIELD: *6 servings*

Calories (kcal): 265; **Total fat:** 25g; **Cholesterol:** 2mg; **Carbohydrate:** 10g; **Dietary fiber:** 3g; **Protein:** 4g; **Sodium:** 241mg; **Potassium:** 95mg; **Calcium:** 12mg; **Iron:** trace; **Zinc:** trace; **Vitamin A:** 14IU.

Erika's Chicken Noodle Soup

gluten milk soy egg corn nuts

- 3 large boneless skinless chicken breasts
- Water
- 8 cups (1.9 L) GFCF organic chicken broth
- 1 pound (455 g) celery, cut into bite-sized pieces
- 1 pound (455 g) carrots, peeled and cut into bite-sized pieces
- 1 large onion, chopped fine
- 2 tablespoons (8 g) chopped parsley
- Salt and ground black pepper to taste
- 1 pound (455 g) GF noodles

Add chicken and broth to a large stock pot and bring to boil. Skim off brown foam and yellow patches. Add celery, carrots, onion, and parsley, cover, reduce heat to low and simmer for at least one hour, stirring occasionally to break chicken up into pieces (or you can remove breasts after 20 minutes and shred with a fork, and then return to the pot).

Meanwhile, boil another large pot of water and cook the noodles according to package directions. Drain and rinse noodles.

When soup is done, add noodles, and season to taste with salt and pepper. Serve.

YIELD: *6 to 8 servings*

Calories (kcal): 373; **Total fat:** 4g; **Cholesterol:** 56mg; **Carbohydrate:** 51g; **Dietary fiber:** 6g; **Protein:** 28g; **Sodium:** 701mg; **Potassium:** 569mg; **Calcium:** 59mg; **Iron:** 2mg; **Zinc:** 1mg; **Vitamin A:** 14380IU.

White Bean Stew with Swiss Chard

gluten   milk   soy   egg   corn   nuts

This is a nice, hearty soup for those cold weather months.

- 2 ounces (55 g) nitrate-free bacon, chopped fine
- 1 small onion, chopped fine
- 1 carrot, chopped fine
- 2 cloves garlic
- 1 bay leaf
- 1 sprig rosemary
- 3 cups (710 ml) GFCF chicken broth
- 2 cans (15.5 ounces, or 450 g each) cannellini beans, rinsed
- 3 cups (165 g) chopped Swiss chard (from about 1 bunch)
- 2 tablespoons (8 g) chopped parsley
- Salt and ground black pepper
- Extra virgin olive oil for drizzling (optional)

Cook bacon in a large pot or Dutch oven over medium-high heat for 3 to 5 minutes, until golden and most of the fat has rendered. Add onion and carrot and cook until softened, 5 minutes. Stir in the garlic, bay leaf, and rosemary and cook for a few seconds, until fragrant. Pour in broth, beans, and chard, and bring to a boil. Reduce heat and simmer for 15 minutes. Remove bay leaf and rosemary, add parsley, and season to taste with salt and pepper. Serve with a drizzle of olive oil if desired.

TIP: *You can use spinach in place of the chard, but use the curly leaf variety, which will stand up to cooking better.*

YIELD: *4 servings*

Calories (kcal): 427; **Total fat:** 10g; **Cholesterol:** 13mg; **Carbohydrate:** 61g; **Dietary fiber:** 21g; **Protein:** 26g; **Sodium:** 642mg; **Potassium:** 1458mg; **Calcium:** 238mg; **Iron:** 9mg; **Zinc:** 3mg; **Vitamin A:** 6079IU.

CHAPTER 18

Fruits, Sweets, and Treats

FRUITS CAN BE SERVED A VARIETY OF WAYS, AND FRESH
is always the healthiest. Fresh fruit cut up is easy to handle
for most children. For those with sensory issues, use pureed
fruits and fruit sauces such as applesauce and pearsauce.
Baby foods are readily available and easy to use.

For an easy, tasty, and healthy "syrup" topping, blend frozen
raspberries or strawberries (organic is the best choice). Spoon
on top of any mix of cut-up fruit.

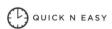

Aunt Fran's Frozen Blueberries

gluten   milk   soy   egg   corn   nuts

Colleen Godbout remembers this as her favorite treat, especially in the summer.

- 1 pint (402 g) fresh blueberries

Wash berries well, then dry on a paper towel. Lay the blueberries flat on a cookie sheet, keeping them separate. Place the cookie sheet in the freezer. Once frozen, place them in resealable plastic bags for storage.

NOTE: *These are also delicious added to cereals.*

For a really Quick N Easy version, buy organic frozen blueberries.

YIELD: *1 pint (402 g), divided in suitable serving sizes*

Calories (kcal): 41; **Total fat:** trace; **Cholesterol:** 0mg; **Carbohydrate:** 10g; **Dietary fiber:** 2g; **Protein:** trace; **Sodium:** 4mg; **Potassium:** 65mg; **Calcium:** 4mg; **Iron:** trace; **Zinc:** trace; **Vitamin A:** 73IU

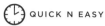

Baked Honey Apple Slices

gluten   milk   soy   egg   corn   nuts

This is very appealing to little ones, and another quick and easy recipe.

- ¹/₄ cup (85 g) honey
- Juice of 1 lemon (fresh or bottled)
- 3 large cooking apples
- ¹/₂ teaspoon cinnamon
- 2 teaspoons ghee

Mix honey and lemon juice in a shallow baking dish or pie pan.

Peel and core apples. Cut apples in quarters, then slices.

Place apples in honey-juice mixture, coating well. Sprinkle with cinnamon.

Melt ghee and pour over the mix.

Bake in a moderate oven, 350°F (180°C, gas mark 4), for 30 to 40 minutes or until tender.

Baste with pan liquid twice during baking.

YIELD: *4 to 6 servings*

Calories (kcal): 149; **Total fat:** 3g; **Cholesterol:** 6mg; **Carbohydrate:** 35g; **Dietary fiber:** 3g; **Protein:** trace; **Sodium:** 2mg; **Potassium:** 153mg; **Calcium:** 16mg; **Iron:** 1mg; **Zinc:** trace; **Vitamin A:** 145IU

Poached Pears

gluten   milk   soy   egg   corn   nuts

Poached fruit is an easy, but elegant dessert for a festive occasion. Serve pears alone or with poaching liquid, warm or chilled, spooned over ice cream, yogurt, or angel-food cake.

- 4 medium pears (about 11/4 pounds, or 560 g), peeled, cored, and quartered
- 2 cups (475 ml) cranberry juice
- 2 cinnamon sticks
- 3 whole cloves
- Zest of 1/2 orange, in strips

Put all ingredients into a large saucepan. Be sure that pan is not too large, so that the juice completely covers the pears. If the juice does not cover the pears and the fruit floats, place a small plate upside down in pot, to weight pears down in liquid. Bring to a simmer over medium heat and cook for 7 (for ripe fruit) to 10 minutes (for less ripe fruit). Pears should pierce easily with a fork.

To make syrup, transfer pears to a bowl. Simmer the poaching liquid until it is reduced by one-third and thickened to desired consistency, 30 to 40 minutes. Pears can be stored in poaching liquid in a covered container in the refrigerator for up to 3 days.

This recipe works well with fruit of the same firmness and ripeness. Try combining apples with pears. Softer fruits such as peaches and plums are also a good option, but you'll need to reduce the cooking time so the fruit does not become mushy.

YIELD: *Makes 4 servings of 4 quarters each.*

Calories (kcal): 204; **Total fat:** 2g; **Cholesterol:** 0mg; **Carbohydrate:** 52g; **Dietary fiber:** 9g; **Protein:** 1g; **Sodium:** 16mg; **Potassium:** 320mg; **Calcium:** 138mg; **Iron:** 4mg; **Zinc:** trace; **Vitamin A:** 84IU

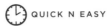 QUICK N EASY

Warm Stewed Fruit

gluten   milk   soy   egg   corn   nuts

This recipe title says it all—a warm, tasty comfort food. It is especially good for those with oral motor difficulties who do not handle raw fruit well and prefer softer textures.

- 6 medium apples (can use different varieties), peeled and chopped
- 1/2 teaspoon cinnamon
- 1/4 teaspoon dried ginger
- 1/4 cup (60 ml) apple juice or white grape juice
- 1/4 cup (60 ml) water
- 1 teaspoon sugar-free mixed berry jam (optional)

Combine all ingredients in a saucepan. Bring to a boil. Reduce heat and simmer, uncovered, until apples are soft.

VARIATION: *Use apples and pears or apples and cranberries. This recipe can also be made with 6 cups (660 g) of fresh strawberries instead of apples—just omit the cinnamon, ginger, and water.*

YIELD: *4 to 6 servings*

Calories (kcal): 87; **Total fat:** 1g; **Cholesterol:** 0mg; **Carbohydrate:** 22g; **Dietary fiber:** 4g; **Protein:** trace; **Sodium:** 1mg; **Potassium:** 173mg; **Calcium:** 13mg; **Iron:** trace; **Zinc:** trace; **Vitamin A:** 74IU

Fruit Clafouti

gluten   milk   soy   egg   corn   nuts

This is a classic French dessert. It falls somewhere between a pancake and a custard, and is surprisingly simple to make. Traditionally, sour cherries are used, but you can use any fresh fruit in season you like (although softer fruits work better than crunchy ones like apples, which require more baking time).

- 1 pound (455 g) fruit (either cherries, berries, or chopped fruit such as peaches, apricots, or plums)
- 1 cup (235 ml) rice milk
- ¹/₂ cup (100 g) sugar
- 3 large eggs
- ¹/₂ cup (70 g) GF flour blend
- 2 teaspoons GFCF vanilla
- 1 teaspoon lemon zest
- ¹/₄ teaspoon salt

Preheat the oven to 350°F (180°C, gas mark 4). Distribute the fruit evenly on the bottom of a greased baking dish or large pie plate. Combine the rice milk, sugar, eggs, flour blend, vanilla, zest, and salt in a blender for 1 minute. Pour over the fruit and bake for 45 to 50 minutes, until edges have puffed and top is lightly browned (center should be set and should not look liquid-y when jiggled). Cool for 5 to 10 minutes, then cut into wedges and serve.

YIELD: *6 servings*

Calories (kcal): 225; **Total fat:** 3g; **Cholesterol:** 112mg; **Carbohydrate:** 44g; **Dietary fiber:** 3g; **Protein:** 6g; **Sodium:** 142mg; **Potassium:** 179mg; **Calcium:** 23mg; **Iron:** 1mg; **Zinc:** trace; **Vitamin A:** 918IU.

Tropical Fruit Salad

gluten   milk   soy   egg   corn   nuts

For the Dressing

- 2 tablespoons (30 ml) lime juice
- 1 teaspoon lime zest
- 1 tablespoon (20 g) agave nectar
- 1 tablespoon (6 g) chopped mint
- 1 teaspoon grated ginger (optional)

In a small bowl, whisk all ingredients until combined.

For the Salad

- ¹/₂ large papaya, peeled and seeded
- 1 mango, peeled and pitted
- ¹/₂ medium pineapple, peeled and cored
- 3 kiwis, peeled
- Grated fresh coconut, toasted (optional)

Cut all the fruit into bite-sized pieces and place in a large bowl. Toss with dressing no more than 2 hours before serving. Garnish with toasted coconut.

YIELD: *4 to 6 servings*

Calories (kcal): 86; **Total fat:** trace; **Cholesterol:** 0mg; **Carbohydrate:** 22g; **Dietary fiber:** 3g; **Protein:** 1g; **Sodium:** 4mg; **Potassium:** 301mg; **Calcium:** 25mg; **Iron:** trace; **Zinc:** trace; **Vitamin A:** 1530IU.

Fried Bananas

gluten   milk   soy   egg   corn   nuts

Small bananas, called baby, finger, or apple bananas, are best for this dish, but slightly green, regular bananas can be used. Just cut them in half lengthwise, and then in half again crosswise.

- 1³/₄ cups (175 g) rice flour
- ¹/₄ cup (20 g) unsweetened shredded coconut
- 1 tablespoon (13 g) sugar
- 1 tablespoon (8 g) sesame seeds
- 1 teaspoon baking powder
- ¹/₄ teaspoon salt
- ¹/₂ cup (120 ml) water
- 3 cups (705 ml) canola oil (or other oil suitable for frying)
- ¹/₂ pound (225 g) slightly green baby bananas, peeled and cut in half lengthwise
- Honey, for drizzling

Mix the rice flour, coconut, sugar, sesame seeds, baking powder, and salt together in a medium bowl. Whisk in the water until the batter is smooth and free of lumps. Heat the oil in a wok or deep pan to 350°F (180°C).

Dip the banana pieces into the batter and then carefully slide them into the hot oil. Cook for 3 minutes, then flip over and cook another 2 minutes, until golden brown all over. Remove with a slotted spoon and drain on a plate lined with paper towels. Drizzle with honey and serve immediately.

YIELD: *2 to 4 servings*

Calories (kcal): 181; **Total fat:** 10g; **Cholesterol:** 30mg; **Carbohydrate:** 19g; **Dietary fiber:** 2g; **Protein:** 3g; **Sodium:** 99mg; **Potassium:** 237mg; **Calcium:** 101mg; **Iron:** 1mg; **Zinc:** 1mg; **Vitamin A:** 30IU.

Sugar-Free Cinnamon Applesauce

gluten   milk   soy   egg   corn   nuts

The trick to omitting the sugar in this recipe is using naturally sweet apples. Try to get fresh apples from a farm stand or a farmer's market, or better yet, pick your own. Supermarket apples may need to be peeled due to the heavy wax coating on the skins.

- 5 pounds (2.2 kg) sweet apples (about 10 medium), such as Jonagold, Golden Delicious, or Braeburns, washed well
- $^1/_4$ teaspoon table salt
- $^1/_8$ to $^1/_4$ teaspoon ground cinnamon
- 1 to $1^1/_2$ cups (235 to 355 ml) water, apple juice, or apple cider
- 1 tablespoon (15 ml) lemon juice

Peel (optional) and core apples, and then cut into slices (an apple-corer works great for this). Toss apples, salt, cinnamon, and liquid in a large pot or Dutch oven. Cover pot and cook apples over medium-high heat until they begin to break down, 15 to 20 minutes, stirring occasionally.

If your apples are unpeeled and/or you want a smooth-textured applesauce, pass cooked apples through food mill fitted with medium disk. Add lemon juice and additional liquid if needed to adjust consistency. For chunkier sauce (and your apples have been peeled), use a potato masher. Sauce can be served warm or chilled, and will keep for up to 5 days in the refrigerator.

NOTE: *Pears can be added to or substituted for the apples, and other seasonings can be added in lieu of the cinnamon. Try 1 tablespoon (6 g) of minced fresh ginger, or 1 teaspoon lemon or orange zest cooked and mashed along with the fruit.*

YIELD: *6 to 8 servings*

With water: Calories (kcal): 155; **Total fat:** 1g; **Cholesterol:** 0mg; **Carbohydrate:** 40g; **Dietary fiber:** 7g; **Protein:** 1g; **Sodium:** 68mg; **Potassium:** 303mg; **Calcium:** 21mg; **Iron:** trace; **Zinc:** trace; **Vitamin A:** 139IU.

With apple juice: Calories (kcal): 177; **Total fat:** 1g; **Cholesterol:** 0mg; **Carbohydrate:** 45g; **Dietary fiber:** 7g; **Protein:** 1g; **Sodium:** 68mg; **Potassium:** 358mg; **Calcium:** 23mg; **Iron:** 1mg; **Zinc:** trace; **Vitamin A:** 139IU.

Chocolate Chip Cookies

gluten   milk   soy   egg   corn   nuts

Almost every child wants to be able to eat a chocolate chip cookie, so we are giving you a recipe for a GFCF version of this favorite treat.

- 1 cup (225 g) ghee, softened
- 2 cups (450 g) Sucanat
- 2 large eggs
- 1/2 teaspoon salt
- 2 tablespoons (28 ml) vanilla
- 1 cup (120 g) almond flour
- 1 cup (140 g) garbanzo flour
- 1 teaspoon baking soda
- 2 cups (350 g) GFCF semisweet chocolate chips
- 2 cups (190 g) ground almonds or walnuts (can substitute with the above almond flour)

Place a rack in the center of the oven. Preheat oven to 375°F (190°C, or gas mark 5). Line several baking sheets with Silpat sheets or parchment paper. With an electric mixer, beat the ghee with the Sucanat until very fluffy. In a separate small bowl, mix together the eggs, salt, and vanilla until well blended. Add to the ghee/Sucanat mixture. Stir until well blended. In a separate large bowl, mix together the almond flour, garbanzo bean flour, and baking soda. Add to the ghee/Sucanat mixture. Stir until well blended. Stir in chocolate chips and the ground almonds or walnuts. If the dough is too stiff to work, add more ghee. Drop onto the baking sheets, spacing the cookies 2 inches (5 cm) apart.

Bake until the cookies are just slightly colored on top and rimmed with brown at the edges (8 to 10 minutes). Be sure to rotate the sheets halfway through the baking time (front to back). Be careful: Since the recipe does not use regular flour, the cookies can burn more quickly than usual. Watch them closely. Remove the sheets to a rack. Let the cookies cool for a few minutes before transferring them to a rack to finish cooling. Can freeze when completely cool. Place wax paper between layers of cookies before freezing them.

YIELD: *48 cookies*

Calories (kcal): 157; **Total fat:** 10g; **Cholesterol:** 19mg; **Carbohydrate:** 15g; **Dietary fiber:** 1g; **Protein:** 3g; **Sodium:** 55mg; **Potassium:** 100mg; **Calcium:** 23mg; **Iron:** 1mg; **Zinc:** trace; **Vitamin A:** 197IU

Cashew Cookies

gluten milk soy egg corn nuts

Every child loves cookies and these protein-packed cookies are sure to win them over.

- 16 ounces (455 g) cashews
- 1 cup (235 ml) sunflower oil plus 2 tablespoons (28 ml) for making cashew butter
- $^3/_4$ cup (170 g) brown sugar
- $^3/_4$ cup (150 g) sugar
- 4 eggs
- $^1/_2$ cup (120 ml) water
- 1 tablespoon (14 g) baking soda
- 1 tablespoon (8 g) xanthan gum
- $^3/_4$ teaspoon salt
- $2^1/_4$ cups (315 g) brown rice flour
- $1^1/_2$ cups (180 g) quinoa flour
- $1^1/_2$ cups (180 g) tapioca starch

Grind cashews in a food processor and add enough sunflower oil to make a smooth nut butter. Mix additional 1 cup (235 ml) sunflower oil and all remaining ingredients. Chill dough at least 1 hour.

Place dough in a cookie press or roll out between 2 sheets of waxed paper and shape with cutters. Bake pressed cookies at 375°F (190°C, or gas mark 5) for 12 to 15 minutes, cut-out cookies for 10 to 12 minutes. This dough can also be rolled into balls and crisscrossed with a fork.

YIELD: *18 to 24 cookies*

Calories (kcal): 480; Total fat: 27g; Cholesterol: 42mg; Carbohydrate: 55g; Dietary fiber: 3g; Protein: 9g; Sodium: 322mg; Potassium: 328mg; Calcium: 32mg; Iron: 3 3mg; Zinc: 2mg; Vitamin A: 62IU

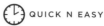 QUICK N EASY

Dark Chocolate Cookies

gluten milk soy egg corn nuts

- $^1/_2$ cup (120 ml) plus 2 tablespoons (28 ml) canola oil
- $^1/_2$ cup (100 g) sugar
- $^1/_2$ cup (115 g) brown sugar
- 1 egg
- $^1/_2$ teaspoon xanthan gum
- $^1/_2$ teaspoon baking powder
- $^3/_4$ teaspoon salt
- $1^1/_4$ cups (125 g) quinoa flakes
- $^1/_2$ cup (70 g) brown rice flour
- $^1/_4$ cup (40 g) potato starch
- $^1/_4$ cup (30 g) tapioca starch
- 6 ounces (170 g) GFCF dark chocolate, broken
- $^2/_3$ cup (66 g) pecan pieces

Cream together first 5 ingredients. Add remaining ingredients and mix. Drop by teaspoonfuls on a cookie sheet. Flatten slightly with a spatula. Bake in 375°F (190°C, or gas mark 5) oven for 15 minutes.

YIELD: *45 cookies*

Calories (kcal): 100; Total fat: 6g; Cholesterol: 4mg; Carbohydrate: 12g; Dietary fiber: 1g; Protein: 1g; Sodium: 44mg; Potassium: 66mg; Calcium: 9mg; Iron: 1mg; Zinc: trace; Vitamin A: 9IU

Maya's Cookies

gluten milk soy egg corn nuts

Extra protein has been added to these cookies, reducing the negative effect on blood sugar. This is also a way to sneak protein into the picky eater.

- ⅞ cup (105 g) almond meal flour
- ⅞ cup (88 g) GF oat flour
- ⅞ cup (125 g) garbanzo and fava bean flour
- 1½ cups (210 g) GF flour
- 1 teaspoon baking soda
- ½ teaspoon salt
- 1 cup (200 g) sugar
- ½ teaspoon cinnamon
- 1¼ cups (295 ml) safflower oil
- ¼ cup (85 g) molasses
- 5 eggs or 3 eggs and 3 egg whites
- 2 teaspoons vanilla

Preheat oven to 350°F (180°C, gas mark 4).

Combine all dry ingredients in a bowl.

In a large bowl, beat the liquid ingredients on medium speed until smooth. Add dry ingredients and mix thoroughly with a wooden spoon.

Drop by rounded teaspoons on an ungreased cookie sheet. Flatten with bottom of a glass that has been dipped in sugar.

Bake 8 minutes, until edges are lightly browned. Transfer to a wire rack to cool. These cookies can be stored in a covered container for up to 3 days or in a sealed freezer bag in the freezer for up to 6 months.

YIELD: *44 cookies*

Calories (kcal): 135; **Total fat:** 8g; **Cholesterol:** 21mg; **Carbohydrate:** 14g; **Dietary fiber:** 1g; **Protein:** 3g; **Sodium:** 61mg; **Potassium:** 105mg; **Calcium:** 21mg; **Iron:** 1mg; **Zinc:** trace; **Vitamin A:** 33IU

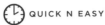 QUICK N EASY

Peanut Butter Truffle Cookies

gluten milk soy egg corn nuts

The yummy taste of this recipe, which has been modified from a Skippy peanut butter recipe, is excellent for hiding nutritional supplements.

- 1 cup (260 g) creamy GFCF peanut butter
- 1 cup (225 g) light brown sugar
- 1 large egg
- 1 teaspoon baking soda
- ½ cup (90 g) GFCF semisweet chocolate chips

Preheat oven to 350°F (180°C, gas mark 4). Cream together all the ingredients, except for the chocolate chips, with a wooden spoon. Add chocolate chips. Drop by rounded teaspoonfuls onto a greased cookie sheet. Bake 9 minutes. Allow to cool for 5 minutes on the sheet before removing to cool completely.

NOTE: *Be sure to read the peanut butter label, some brands contain soy.*

YIELD: *36 cookies*

Calories (kcal): 71; **Total fat:** 4g; **Cholesterol:** 5mg; **Carbohydrate:** 7g; **Dietary fiber:** 1g; **Protein:** 2g; **Sodium:** 72mg; **Potassium:** 72mg; **Calcium:** 7mg; **Iron:** trace; **Zinc:** trace; **Vitamin A:** 13IU

Gingersnap Cookies

gluten milk soy egg corn nuts

Perfect with a cup of tea for mom, or try sandwiching vanilla CF ice cream between cookies to make a kid's dessert.

- ³/₄ cup (100 g) arrowroot flour
- ³/₄ cup (90 g) tapioca flour
- ¹/₂ cup (70 g) garbanzo and fava bean flour
- ¹/₄ cup (35 g) sorghum flour
- ³/₄ teaspoon xanthan gum
- 2 teaspoons baking soda
- 1 teaspoon ground cinnamon
- 1 teaspoon ground cloves
- 3 teaspoons ground ginger
- ³/₄ teaspoon sea salt
- ³/₄ cup (135 g) crystallized ginger, chopped
- ¹/₂ cup (112 g) non-dairy shortening
- ¹/₄ cup (55 g) non-dairy spread
- 1 cup (225 g) light brown sugar
- ¹/₂ tablespoon flax seeds, ground
- 1 tablespoon (15 ml) water
- ¹/₄ cup (85 g) molasses
- ¹/₂ cup (100 g) sugar

Mix the flours, xanthan gum, baking soda, spices, salt, and crystallized ginger together with a whisk and set aside. Cream the shortening, spread, and brown sugar together. Mix the flax seeds and water together and add it to the molasses. Pour the molasses mixture into the creamed sugar mixture and mix on low speed with an electric mixer until combined. Add the flour mixture into the sugar-molasses mixture and mix on low until well combined. Chill 1 hour.

Wet your hands and roll dough into walnut-size balls and roll in sugar. Place on a greased cookie sheet 2 inches (5 cm) apart. Bake for 12 minutes in a 350°F (180°C, gas mark 4) oven.

YIELD: *about 48 cookies*

Calories (kcal): 82; **Total fat:** 3g; **Cholesterol:** 0mg; **Carbohydrate:** 13g; **Dietary fiber:** trace; **Protein:** trace; **Sodium:** 97mg; **Potassium:** 121mg; **Calcium:** 15mg; **Iron:** 1mg; **Zinc:** trace; **Vitamin A:** 43IU

Welby's 3-in-1 Cookie Recipe

 gluten milk soy egg corn nuts

Working from one standard dry mix, Welby Griffin has come up with 3 great cookie variations. The addition of almond meal and sorghum also makes these cookies high in protein (just another excuse to make them!).

Dry Mix

- ¹/₂ cup (60 g) tapioca flour
- ¹/₂ cup (70 g) sorghum flour
- ¹/₂ cup (60 g) almond meal
- ¹/₄ cup (40 g) potato starch
- 1 teaspoon baking powder
- ¹/₂ teaspoon baking soda
- ¹/₄ teaspoon salt
- ¹/₄ teaspoon xanthan gum

For Chocolate Chip Cookies

- ¹/₂ cup (120 g) GFCF Spread (such as Earth Balance)
- ³/₄ cup (170 g) brown sugar
- ¹/₄ cup (50 g) granulated sugar
- 1 large egg
- 1¹/₂ teaspoon GF vanilla
- 6 ounces (170 g) GFCF chocolate chips

For Peanut Butter Cookies

- ¹/₃ cup (80 g) GFCF Spread
- ¹/₃ cup (87 g) peanut butter
- ³/₄ cup (150 g) granulated sugar
- 1 large egg
- 1 teaspoon honey
- 1 teaspoon GF vanilla
- ¹/₂ cup (72.5 g) chopped peanuts (optional)

For Sugar Cookies

- ¹/₂ cup (120 g) GFCF Spread
- 1 cup granulated sugar
- 1 large egg
- 1¹/₂ teaspoons GF vanilla extract
- Dash of nutmeg

To make dry mix

Blend all dry mix ingredients in a bowl and set aside.

To make all cookies

Preheat oven to 350°F (180°C, gas mark 4). Spray a baking sheet with cooking spray or line with parchment paper and set aside.

In a large bowl, cream together the GFCF spread and sugar(s). (For the peanut cookie variation, also add in the peanut butter.) Then add the remaining ingredients for your chosen recipe, except for any chocolate chip or nut additions. Stir in the dry mix, and then gently fold in the nuts or chips. Chill dough until firm.

Roll dough into 1-inch (2.5 cm) balls and place 2 to 3 inches (5 to 7.5 cm) apart on the prepared cookie sheet (if dough becomes too warm, place cookie sheet in refrigerator for 10 minutes to firm it up). Bake cookies for 10 to 15 minutes (depending on whether you like your cookies chewy or crispy). Allow cookies to cool on sheet for 5 minutes before moving to a cooling rack.

NOTE: *Peanut butter cookies may be flattened with a fork or the back of a slotted spatula halfway through baking, to achieve a more classic look.*

TIP: *Make a several batches of dry mix at a time, and then store them in separate, labeled, zipper lock bags in the freezer. Then, when the urge strikes, whipping up a batch of these cookies is quick and easy.*

Sugar cookie variations: Roll balls of cookie dough in cinnamon sugar to make Snickerdoodles or in colored sugar for a holiday look.

YIELD: *3¹/₂ dozen cookies*

Dry Mix: Calories (kcal): 20; **Total fat:** trace; **Cholesterol:** 0mg; **Carbohydrate:** 4g; **Dietary fiber:** trace; **Protein:** 1g; **Sodium:** 39mg; **Potassium:** 23mg; **Calcium:** 13mg; **Iron:** trace; **Zinc:** trace; **Vitamin A:** 0IU.

Chocolate Chip Cookies: Calories (kcal): 76; **Total fat:** 4g; **Cholesterol:** 5mg; **Carbohydrate:** 10g; **Dietary fiber:** trace; **Protein:** 1g; **Sodium:** 42mg; **Potassium:** 34mg; **Calcium:** 22mg; **Iron:** 1mg; **Zinc:** trace; **Vitamin A:** 8IU.

Peanut Butter Cookies: Calories (kcal): 62; **Total fat:** 4g; **Cholesterol:** 5mg; **Carbohydrate:** 6g; **Dietary fiber:** trace; **Protein:** 2g; **Sodium:** 51mg; **Potassium:** 51mg; **Calcium:** 16mg; **Iron:** trace; **Zinc:** trace; **Vitamin A:** 8IU.

Sugar Cookies: Calories (kcal): 60; **Total fat:** 3g; **Cholesterol:** 5mg; **Carbohydrate:** 8g; **Dietary fiber:** trace; **Protein:** 1g; **Sodium:** 41mg; **Potassium:** 25mg; **Calcium:** 14mg; **Iron:** trace; **Zinc:** trace; **Vitamin A:** 8IU.

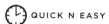 QUICK N EASY

Chocolate Date Balls

gluten   milk   soy   egg   corn   nuts

From Susan Lyttek, Springfield, VA

- 1¹/₂ cups (267 g) pitted, chopped dates
- 1¹/₂ cups (180 g) chopped walnuts, toasted
- ¹/₂ cup (40 g) GFCF unsweetened cocoa powder
- 1 teaspoon cinnamon
- ¹/₄ cup (60 ml) coconut milk

Pulse dates, walnuts, cocoa powder, and cinnamon in food professor until finely ground. Add coconut milk and process until combined. Form into 1-inch balls and freeze.

YIELD: *3¹/₂ dozen balls*

Calories (kcal): 51; **Total fat:** 3g; **Cholesterol:** 0mg; **Carbohydrate:** 6g; **Dietary fiber:** 1g; **Protein:** 1g; **Sodium:** 7mg; **Potassium:** 69mg; **Calcium:** 6mg; **Iron:** trace; **Zinc:** trace; **Vitamin A:** 17IU.

Meringue Cookies

gluten milk soy egg corn nuts

These cookies are lighter than air, chewy on the inside, and crunchy on the outside. They are portable and a favorite for many. A protein treat that will please the kids who love something crunchy.

- 4 egg whites, at room temperature
- ¹/₄ teaspoon salt
- ¹/₄ teaspoon cream of tartar
- 1¹/₂ cups (300 g) sugar
- 1¹/₂ teaspoons vanilla

Basics

Use a clean, dry bowl that is absolutely grease-free. Glass, ceramic, stainless steel are best. Avoid copper. Plastic bowls should be avoided because they can have may appear trace amounts of oil.

Cold eggs separate easily, but eggs whip to a higher volume when at room temperature. Separate the cold eggs, and then set them aside for 10 or 15 minutes. There can be absolutely no yolk mixed in the whites. Save the yolks for another dish.

Superfine sugar is best. Simply process granulated sugar in the food processor.

Beat egg whites with salt and cream of tartar until stiff. Add sugar 1 tablespoon (13 g) at a time, beating well after each addition. Add vanilla. Adding sugar early in the beating process results in a firmer, finer-textured meringue. When the mixture becomes stiff and shiny like satin, stop mixing, the meringue is ready.

If making a variation, add extra ingredient.

Line large baking sheets with parchment paper. Drop meringue by tablespoonful 1¹/₂ inches (3.75 cm) apart onto prepared baking sheets.

Bake at 250°F (120°C, or gas mark ¹/₂) for 30 to 40 minutes (until they crack). Turn off oven and let them cool down (15 minutes).

VARIATIONS:

- **ALMOND MERINGUES:** *1 teaspoon GFCF almond extract*
- **CINNAMON MERINGUES:** *¹/₈ teaspoon ground cinnamon*
- **CHOCOLATE CHIP:** *1 cup (85 g) GFCF chocolate chips*
- **CHOCOLATE MERINGUES:** *1 cup (85 g) GFCF chocolate chips, melted*

YIELD: *2 dozen*

Calories (kcal): 52; **Total fat:** 0g; **Cholesterol:** 0mg; **Carbohydrate:** 13g; **Dietary fiber:** 0g; **Protein:** 1g; **Sodium:** 31 mg; **Potassium:** 13mg; **Calcium:** 1mg; **Iron:** trace ; **Zinc:** trace ; **Vitamin A:** 0IU

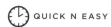 QUICK N EASY

Apple Pie Cake

gluten milk soy egg corn nuts

This recipe combines the best of two family favorites into one really fantastic dessert.

- $^1/_3$ cup (40 g) quinoa flour
- $^1/_3$ cup (45 g) brown rice flour
- $^1/_3$ cup (40 g) tapioca starch
- $^2/_3$ cup (135 g) sugar
- 1 teaspoon baking soda
- 1 teaspoon xanthan gum
- $^1/_2$ teaspoon cinnamon
- 1 pinch salt
- 2 tablespoons (28 ml) oil
- 1 egg
- 1 tablespoon (15 ml) hot water
- 4 apples, sliced thin
- $^1/_4$ cup (35 g) crushed nuts (optional)

Mix all ingredients except crushed nuts, adding apples last. Pour into ungreased 9-inch (22.5-cm) pie pan. Sprinkle with nuts (optional). Bake in a 350°F (180°C, gas mark 4) oven for 35 minutes.

YIELD: *8 servings*

Calories (kcal): 238; **Total fat:** 7g; **Cholesterol:** 23mg; **Carbohydrate:** 43g; **Dietary fiber:** 3g; **Protein:** 3g; **Sodium:** 184mg; **Potassium:** 184mg; **Calcium:** 19mg; **Iron:** 1mg; **Zinc:** 1mg; **Vitamin A:** 73IU

Chocolate Almond Cake

gluten　milk　soy　egg　corn　nuts

This is a treat everyone will like.

- 2 cups (280 g) GF flour blend
- 1/2 cup (60 g) almond flour
- 1 cup (225 g) light brown sugar
- 1/2 cup (40 g) GFCF unsweetened cocoa
- 1 1/2 teaspoons GF baking powder
- 1/8 teaspoon baking soda
- 1/4 teaspoon xanthan gum
- 1/8 teaspoon salt
- 1 1/2 cups (355 ml) rice milk, warmed
- 1/2 cup (120 ml) almond oil
- 1 teaspoon (5 ml) vanilla
- 1/4 teaspoon almond extract
- 1/2–1 cup (85–170 g) GFCF chocolate chips

Preheat oven to 350°F (180°C, gas mark 4).

Lightly grease a 9-inch (22.5-cm) round cake pan or an 11 x 7-inch (27.5 x 17.5-cm) pan and line it with parchment.

Mix together the flour blend, almond flour, brown sugar, cocoa, baking powder, baking soda, xanthan gum, and salt.

Whisk in rice milk and almond oil. Then stir in vanilla and almond extract. Fold in chocolate chips.

Pour mixture into prepared pan. Let it sit for 5 minutes before placing in oven on the middle rack.

Bake 20 to 25 minutes or until done. Allow it to sit for 10 minutes, then turn it out on a rack.

Dust with confectioners' sugar or frost with GFCF icing.

YIELD: *8 servings*

Calories (kcal): 528; **Total fat:** 25g; **Cholesterol:** 0mg; **Carbohydrate:** 75g; **Dietary fiber:** 4g; **Protein:** 8g; **Sodium:** 158mg; **Potassium:** 401 mg; **Calcium:** 125mg; **Iron:** 3 3mg; **Zinc:** 1mg; **Vitamin A:** 7IU

Carrot Cake

gluten   milk   soy   egg   corn   nuts

- 1 package (10.5 ounces, or 294 g) extra-firm silken tofu
- 1½ ounces (42 ml) canola oil
- 2¼ cups (450 g) sugar
- 1½ cups (355 ml) canola oil
- 6 cups (720 g) shredded carrots
- 1½ cups (180 g) tapioca flour
- 1½ cups (180 g) arrowroot flour
- 1 cup (140 g) garbanzo and fava bean flour
- ½ cup (70 g) sorghum flour
- 1 teaspoon xanthan gum
- 1 tablespoon (14 g) baking powder
- 1 tablespoon (14 g) baking soda
- 1 tablespoon (7 g) ground cinnamon
- ¾ teaspoon ground nutmeg
- ¾ teaspoon ground clove
- 1 teaspoon salt
- Frosting, recipe follows
- 3 cups (315 g) toasted, finely chopped walnuts

Preheat oven to 350°F (180°C, gas mark 4). Spray two 9-inch (22.5-cm) cake pans with canola oil, line bottom with parchment paper, and spray again. Lightly flour the pans with white rice flour. In a food processor, puree the tofu and 1½ ounces (42 ml) canola oil until very smooth and set aside. Beat together in a mixer with the paddle attachment (or by hand) the sugar and the tofu mixture for about 3 minutes; add in the shredded carrot. While the oil and sugar are mixing, combine together with a whisk in a separate bowl the flours, xanthan gum, baking powder, baking soda, spices, and salt. Add this mixture to the carrot mixture and mix until combined. Do not overmix, as it will result in a dense, unleavened cake. Divide mixture between prepared cake pans and bake for about 50 to 60 minutes or until a toothpick comes out clean.

After the cake is completely cool, you can cut each cake into 2 layers to make a 4-layer cake (or do not cut the cakes, to make a 2-layer cake). Frost the top of the first layer and lightly sprinkle with walnuts. Place the second layer on top of the first, frost, and sprinkle with walnuts. Do this for all 4 layers, omitting the walnuts on the top layer. Frost the sides of the cake and then press the remainder of the nuts onto the sides and top of the frosting.

YIELD: *8 to 16 servings*

Calories (kcal): 835; **Total fat:** 55g; **Cholesterol:** 0mg; **Carbohydrate:** 81g; **Dietary fiber:** 4g; **Protein:** 11g; **Sodium:** 735mg; **Potassium:** 321 mg; **Calcium:** 109mg; **Iron:** 2 2mg; **Zinc:** 1mg; **Vitamin A:** 12956IU

Frosting

gluten   milk   soy   egg   corn   nuts

- 2¼ pounds (1 kg) vegan cream cheese
- 1 tablespoon (1 ml) vanilla
- 1½ tablespoons (23 ml) lemon juice
- 9 ounces (255 g) confectioners' sugar, sifted

In a mixer, soften cream cheese by beating with the paddle attachment. Add the vanilla and lemon juice until combined. Add the confectioners' sugar and mix until there are no lumps.

Travis Martin's Favorite Flourless Chocolate Mousse Cake

gluten   milk   soy   egg   corn   nuts

Using bittersweet chocolate avoids the dairy-based milk chocolate and lessens the glucose effect without sacrificing taste. Serve sweet things in small half portions and do so after a meal of protein and fiber. This will slow the entry of sugar into the bloodstream and avoid the glucose rise and fall that can trigger behavior and attention problems.

- 8 ounces (225 g) GFCF bittersweet chocolate, finely chopped
- 6 tablespoons (90 g) non-dairy spread (nonhydrogenated)
- 6 large eggs, separated
- $^1/_2$ cup (100 g) sugar

Preheat oven to 275°F (140°C, or gas mark 1) and place rack in center of oven. Grease a 9-inch (22.5-cm) springform pan.

Place chopped chocolate and spread in a large, microwave-safe bowl and microwave on high in 30-second increments. Stir after each increment, continuing until the chocolate is completely melted. Allow to cool slightly, then whisk in the egg yolks.

Beat egg whites to soft peaks. Gradually add sugar, beating until stiff and glossy.

Whisk one-fourth of the egg whites into the chocolate mixture to lighten it.

Using a rubber spatula, gently fold the chocolate mixture into the rest of the egg whites.

Pour mixture into the prepared pan and smooth the top.

Bake 40 to 50 minutes. The thin mousse cake will have pulled away from the pan side.

Allow to cool.

To serve, dust the top of the cake with confectioners' sugar or spread with raspberry fruit spread.

YIELD: *8 servings*

Calories (kcal): 322; **Total fat:** 27g; **Cholesterol:** 140mg; **Carbohydrate:** 21g; **Dietary fiber:** 4g; **Protein:** 7g; **Sodium:** 146mg; **Potassium:** 281 mg; **Calcium:** 40mg; **Iron:** 2 2mg; **Zinc:** 1mg; **Vitamin A:** 616IU

QUICK N EASY

Strawberry "Cheesecake"

gluten   milk   soy   egg   corn   nuts

*You and I know it's not cake, but the name really helps the cause. This fast and
fun treat makes a great, quick school-day breakfast.*

- $1/2$ cup (115 g) Tofutti Better Than Cream Cheese
- 4 GFCF rice cakes
- 1 cup (170 g) sliced fresh strawberries

Spread 2 tablespoons (30 g) Tofutti Better Than Cream Cheese evenly
onto each rice cake. Arrange one-quarter of the sliced strawberries on
top of each and serve.

YIELD: *4 servings*

Calories (kcal): 181; **Total fat:** 10g; **Cholesterol:** 30mg; **Carbohydrate:** 19g; **Dietary fiber:** 2g; **Protein:** 3g;
Sodium: 99mg; **Potassium:** 132mg; **Calcium:** 26mg; **Iron:** trace; **Zinc:** trace; **Vitamin A:** 208IU.

Hot Chocolate Pudding Cake

gluten   milk   soy   egg   corn   nuts

This is a great rustic treat for a cold winter's night, and delicious with served GFCF vanilla ice cream.

- $^2/_3$ cup (54 g) GFCF unsweetened cocoa powder, divided
- $^1/_3$ cup (75 g) brown sugar
- $^1/_4$ cup (22 g) GFCF chocolate chips
- $^3/_4$ cup (105 g) GF flour blend
- 1 teaspoon baking powder
- $^1/_4$ teaspoon salt
- 6 tablespoons (85 g) ghee, melted
- 1 large egg yolk
- 1 cup (200 g) sugar
- $^1/_3$ cup (80 ml) rice milk
- 2 teaspoons GFCF vanilla
- $1^1/_2$ cups (355 ml) hot water

Preheat oven to 325°F (170°C, gas mark 3), and grease an 8-inch square baking dish. In a small bowl, combine $^1/_3$ cup (27 g) cocoa powder, brown sugar, and chocolate chips and set aside. In another bowl, whisk together flour, baking powder, and salt, and set aside.

In a medium bowl, whisk together the ghee and remaining cocoa powder until smooth. Add yolk, sugar, rice milk, and vanilla and whisk to combine. Stir in flour mixture until just combined. Spread batter evenly into baking dish, and then sprinkle with reserved cocoa-brown sugar mixture. Pour hot water evenly over batter and bake for 40 to 45 minutes, until edges have puffed up and begun to pull away from the sides of the pan (center will still jiggle slightly). Cool on wire rack 20 minutes; serve warm.

YIELD: *6 to 8 servings*

Calories (kcal): 347; **Total fat:** 14g; **Cholesterol:** 54mg; **Carbohydrate:** 55g; **Dietary fiber:** 4g; **Protein:** 3g; **Sodium:** 192mg; **Potassium:** 31mg; **Calcium:** 52mg; **Iron:** 1mg; **Zinc:** trace; **Vitamin A:** 424IU.

Angel Food Cake

gluten   milk   soy   egg   corn   nuts

Adapted from Natalie Naramor (http://glutenfreemommy.com)

Naturally casein free, angel food cake can be easily adapted to become gluten-free as well. A simple garnish of fresh berries is all this cake needs to turn it into a delicious dessert.

- 1 cup (140 g) GF flour blend
- 1 teaspoon xanthan gum
- $^1/_4$ teaspoon salt
- $1^1/_2$ cups (300 g) granulated sugar, divided
- 12 egg whites, room temperature
- 1 teaspoon cream of tartar
- 2 teaspoons GFCF vanilla

Preheat oven to 325°F (170°C, gas mark 3). In a medium bowl, combine the flour blend, xanthan gum, salt, and $^3/_4$ cup (150 g) sugar.

With an electric mixer, beat the egg whites, cream of tartar, and vanilla until they become foamy and the lines of the whisk leave a trail. With the mixer running, add the remaining sugar one tablespoon at a time. Continue beating until egg whites are glossy and hold soft peaks. Sift flour mixture in thirds over the top of the egg whites, gently folding in after each addition.

Scrape the batter into an ungreased tube pan with a removable bottom (or line bottom with parchment paper). Bake for 50 to 60 minutes, until top is golden and sides begin to pull away. Cool for 10 minutes on wire rack, then invert, propped on a bottle or a funnel, and cool completely. Loosen the cake from the pan by running a knife around the edge, invert over a plate, and then slide pan off. Carefully remove cake bottom, gently slice with a serrated knife, and serve.

TIP: *Angel food freezes well—Wrap leftovers into individual portions, or have a whole cake on hand for when you need it! (Thaw the cake in its wrapping at room temperature.)*

YIELD: *10 to 12 servings*

Calories (kcal): 225; **Total fat:** 3g; **Cholesterol:** 112mg; **Carbohydrate:** 44g; **Dietary fiber:** 3g; **Protein:** 6g; **Sodium:** 142mg; **Potassium:** 91mg; **Calcium:** 3mg; **Iron:** trace; **Zinc:** trace; **Vitamin A:** 0IU.

Banana Cake or Muffins

gluten   milk   soy   egg   corn   nuts

Besides being downright delicious, this versatile treat can be made as a cake or muffins.

- 1 cup (120 g) quinoa flour
- $^2/_3$ cup (90 g) brown rice flour
- $^1/_3$ cup (40 g) tapioca starch
- 1 cup (200 g) sugar
- 1 teaspoon xanthan gum
- $^1/_2$ tablespoon (7 g) baking soda
- 2 teaspoons baking powder
- $^3/_4$ teaspoon salt
- 2 eggs + 1 egg white
- 1 cup (225 g) mashed banana
- $^1/_2$ cup (120 ml) oil (safflower, almond, sunflower, canola)
- $^1/_2$ cup (120 ml) rice milk

Combine dry ingredients in a mixing bowl. Add remaining ingredients and mix on low speed of an electric mixer until blended. Mix on medium-high speed for 2 minutes. Oil a 9 x 13-inch (22.5 x 32.5-cm) pan and cover with parchment paper or use cupcake papers. Bake in a 350°F (180°C, gas mark 4) oven; cake bakes for 45 minutes, muffins for 20 minutes.

NOTE: *Nut butter makes a great, healthy frosting for this recipe.*

YIELD: *8 cake servings or 12 medium muffins*

Calories (kcal): 393; **Total fat:** 16g; **Cholesterol:** 47mg; **Carbohydrate:** 58g; **Dietary fiber:** 3g; **Protein:** 6g; **Sodium:** 585mg; **Potassium:** 328mg; **Calcium:** 91mg; **Iron:** 3 3mg; **Zinc:** 1mg; **Vitamin A:** 93IU

Ian's Cranberry Muffins

gluten   milk   soy   egg   corn   nuts

- $^3/_4$ cup (90 g) tapioca flour
- $^2/_3$ cup (80 g) quinoa flour
- $^2/_3$ cup (100 g) potato starch
- $^1/_2$ teaspoon xanthan gum
- $^1/_2$ teaspoon salt
- $2^1/_2$ teaspoons baking powder
- 1 tablespoon egg replacer powder
- $^1/_4$ cup (50 g) sugar
- 1 cup (235 ml) potato milk, constituted
- $^1/_4$ cup (60 ml) canola oil
- $^1/_2$ teaspoon vanilla
- $^2/_3$ cup (80 g) dried cranberry pieces

Preheat oven to 400°F (200°C, or gas mark 6). Mix dry ingredients. Stir in liquids. Add cranberries. Spoon batter into a greased muffin tin. Bake for 20 to 25 minutes. Remove muffins from tin and cool on a wire rack.

YIELD: *12 muffins*

Calories (kcal): 178; **Total fat:** 5g; **Cholesterol:** 0mg; **Carbohydrate:** 34g; **Dietary fiber:** 1g; **Protein:** 1g; **Sodium:** 246mg; **Potassium:** 92mg; **Calcium:** 79mg; **Iron:** 1mg; **Zinc:** trace; **Vitamin A:** 33IU

Pie Crusts and Crumble Desserts

These recipes include ready-to-eat GFCF cookies as a substitute for flours. This is a quick and delicious way of making a pie crust or crumble dessert.

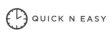 QUICK N EASY

Pie Crust

gluten   milk   soy   egg   corn   nuts

- 1 package (6 ounces, or 170 g) Snickerdoodle cookies
- 3 tablespoons (45 g) nondairy margarine, melted
- 1 teaspoon (5 ml) vanilla
- 1/4 teaspoon cinnamon
- 1/3 cup (75 g) brown sugar
- 1/2 cup (35 g) coconut or (60 g) chopped nuts (optional)

Process all ingredients in a food processor until well combined.

Place in a 9-inch (22.5-cm) pie shell. Press down and smooth crumbs up the sides.

Bake at 350°F (180°C, gas mark 4) for 8 minutes. Let cool.

Fill as desired—works great for pumpkin or pecan pies!

YIELD: *One 9-inch (22.5-cm) pie shell*

Calories (kcal): 120 9; **Total fat:** 65g; **Cholesterol:** 0mg; **Carbohydrate:** 146g; **Dietary fiber:** 15g; **Protein:** 13g; **Sodium:** 427mg; **Potassium:** 330mg; **Calcium:** 180mg; **Iron:** 66mg; **Zinc:** 1mg; **Vitamin A:** 2649IU

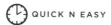 QUICK N EASY

Baked Apple Crumble

gluten   milk   soy   egg   corn   nuts

- 5 large apples, peeled and cut into chunks
- 3 tablespoons (45 ml) lemon juice
- 1/2 cup (100 g) sugar
- 1/2 teaspoon cinnamon
- 1/4 teaspoon nutmeg
- 1 package (6 ounces, or 170 g) No-oats "Oatmeal" cookies
- 1/2 cup (115 g) brown sugar
- 6 tablespoons (90 g) nondairy spread
- 1/4 teaspoon vanilla
- Pinch of salt

Put apples in a bowl with the lemon juice. Combine apples with the sugar, cinnamon, and nutmeg. Toss to coat.

Spray an 8 x 8-inch (20 x 20-cm) pan with GFCF cooking spray. Spread apples in the bottom of the pan. Place the cookies, brown sugar, margarine, vanilla, and salt in a food processor and process until well combined. Spread the cookie mixture over the apples and bake in a 350°F (180°C, gas mark 4) oven for 40 minutes.

Can be served warm or at room temperature.

NOTE: *Read the label on the margarine—some brands may contain soy or corn.*

YIELD: *12 servings of 1/2 cup (125 g) each*

Calories (kcal): 189; **Total fat:** 7g; **Cholesterol:** 0mg; **Carbohydrate:** 31g; **Dietary fiber:** 3g; **Protein:** 1g; **Sodium:** 80mg; **Potassium:** 96mg; **Calcium:** 22mg; **Iron:** 1mg; **Zinc:** trace; **Vitamin A:** 378IU

American Apple Pie

gluten   milk   soy   egg   corn   nuts

This is adapted from www.gfutah.org recipes online.

- 1 teaspoon ground cinnamon
- 3 tablespoons (24 g) cornstarch
- 3/4 cup (150 g) sugar
- 5 cups (750 g) peeled, cored, and sliced baking apples
- Unbaked 8-inch (20-cm) double Pie Crust (page 226)

Mix cinnamon, cornstarch, and sugar together in a medium bowl and stir in apples.

Spread apple mixture in an unbaked pie shell.

Cover with top crust and crimp edges with your fingers to seal. Cut slits in top.

Bake in preheated 400°F (200°C, or gas mark 6) for 10 minutes. Turn oven to 350°F (180°C, gas mark 4) and continue cooking for 30 to 40 minutes or until crust is lightly brown.

VARIATION: *Omit top crust and sprinkle pie with Walnut Streusel (recipe follows).*

NOTE: *This recipe can also be made with peaches or pears.*

YIELD: *8 servings*

Calories (kcal): 287; **Total fat:** 8g; **Cholesterol:** 0mg; **Carbohydrate:** 53g; **Dietary fiber:** 4g; **Protein:** 2g; **Sodium:** 54mg; **Potassium:** 142mg; **Calcium:** 32mg; **Iron:** 1mg; **Zinc:** trace; **Vitamin A:** 378IU

Walnut Streusel

gluten   milk   soy   egg   corn   nuts

- 1/2 cup (80 g) rice flour
- 1/4 cup (50 g) sugar
- 1/4 cup (60 g) brown sugar
- 1/4 teaspoon ground cinnamon
- 1/4 teaspoon ground nutmeg
- 1/4 cup (55 g) nondairy spread
- 1/2 cup (65 g) walnuts, chopped fine

Combine flour, sugars, and spices.

Cut in cold spread with knives or pastry blender until coarse and crumbly. Add in walnuts. Sprinkle over pie; bake until topping is golden brown.

YIELD: *1 1/2 cups (310 g)*

Calories (kcal): 140; **Total fat:** 82g; **Cholesterol:** 0mg; **Carbohydrate:** 157g; **Dietary fiber:** 5g; **Protein:** 20g; **Sodium:** 549mg; **Potassium:** 543mg; **Calcium:** 100mg; **Iron:** 3mg; **Zinc:** 3mg; **Vitamin A:** 2205IU

Tracey's Pie Crust

gluten   milk   soy   egg   corn   nuts

- $^1/_2$ cup (70 g) brown rice flour
- $^1/_2$ cup (60 g) quinoa flour
- $^1/_2$ cup (60 g) tapioca starch
- $^1/_2$ cup (80 g) sweet rice flour
- $^1/_4$ cup (35 g) garbanzo bean flour
- 2 teaspoons xanthan gum
- 1 teaspoon salt
- $^1/_2$ cup (120 ml) + 2 tablespoons (28 ml) oil (sunflower, almond, safflower, canola)
- $^1/_4$ cup (60 ml) milk substitute
- $^1/_2$ cup (120 ml) water

Stir together dry ingredients. Add oil, milk substitute, and water and mix thoroughly. Divide dough in half and roll out bottom crust between two pieces of floured parchment paper. Lift parchment paper and dough and place both in bottom of an ungreased pie pan. Roll out second pie crust. Loosely roll together crust with parchment paper and unroll carefully over filled pie crust. Bake per pie's instructions.

TIP: *A small, one-handled roller works well.*

VARIATION: *For pot pies, replace flours with the following mixture: 3/4 cup (105 g) brown rice flour, 1/2 cup (60 g) quinoa flour, 1/2 cup (60 g) tapioca starch, 1/2 cup (70 g) garbanzo bean flour.*

YIELD: *1 double pie crust or 2 single pie crusts*

Calories (kcal): 119 9; **Total fat:** 73g; **Cholesterol:** 0mg; **Carbohydrate:** 125g; **Dietary fiber:** 7g; **Protein:** 14g; **Sodium:** 1088mg; **Potassium:** Calcium: 558mg 48mg; **Iron:** 5mg; **Zinc:** 3 3mg; **Vitamin A:** 5IU

Pumpkin Pie (Pareve)

gluten   milk   soy   egg   corn   nuts

This is Travis Martin's favorite Kosher recipe, and it is as good as the usual version. Enjoy!

- 3 cups (675 g) canned pumpkin
- 1 cup (225 g) brown sugar
- 1 cup (200 g) granulated sugar
- 1 teaspoon salt
- 1 teaspoon nutmeg
- 1 teaspoon cinnamon
- 1 teaspoon ginger
- $^1/_4$ teaspoon cloves
- $^1/_4$ teaspoon allspice
- 4 eggs, beaten
- $^1/_4$ cup (55 g) margarine, ghee, or nondairy shortening, melted
- 1 unbaked (10-inch, or 25-cm) pie shell In a large bowl, mix together pumpkin, sugars, salt, and spices.

In a small bowl, mix together eggs and margarine or ghee. Add to pumpkin mixture.

Pour mixture into a pie shell. Bake for 10 minutes in a preheated 450°F (230°C, or gas mark 8) oven.

Reduce heat to 350°F (180°C, gas mark 4) and bake 40 minutes longer or until a knife inserted into center comes out clean.

YIELD: *8 servings*

Calories (kcal): 443; **Total fat:** 17g; **Cholesterol:** 111mg; **Carbohydrate:** 69g; **Dietary fiber:** 5g; **Protein:** 5g; **Sodium:** 362mg; **Potassium:** 329mg; **Calcium:** 80mg; **Iron:** 3mg; **Zinc:** 1 1mg; **Vitamin A:** 20992IU

Blender Pecan Pie

gluten   milk   soy   egg   corn   nuts

This is a simple way to make a holiday favorite.

- 2 cups (200 g) pecan halves, divided
- 2 large eggs
- $2/3$ cup (135 g) sugar
- $1/2$ teaspoon salt
- $1/2$ cup (170 g) agave nectar
- 2 tablespoons (28 g) ghee, melted
- 1 teaspoon GFCF vanilla extract
- 1 9-inch prebaked GFCF pie crust

Preheat oven to 425°F (220°C, gas mark 7). Select 1 cup (100 g) of the best looking pecan halves and reserve for top. Combine the remaining filling ingredients in a blender and puree until smooth. Pour into prebaked crust, top with reserved pecan halves and bake for 15 minutes. Reduce oven temperature to 350°F (180°C, gas mark 4) and bake for another 30 minutes, until center of pie is set. Cool completely on a wire rack, 2 to 3 hours. Serve.

YIELD: *8 servings*

Calories (kcal): 398; **Total fat:** 26g; **Cholesterol:** 70mg; **Carbohydrate:** 42g; **Dietary fiber:** 3g; **Protein:** 4g; **Sodium:** 43mg; **Potassium:** 123mg; **Calcium:** 16mg; **Iron:** 1mg; **Zinc:** 2mg; **Vitamin A:** 242IU.

Apple, Pear, and Cranberry Crisp

gluten milk soy egg corn nuts

This is a great, simple-to-make, holiday dessert. If you can't find fresh cranberries, frozen ones can be thawed and used instead. Or, if cranberries are too tart for your taste, try substituting an equal amount of raspberries or blueberries.

For Topping

- $^1/_2$ cup (70 g) GF flour blend
- $^1/_2$ cup (55 g) chopped pecans
- $^1/_2$ cup (120 g) brown sugar
- 1 teaspoon ground ginger
- $^1/_2$ teaspoon ground cinnamon
- $^1/_8$ teaspoon salt
- 4 tablespoons (56 g) Spectrum Palm Shortening, chilled

For Filling

- 3 medium tart apples, peeled, cored, and cut into $^1/_2$-inch pieces
- 3 semi-firm pears, such as Bosc or Bartlett, peeled, cored, and cut into $^1/_2$-inch pieces
- 1 cup (100 g) fresh cranberries
- $^1/_2$ cup (100 g) sugar
- $^1/_2$ teaspoon lemon zest
- Pinch salt

TO MAKE THE TOPPING: In food processor, pulse dry ingredients until combined. Add shortening and continue pulsing until small clumps form and mixture appears sandy. Set aside in the refrigerator until ready to use.

TO MAKE THE FILLING: Preheat oven to 350°F (180°C, gas mark 4). In large bowl, toss apples, pears, and cranberries with sugar, salt, and lemon zest until evenly coated. Transfer mixture to an 8- or 9-inch square baking dish and sprinkle evenly with chilled topping. Bake for 40 to 45 minutes, until fruit is bubbling and topping is golden brown.

YIELD: *6 servings*

Calories (kcal): 414; **Total fat:** 16g; **Cholesterol:** 0mg; **Carbohydrate:** 70g; **Dietary fiber:** 7g; **Protein:** 3g; **Sodium:** 56mg; **Potassium:** 281mg; **Calcium:** 32mg; **Iron:** 1mg; **Zinc:** 1mg; **Vitamin A:** 74IU.

Apricot Almond Torte

gluten   milk   soy   egg   corn   nuts

You can substitute sliced peaches or plums in place of the apricots.

- $^1/_3$ cup (37 g) slivered almonds
- $^3/_4$ cup (150 g) sugar, plus 2 tablespoons (26 g) for sprinkling
- $^3/_4$ cup (105 g) GF flour blend, plus more for dusting pan
- $^1/_2$ teaspoon baking powder
- $^1/_4$ teaspoon xanthan gum
- $^1/_4$ teaspoon salt
- 6 tablespoons (83 g) Spectrum Palm Shortening, plus more for greasing pan
- 1 large egg
- 1 large egg yolk
- 1 teaspoon GFCF vanilla extract
- $^1/_4$ teaspoon GFCF almond extract
- 1 pound (455 g) fresh apricots, halved and pitted

Preheat oven to 350°F (180°C, gas mark 4). Grease and flour a 9-inch springform pan. In the bowl of a food processor, grind nuts and $^3/_4$ cup sugar together until fine. Add flour blend, baking powder, xanthan gum and salt and continue processing until combined. Add shortening and pulse until all the nut mixture is coated. Add the egg, yolk, and extracts and process until smooth, scraping sides if necessary. Spread batter evenly in the prepared pan, and then arrange apricots cut side-up on top. Sprinkle apricots with the remaining sugar and bake for 55 to 60 minutes. Cool for 30 minutes on wire rack; serve warm or at room temperature.

YIELD: *6 to 8 servings*

Calories (kcal): 321; **Total fat:** 14g; **Cholesterol:** 54mg; **Carbohydrate:** 45g; **Dietary fiber:** 4g; **Protein:** 5g; **Sodium:** 115mg; **Potassium:** 212mg; **Calcium:** 46mg; **Iron:** 1mg; **Zinc:** trace; **Vitamin A:** 1459IU.

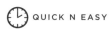

Grandma Lillie's Apple Dumplings

gluten   milk   soy   egg   corn   nuts

A cross between an omelet and a pancake.

- 3–4 tablespoons (45–60 ml) oil (safflower, sunflower, almond, canola)
- 2 apples, peeled and cored and thinly sliced into rings
- 6–8 eggs
- 4 tablespoons (35 g) brown rice flour
- Cinnamon

Heat oil in a medium/large skillet and sauté apples until soft. Beat eggs with flour and pour batter on top of apples in skillet and heat on medium heat until bubbly. Sprinkle cinnamon on top. Put in a pie plate or pan under broiler until it fluffs up.

Cut into wedges and serve with syrup, almond butter, or jam.

YIELD: *8 servings*

Calories (kcal): 164; **Total fat:** 11g; **Cholesterol:** 187mg; **Carbohydrate:** 10g; **Dietary fiber:** 1g; **Protein:** 6g; **Sodium:** 56mg; **Potassium:** 108mg; **Calcium:** 25mg; **Iron:** 1mg; **Zinc:** 1mg; **Vitamin A:** 298IU

Chocolaty Pumpkin Bars

gluten   milk   soy   egg   corn   nuts

These bars are for those who love chocolate! Calcium and magnesium powders can be hidden in this recipe.

- 2 cups (280 g) GF flour blend
- $1/2$ teaspoon xanthan gum
- $3/4$ cup (150 g) sugar
- 1 cup (125 g) finely chopped pecans (optional)
- 2 teaspoons baking powder
- 1 teaspoon ground cinnamon
- $1/2$ teaspoon baking soda
- $1/2$ teaspoon salt
- 4 large eggs, beaten
- 1 can (15 ounces, or 420 g) pumpkin puree
- $1/2$ cup (120 ml) canola oil
- $1/4$ cup (60 ml) milk substitute
- $1/2$ cup (80 g) GFCF mini chocolate chips

Preheat oven to 350°F (180°C, gas mark 4). Whisk together the flour, xanthan gum, sugar, pecans, baking powder, cinnamon, baking soda and salt in a large bowl. In a separate bowl, combine the eggs, pumpkin, oil, and milk substitute. Stir the wet and dry mixtures together, then add chocolate chips. Spread the batter evenly into a greased 15 x 10 x 1-inch (37.5 x 25 x 2.5-cm) pan (a jellyroll pan with an edge) that has been sprayed with nonstick spray.

Bake 25 minutes. Check with a toothpick in the middle—it is done when the toothpick comes out clean. Cool completely on a wire rack in the pan before cutting and serving.

YIELD: *2 dozen bars*

Calories (kcal): 186; **Total fat:** 10g; **Cholesterol:** 31mg; **Carbohydrate:** 22g; **Dietary fiber:** 2g; **Protein:** 2g; **Sodium:** 122mg; **Potassium:** 93mg; **Calcium:** 37mg; **Iron:** 1mg; **Zinc:** 1mg; **Vitamin A:** 3962IU

Coconut Lime Bars

gluten   milk   soy   egg   corn   nuts

Another recipe using the versatile and healthful coconut! Our recipe for crumb crust calls for GFCF Snickerdoodle cookies, but you can substitute an equal amount of another type of GFCF cookie.

- 1 recipe Pie Crust (see page 311), including the coconut and omitting the cinnamon
- 1¹/₂ cups (300 g) sugar
- 3 tablespoons (24 g) tapioca flour
- 1 teaspoon baking powder
- 4 large eggs
- 1 tablespoon (6 g) grated lime zest
- ¹/₂ cup (120 ml) fresh lime juice

Preheat the oven to 350°F (180°C, gas mark 4). Grease an 8 or 9-inch (20 to 23 cm) square baking pan and line with an 8 or 9-inch (20 to 23 cm) wide strip of parchment that hangs over the edges. Press pie crust firmly into an even layer on the bottom of the pan and bake for 8 minutes.

Meanwhile, in a small bowl, whisk the sugar, flour, and baking powder together. In a larger bowl, beat the eggs lightly. Whisk in the sugar mixture and then add the lime zest and juice, whisking until well combined. Pour the filling onto the warm crust and bake for 30 minutes, until top is pale golden and set. Cool on wire rack completely, and then chill in the refrigerator at least 2 hours. When ready to serve, lift edges of parchment and transfer bars to a cutting board. Cut into 16 squares.

YIELD: *16 pieces*

Calories (kcal): 98; **Total fat:** 1g; **Cholesterol:** 54mg; **Carbohydrate:** 21g; **Dietary fiber:** trace; **Protein:** 2g; **Sodium:** 47mg; **Potassium:** 25mg; **Calcium:** 24mg; **Iron:** trace; **Zinc:** trace; **Vitamin A:** 80IU.

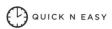

Chocolate Mousse

gluten milk soy egg corn nuts

It doesn't get easier than this! A sweet source of protein and a terrific way to hide supplements.

- 1 bag (12 ounces, or 340 g) or 2 cups GFCF chocolate chips
- 1 package (12 ounces, or 340 g) silken tofu

Melt the chocolate chips. Drain the tofu of its water. Combine chocolate and tofu in food processor. Blend until smooth (this may take several minutes). Chill in the refrigerator for at least a few hours.

YIELD: *4 to 6 servings*

Calories (kcal): 599; **Total fat:** 37g; **Cholesterol:** 0mg; **Carbohydrate:** 73g; **Dietary fiber:** 8g; **Protein:** 12g; **Sodium:** 18mg; **Potassium:** 512mg; **Calcium:** 125mg; **Iron:** 8mg; **Zinc:** 2mg; **Vitamin A:** 96IU

Chocolate-Almond Truffles

gluten milk soy egg corn nuts

The better-quality chocolate used, the richer and more delectable these simple, not-too-sweet truffles will taste. This is also a good way to hide supplements

- 1 cup (235 ml) vanilla soy milk
- 16 ounces (455 g) GFCF semisweet chocolate, chips or chopped
- 6 ounces (170 g) GFCF unsweetened chocolate, chopped
- $1/2$ teaspoon almond extract (optional)
- 1 cup (145 g) raw almonds
- Pinch of salt

Heat soy milk in a saucepan until hot but not boiling. Remove from heat and whisk in chocolates until smooth. Add almond extract, if desired, and whisk. Place in refrigerator and cool for 2 hours or until firm.

Preheat oven to 300°F (150°C, or gas mark 2). Toast almonds for 10 minutes or until lightly browned and fragrant. Cool. Transfer almonds to a food processor and add a pinch of salt. Grind until fine.

When chocolate is firm, scoop out portions and roll quickly between the palms, forming walnut-size balls. Roll each ball in crushed almonds, pressing into sides. Transfer to a parchment-lined baking sheet and keep cool until ready to serve.

YIELD: *36 truffles*

Calories (kcal): 111; **Total fat:** 9g; **Cholesterol:** 0mg; **Carbohydrate:** 10g; **Dietary fiber:** 2g; **Protein:** 2g; **Sodium:** 7mg; **Potassium:** 124mg; **Calcium:** 18mg; **Iron:** 1mg; **Zinc:** 1mg; **Vitamin A:** 33IU

Healthy Truffles

gluten   milk   soy   egg   corn   nuts

A tasty, high-protein snack and a good way to hide supplements.

- 1¹⁄₃ cups (230 g) pitted dates
- ¹⁄₂ cup (85 g) flaxseed
- ¹⁄₂ cup (70 g) peanuts
- ¹⁄₂ cup (60 g) dried cranberries
- ¹⁄₄ teaspoon cinnamon
- ¹⁄₂ – ³⁄₄ cup (130–195 g) GFCF peanut butter
- 1–2 tablespoons (15–30 ml) flaxseed oil (optional)
- Cinnamon or unsweetened shredded coconut (optional)

Mash dates in a bowl with the back of a spoon (or chop dates if too hard to mash). Grind flaxseed, and then add peanuts, to form a fine meal (use short bursts in the food processor to avoid an oily paste). Add to the dates and combine with a spoon or fingers. Add cranberries and cinnamon and combine. Add peanut butter and flax oil and mix well.

Shape the mixture into small balls. Roll in cinnamon or coconut, if desired. Place in an airtight container and refrigerate or freeze immediately. Eat at room temperature, cold, or frozen.

YIELD: *12 to 24 (depending on the size)*

Calories (kcal): 216; **Total fat:** 13g; **Cholesterol:** 0mg; **Carbohydrate:** 21g; **Dietary fiber:** 5g; **Protein:** 7g; **Sodium:** 79mg; **Potassium:** 323mg; **Calcium:** 31mg; **Iron:** 1mg; **Zinc:** 1mg; **Vitamin A:** 10IU

Lemon Pudding

gluten   milk   soy   egg   corn   nuts

This is another good food for hiding mild-tasting supplement powders.

- 6 egg yolks
- ¹⁄₂ cup (65 g) cornstarch
- 1¹⁄₂ cups (300 g) sugar
- 2 cans (14 ounces, or 425 ml, each) coconut milk
- 3 cups (710 ml) dairy-free milk substitute
- Rind from 1 lemon
- 2 cinnamon sticks
- Juice from 1¹⁄₂ lemons

Beat egg yolks. Mix all ingredients together. Heat on medium to a boil. Continue cooking on low, stirring constantly, until thickened. Refrigerate for at least 2 hours or until firm.

YIELD: *6 servings*

Calories (kcal): 644; **Total fat:** 37g; **Cholesterol:** 213mg; **Carbohydrate:** 79g; **Dietary fiber:** 6g; **Protein:** 7g; **Sodium:** 34mg; **Potassium:** 411mg; **Calcium:** 107mg; **Iron:** 5 5mg; **Zinc:** 2mg; **Vitamin A:** 337IU

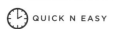 QUICK N EASY

Coconut/Flax Protein Pudding

gluten   milk   soy   egg   corn   nuts

Depending on diet restrictions and choice of protein powder (we use Ultraclear Sustain, which is rice-based), this can be GFCFSF. It is not SCD-compliant, because of the flax and rice.

- 1 cup (170 g) flaxseed
- 1 cup (235 ml) unrefined coconut oil
- 1 cup (120 g) protein powder (soy or rice)

In a coffee grinder, grind flaxseed (in batches) until powdery. Put flax meal in a food processor. Add coconut oil and mix. Add tolerated protein powder.

Mix until consistency is smooth. Adjust ingredient ratios to taste/texture preference.

Spoon into containers and freeze.

YIELD: *2 to 4 servings*

Calories (kcal): 762; **Total fat:** 69g; **Cholesterol:** 0mg; **Carbohydrate:** 16g; **Dietary fiber:** 13g; **Protein:** 32g; **Sodium:** 315mg; **Potassium:** 288mg; **Calcium:** 131mg; **Iron:** 7 7mg; **Zinc:** 3mg; **Vitamin A:** 0IU

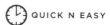

Banana Mango "Pudding"

   gluten   milk   soy   egg   corn   nuts

This recipe is not just tasty, it is a good way to hide supplements.

- 1⅓ cups (315 ml) water
- ¼ cup (50 g) basmati or white rice
- 2 juicy ripe mangos
- 2 large bananas
- 1 teaspoon (5 ml) vanilla
- ⅛ teaspoon cinnamon, to taste (optional)

Bring the water to a boil in a small pan. Add the rice and cover. Simmer gently for 10 minutes, stirring occasionally to prevent sticking. Remove from the heat and set aside to cool to just above room temperature.

Puree the mangos, bananas, and rice in the blender. Add vanilla and cinnamon to taste.

YIELD: *2½ cups (500 g)*

Calories (kcal): 668; **Total fat:** 3g; **Cholesterol:** 0mg; **Carbohydrate:** 164g; **Dietary fiber:** 16g; **Protein:** 8g; **Sodium:** 23mg; **Potassium:** 1635mg; **Calcium:** 78mg; **Iron:** 3mg; **Zinc:** 1mg; **Vitamin A:** 16313IU

Autumn Sweet Cake

gluten   milk   soy   egg   corn   nuts

"This is a 'must' at our house for every Thanksgiving. Everyone loves it. There is no pumpkin in this pudding!"

- 2 pounds (910 g) sweet potatoes (garnet or white Japanese)
- 2 pounds (910 g) butternut squash
- 3 quarts (2.8 L) + $^1/_2$ cup (120 ml) water
- 1 teaspoon salt
- 1 thin slice fresh ginger, peeled
- 1 cinnamon stick
- 5 cloves
- 1 cup (235 ml) Thai coconut milk
- $^1/_4$ cup (40 g) rice flour
- 1 teaspoon xanthan gum
- 2 ounces (55 g) GFCF buttery sticks, room temperature
- 3 eggs
- $1^3/_4$ cups (350 g) sugar
- $^1/_4$ teaspoon salt

Peel, seed, and cut squash into large chunks. Peel sweet potatoes and cut into chunks. In a very large pot, bring 3 quarts (2.8 L) water to a boil. Add salt. Add squash and sweet potato chunks. Cook until soft.

In a separate small saucepan, add spices to $^1/_2$ cup (120 ml) water. Bring to a boil. Cook on medium for 5 minutes.

Meanwhile, preheat oven to 400°F (200°C, or gas mark 6) and grease a 9-inch (22.5-cm) round cake pan.

Mix coconut milk with flour and xanthan gum.

Mash squash and sweet potatoes after draining, while still hot. (Tip: Save some of the liquid to drink warm as a vegetable broth. It is delicious and packed with vitamins.)

Add buttery sticks, eggs, coconut milk mixture, sugar, salt, and the liquid in which the spices were boiled. This liquid should have been significantly reduced.

Mix everything. Pour mixture into a greased pan. Bake for $1^1/_2$ hours or until a knife inserted in the center comes out clean. Let cool before turning over. This can also be served warm out of the baking dish.

YIELD: *8 servings*

Calories (kcal): 490; **Total fat:** 17g; **Cholesterol:** 88mg; **Carbohydrate:** 84g; **Dietary fiber:** 7g; **Protein:** 6g; **Sodium:** 397mg; **Potassium:** 662mg; **Calcium:** 135mg; **Iron:** 3mg; **Zinc:** 11mg; **Vitamin A:** 24229IU

Rice Cream

gluten milk soy egg corn nuts

"I scream, you scream, we all scream for rice cream."

- 2 cups (475 ml) rice milk
- $1/4$ cup (50 g) sugar
- 1 tablespoon (8 g) powdered egg whites
- 1 tablespoon (15 ml) oil
- $1/4$ teaspoon salt
- $1/2$ cup (75 g) fruit, optional

Put all ingredients in a blender. Add additional rice milk to 4-cup (945 ml) mark and blend. Pour into an ice cream maker and mix.

This has a texture like ice milk.

YIELD: *4 servings*

Calories (kcal): 112; **Total fat:** 3g; **Cholesterol:** 0mg; **Carbohydrate:** 19g; **Dietary fiber:** trace; **Protein:** 1g; **Sodium:** 144mg; **Potassium:** 15mg; **Calcium:** 6mg; **Iron:** trace; **Zinc:** trace; **Vitamin A:** 0IU

Aidan's Avocado Fruit Surprise

gluten milk soy egg corn nuts

Carla and Aidan provide this dessert, which is like a creamy mousse. The raspberries add a nice tang; however, if lumps are a problem, they can be eliminated.

- 1 ripe avocado (soft but not discolored)
- 1 cup (155 g) frozen blueberries
- 1 cup (135 g) frozen raspberries
- 1 teaspoon (5 ml) lemon juice

Peel and pit the avocado and place in a food processor or blender along with the berries and lemon juice. Blend until smooth.

Store in the freezer in one container or separately in $1/4$ cup (125 g) servings.

NOTE: *If omitting raspberries because they are too "lumpy," double the amount of blueberries for a total of 2 cups (310 g) frozen berries.*

YIELD: *1 cup (4 servings, $1/4$ cup [125 g] each)*

Calories (kcal): 165; **Total fat:** 8g; **Cholesterol:** 0mg; **Carbohydrate:** 25g; **Dietary fiber:** 5g; **Protein:** 2g; **Sodium:** 6mg; **Potassium:** 395mg; **Calcium:** 18mg; **Iron:** 1mg; **Zinc:** trace; **Vitamin A:** 377IU

Creamy Fruit Ice Cream

gluten   milk   soy   egg   corn   nuts

The basics of these ice cream recipes are listed first, and the additions are listed last. There are directions for making the recipes without an ice cream machine. If making these using an ice cream machine, follow the manufacturer's instructions. This is also a good source for hiding some supplements.

AUTHORS' NOTE: *Palm shortening has no trans-fatty acids. Palm and coconut oils are excellent for baking and for making ice cream. The taste is mild. If you want an ice cream that is as tasty as the "real thing"—the palm oil shortening will work well.*

Ice cream machines are the easiest way to achieve a good, smooth ice cream.

Basics

- 1 cup (125 g) potato milk powder
- 1 cup (100 g) confectioners' sugar (pure)
- 1 cup (235 ml) very hot water
- 2 tablespoons (28 g) palm shortening
- 1/2 tablespoon guar gum
- 1/4 teaspoon vanilla

Fruit choices

- 1 1/2 cups (165 g) fresh strawberries
- 4 ripe medium bananas

Combination of fruits:

- 3/4 cup (85 g) fresh strawberries
- 2 ripe medium bananas

Combine the basic ingredients and the fruit choice(s). Blend all ingredients thoroughly in a blender (medium to medium-high speed). Place into a tightly lidded plastic container. Place in freezer until frozen.

　　If using an ice cream maker, follow the manufacturer's instructions.

YIELD: *6 servings*

Calories (kcal): 230; **Total fat:** 4g; **Cholesterol:** 0mg; **Carbohydrate:** 51g; **Dietary fiber:** 0g; **Protein:** 0g; **Sodium:** 108mg; **Potassium:** 45mg; **Calcium:** 1mg; **Iron:** trace ; **Zinc:** trace ; **Vitamin A:** 0IU

Thai Ice Cream

gluten   milk   soy   egg   corn   nuts

This ice cream has a very creamy texture. Yum!

- 2 cans (14 ounces, or 425 ml, each) coconut milk
- 2 tablespoons (25 g) sugar
- 1 tablespoon + 1 teaspoon egg whites
- 1/4 teaspoon salt

Blend all ingredients and pour into an ice cream maker and mix.

YIELD: *4 servings*

Calories (kcal): 483; **Total fat:** 47g; **Cholesterol:** 0mg; **Carbohydrate:** 17g; **Dietary fiber:** 4g; **Protein:** 5g; **Sodium:** 171mg; **Potassium:** 529mg; **Calcium:** 33mg; **Iron:** 3mg; **Zinc:** 1mg; **Vitamin A:** 0IU

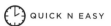 QUICK N EASY

Banana Peanut Butter Mush

gluten   milk   soy   egg   corn   nuts

This guilt-free nutritious ice-cream alternative. It is also a superior food for hiding nutritional supplements, even those that have a stronger taste.

- 2 ripe bananas, sliced and frozen
- 1/2 cup (130 g) GFCF peanut butter
- 1/4 cup (60 ml) milk substitute
- Dash of cinnamon
- 1/8 teaspoon vanilla

Blend in a food processor until smooth. Eat immediately or put in freezer for 10 minutes to set.

VARIATION: *Use almond butter and almond extract instead of GFCF peanut butter and vanilla.*

YIELD: *2 cups (about 450 g)*

Calories (kcal): 250; **Total fat:** 17g; **Cholesterol:** 0mg; **Carbohydrate:** 21g; **Dietary fiber:** 3g; **Protein:** 9g; **Sodium:** 152mg; **Potassium:** 451 mg; **Calcium:** 17mg; **Iron:** 1mg; **Zinc:** 1mg; **Vitamin A:** 48IU

Lemon Strawberry Ice

gluten   milk   soy   egg   corn   nuts

Try adding ¹/₄ cup soy or rice protein powder to this recipe. Adding some protein is both nutritious and helps to reduce the glucose-raising effect of foods which are glycemic.

- 1 cup (170 g) sliced strawberries
- ³/₄ cup (180 ml) fresh-squeezed lemon juice
- ³/₄ cup (255 g) agave nectar
- 2 cups (475 ml) water
- Pinch of salt

Puree all ingredients in a blender or food processor. Pour mixture into 2 ice cube trays and freeze completely, at least 3 hours. Process one tray of ice cubes in the food processor at a time, transferring slush to a container in the freezer before proceeding with the remaining cubes. Serve immediately. Alternatively, freeze mixture using an ice cream machine.

TIP: *Try substituting fresh raspberries or blackberries for the strawberries, or lime juice for lemon juice (you may want to reduce the agave nectar to taste).*

YIELD: *6 servings*

Calories (kcal): 127; **Total fat:** trace; **Cholesterol:** 0mg; **Carbohydrate:** 34g; **Dietary fiber:** 3g; **Protein:** trace; **Sodium:** 3mg; **Potassium:** 84mg; **Calcium:** 8mg; **Iron:** trace; **Zinc:** trace; **Vitamin A:** 14IU.

Honey Peach Sorbet

gluten   milk   soy   egg   corn   nuts

Nectarines can be substituted for the peaches.

- 2 pounds (910 g) ripe peaches
- ³/₄ cup (255 g) mild honey
- 2 tablespoons (30 ml) lemon juice
- 1¹/₂ cups (355 ml) water, divided
- Pinch salt

Preheat oven to 375°F (190°C, gas mark 5). Halve and pit peaches, but leave skins on. Place cut-side down in a roasting pan or baking dish, drizzle with honey, and add ¹/₂ cup (120 ml) water. Cover with foil, bake for 20 minutes, flip peaches over, and continue baking uncovered for 20–40 minutes, until peaches are very tender. Let peaches sit until cool enough to handle, and then slip off their skins and discard. Puree peaches, their roasting juices, lemon juice, salt, and remaining water until smooth. Freeze in an ice cream machine according to the manufacturer's instructions.

YIELD: *8 servings*

Calories (kcal): 135; **Total fat:** trace; **Cholesterol:** 0mg; **Carbohydrate:** 36g; **Dietary fiber:** 2g; **Protein:** 1g; **Sodium:** 3mg; **Potassium:** 191mg; **Calcium:** 7mg; **Iron:** trace; **Zinc:** trace; **Vitamin A:** 462IU.

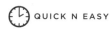

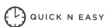

 QUICK N EASY

Easy Ice Cream Pie

gluten   milk   soy   egg   corn   nuts

Some GFCF ice cream and sorbet contain eggs, soy, and/ or nuts. Be sure to carefully read the ingredient list if you are trying to avoid any of those food items.

- 1 quart (1 litre) GFCF ice cream or sorbet of choice, softened slightly
- 4 cups (about 600 g) diced fresh fruit of choice
- 1 prebaked GFCF crumb pie crust

In a standing mixer with the paddle attachment, mix ice cream on low speed until soft. Gently but quickly fold in the diced fruit. Scrape into the crumb crust, mounding the mixture in the center and then smoothing it to the sides with a spatula. Freeze until firm, about 2 hours. Serve right away or cover with plastic wrap and store in the freezer until needed.

YIELD: *8 to 10 servings*

Calories (kcal): 333; **Total fat:** 14g; **Cholesterol:** 24mg; **Carbohydrate:** 49g; **Dietary fiber:** 3g; **Protein:** 4g; **Sodium:** 279mg; **Potassium:** 335mg; **Calcium:** 104mg; **Iron:** 2mg; **Zinc:** 1mg; **Vitamin A:** 736IU.

 QUICK N EASY

Frozen Melon-Ball Pops

gluten   milk   soy   egg   corn   nuts

- 1 cantaloupe or honey dew melon, or ¹/₂ seedless watermelon

Make small balls of the melon of your choice with a melon baller (or make a medley of different melons). Arrange them on a baking sheet or large plate, skewer them with a fun toothpick, and then freeze. Serve.

YIELD: *8 servings*

Calories (kcal): 24; **Total fat:** trace; **Cholesterol:** 0mg; **Carbohydrate:** 6g; **Dietary fiber:** 1g; **Protein:** 1g; **Sodium:** 6mg; **Potassium:** 213mg; **Calcium:** 8mg; **Iron:** trace; **Zinc:** trace; **Vitamin A:** 2225IU.

Quick N Easy:
If You Can't Make It, Buy It!

ICE CREAM

There are excellent GFCF sorbets on the market. Check out Häagen-Dazs and Ben & Jerry's. They are tasty.

ICE CREAM CONES

No childhood is complete without ice cream cones. These can be easily purchased in the stores carrying GFCF items. Brands include Barkat, Cerrone, Glutano, Schar, and others. Check the Gluten Free Pantry at www.glutenfree.com and product resources at www.gfcfdiet.com/directory.htm.

Appendix: Resources

GFCF AND ALLERGY-BASED COOKBOOKS

Dumke, Nicolette (forward by William Crook)
Allergy Cooking with Ease (no wheat, milk, egg, corn, soy, yeast, sugar)
Easy Bread Making for Special Diets

Fenster, Carol
Cooking Free
Special Diet Celebrations
Special Diet Solutions
Gluten-Free Quick & Easy: From Prep to Plate Without the Fuss
1000 Gluten-Free Recipes

Gates, Donna
The Body Ecology Diet and Autism

Gottschall, Elaine
Breaking the Vicious Cycle
(SCD recipes)

Hagman, Bette
The Gluten-Free Gourmet
The Gluten-Free Gourmet Bakes Bread
The Gluten-Free Gourmet Cooks Comfort Foods
The Gluten-Free Gourmet Cooks Fast and Healthy

Hammond, Leslie and Rominger, Marie
The Kid-Friendly Food Allergy Cookbook

Hills, Hilda
Good Food, Milk Free, Grain Free

Jackson, Luke
A User Guide to the GF/CF Diet for Autism, Asperger Syndrome and ADHD

Korn, Danna
Wheat-Free Worry-Free

Kruszka, Bonnie
Eating Gluten-Free with Emily

Lewis, Lisa
Special Diets for Special Kids
Special Diets for Special Kids, Two

Matthews, Julie
Cooking to Heal (www.NourishingHope.com)

Prasad, Ramen
Recipes for the Specific Carbohydrate Diet

Robertson, Robin
366 Simply Delicious Dairy-Free Recipes

Segersten, Alissa and Malterre, Tom
The Whole Life Nutrition Cookbook 2ⁿᵈ edition

Semon, Bruce and Kornblum, Lori
Feast Without Yeast: 4 Stages to Better Healthy

Vess, Sueson
Special Eats: Simple, Delicious Solutions for Gluten-Free & Dairy-Free Cooking

OTHER COOKBOOKS WITH EASY-TO-ADAPT RECIPES

Barnes, Lisa
The Petit Appetit Cookbook

Fallon, Sally, and Enig, Mary
Nourishing Traditions
www.newtrendspublishing.com (877) 707-1776

Katzen, Mollie
Salad People and More Real Recipes

Olson, Cathe
Simply Natural Baby Food

Vann, Lizzie
Organic Baby & Toddler Cookbook

Yaron, Ruth
Super Baby Food

Young, Nicole
Blender Baby Food

SOURCES ON ADHD AND AUTISM

Adams, Christina
A Real Boy (discusses GFCF; child recovered)

Barkley, Russell
Taking Charge of ADHD: The Complete, Authoritative Guide for Parents

Bock, Kenneth and Stauth, Cameron
Healing the New Childhood Epidemics: Autism, ADHD, Asthma and Allergies. The Groundbreaking Program for the 4-A Disorders

Bell, Rachel, and Peiper, Howard
ADD and ADHD Diet

Campbell-McBride, Natasha
Gut and Psychology Syndrome (GAPS)

Crook, William
Help for the Hyperactive Child

DeFelice, Karen
Enzymes for Autism and Other Neurological Conditions

Edelson, Stephen, and Rimland, Bernard
Treating Autism: Parent Stories Recovering Autistic Children

Grandin, Temple
Emergence: Labeled Autistic
Thinking in Pictures: And Other Reports from My Life with Autism

Hallowell, Edward, and Ratey, John
Delivered from Distraction: Getting the Most out of Life with Attention Deficit Disorder
Driven to Distraction: Recognizing and Coping with Attention Deficit Disorder from Childhood Through Adulthood

Hamilton, Lynn
Facing Autism: Giving Parents Reason for Hope and Guidance for Help

Hart, Charles
A Parent's Guide to Autism

Jepson, Bryan; Wright Katie, and Johnson, Jane
Changing the Course of Autism: A Scientific Approach for Parents and Physicians.

Kaplan, Lawrence, and Burstein, Jay
Diagnosis Autism—Now What?

Kranowitz, Carol
The Out-of-Sync Child
The Out-of -Sync Child Has Fun

Lemer, Patricia
Envisioning A Bright Future Interventions that Work for Children and Adults with Autism Spectrum Disorders

Lewis, Lisa
The Encyclopedia of Dietary Interventions for the Treatment of Autism and Related Disorders (with Karyn Seroussi)

Matthews, Julie
Nourishing Hope (www.NourishingHope.com)

McCandless, Jaquelyn
Children with Starving Brains: a Medical Treatment Guide for Autism Spectrum Disorder 3ʳᵈ edition.

McCarthy, Jenny
Mother Warriors: A Nation of Parents Healing Autism Against All Odds (2008)

Pangborn, Jon, and Baker, Sidney
Autism: Effective Biomedical Treatments and 2007 Supplement [Video] A Piece of the Puzzle— Autism, Recovery & The GFCF Diet Interviews with parents and doctors, including Jerry Kartzinel, MD

Rapp, Doris
Is This Your Child?
Our Toxic World: A Wake Up Call
Is This Your Child's World?

Rimland, Bernard
Infantile Autism
Nutrition and Behavior Problems
Recovering Autistic Children

Seroussi, Karyn
Unraveling the Mystery of Autism and Pervasive Developmental Disorder
The Encyclopedia of Dietary Interventions for the Treatment of Autism and Related Disorders (with Lisa Lewis)

Shaw, William
Biological Treatments for Autism and PDD

Wiseman, Nancy
Could It Be Autism?

Zimmerman, Marcia
The A.D.D. Nutrition Solution: A Drug-Free 30 Day Plan

GENERAL HEALTH CARE AND CHILD CARE BOOKS

Baker, Sidney McDonald
Detoxification and Healing

Balch, Phyllis and James
Prescription for Nutritional Healing

Crook, William
Yeast Connection Handbook

Dadd, Debra
Home Safe Home
Nontoxic, Natural and Earthwise

Dodt, Colleen
Natural Baby Care

Kahan, Barbara
Healthier Children

Phelan, Thomas
1-2-3 Magic

Pottkotter, Louis
The Natural Nursery

Price, Weston A.
Nutrition and Physical Degeneration

Schmidt, Michael
Healing Childhood Ear Infections
Beyond Antibiotics

Smith, Lendon
How to Raise a Healthy Child
The Infant Survival Guide

Zand, Janet, and Roundtree, Robert
Smart Medicine for a Healthier Child

MAGAZINES AND NEWSLETTERS

This is just an abbreviated listing. Most organizations offer newsletters. Check their Web sites for information.

ADDitude Magazine
www.additudemag.com
Information on ADD symptoms, medication, treatment, diagnosis and parenting ADD children.
39 West 37th St., 15th Floor
New York, NY 10018
1-646-366-0830

ANDI Newsletter
www.AutismNDI.com
P.O. Box 335
Pennington, NJ 08534-0335
Fax: (609) 737-8453

Developmental Delay Resources (DDR)
www.devdelay.org
5801 Beacon Street
Pittsburgh, PA 15217
(800) 497-0944
Newsletter and complete resources

Gluten-Free Living (newsletter)
www.glutenfreeliving.com
19A Broadway
Hawthorne, NY 10532
(914) 741-5420

Glutenfreeda
www.glutenfreeda.com
Online cooking magazine and recipe book.
Includes resources, links, products, product testing, and updates.

Living Without
www.livingwithout.com
1202 N 75ᵗʰ Street, Suite 294
Downers Grove, IL 60516
(630) 415-3378

Mothering Magazine
www.mothering.com

Shafer Autism Report
www.sarnet.org
Latest updates on anything about autism; newsletter.

ORGANIZATIONS AND INFORMATION ONLINE

Autism Diet Online
www.autism-diet-online.com
Information, guidelines, avoidances, substitutes

Autism Network for Dietary Intervention (ANDI)
www.AutismNDI.com
P.O. Box 335 Pennington, NJ 08534-0335
Fax: (609) 737-8453

Autism One
www.autismone.org

Autism Research Institute and Defeat Autism Now! (ARI)
www.autism.com
4182 Adams Avenue
San Diego, CA 92116 USA
1-866-366-3361

Autism Society of America (ASA)
www.autism-society.org
7910 Woodmont Avenue, Suite 300
Bethesda, Maryland 20814-3067
301.657.0881 or 800.328.8476

Autism Speaks USA
www.autismspeaks.org
US 2 Park Avenue
11th Floor
New York, NY 10016
Phone: (212) 252-8584
Fax: (212) 252-8676

Autism Speaks Canada
www.walknowforautism.org/site/c.
ghKKIUPFluE/b.3948809/
1243 Islington Avenue, Suite 504
Toronto, ON M8X 1Y9

Autism Speaks: United Kingdom
www.autismspeaks.org.uk

Celiac Disease Foundation
www.celiac.org
13521 Ventura Boulevard, Suite 3
Studio City, CA 91604-2379
(818) 990-2354

Celiac Sprue Association of America, Inc.
www.csaceliacs.org
P.O. Box 31700
Omaha, NE 68131-0700
(877) CSA-4CSA

Children and Adults With Attention Deficit Hyperactivity Disorder (CHADD)
www.chadd.org
8181 Professional Place, Suite 150
Landover, MD 20785
(800) 233-4050

Dana's View
www.danasview.net

Developmental Delay Resources (DDR)
www.devdelay.org
5801 Beacon Street
Pittsburgh, PA 15217
(800) 497-0944
Complete information on resources, referrals, publications, books, practitioners, and newsletter.

Families for Early Autism Treatment (FEAT)
www.feat.org
P.O. Box 255722
Sacramento, CA 95865-5722
(916) 843-1536

Feingold Association
www.feingold.org
Diet information for ADHD through Autism

Generation Rescue
www.generationrescue.org
(Jenny McCarthy)

The GF/CF Diet
www.gfcfdiet.com
Complete information, diet guidelines, newsletter, recipes, product information, acceptable and unacceptable foods. Includes the GFCF Kids Forum (http://health.groups.yahoo.com/group/GFCFKids/)

Gluten Intolerance Group
www.gluten.net
31214 124th Ave SE
Auburn, WA 98092-3667
Phone: 253-833-6655
Fax: 253-833-6675

Gluten Intolerance Group of North America
www.gluten.net
15110 10ʰ Avenue SW Suite A
Seattle, WA 98166-1820
(206) 246-6652

Low Oxalate Diet
www.lowoxalate.info/
www.branwen.com/rowan/oxalate.htm

Mindd Foundation
www.mindd.org
PO Box 151 Vaucluse
NSW 2030 Australia

National Autism Association
www.nationalautismassociation.org
1330 W. Schatz Road
Nixa, MO 65714
(877) NAA-Autism

Nourishing Hope
www.nourishinghope.com
Julie Matthews

Pathfinders For Autism
www.pathfindersforautism.org
Help line: (866) 806-8400

Rotation Diets
www.drsallyrockwell.com
PO Box 31065
Seattle, WA 98103
1-888-343-8482

Safe Minds
www.safeminds.org
16033 Bolsa Chica St #104-142
Huntington Beach, CA 92649
404 934-0777

SCD Websites:
www.breakingtheviciouscycle.info
www.scdiet.com
www.pecanbread.com

Talk About Curing Autism (TACA)
www.talkaboutcuringautism.org
3070 Bristol Street, Suite 340
Costa Mesa, CA 92626
949-640-4401

Thoughtful House Center for Children
www.thoughtfulhouse.org
3001 Bee Caves Road
Austin, TX 78746
Telephone: 512-732-8400
Fax: 512-732-8353

Unlocking Autism
www.unlockingautism.org
P.O. Box 208
Tyrone, GA 30290
1-866-366-3361

Weston A. Price Foundation
www.westonaprice.org
4200 Wisconsin Ave., NW
Washington DC 20016
Phone: (202) 363-4394 | Fax: (202) 363-4396

PRODUCT SOURCES—GFCF AND HYPOALLERGENIC

There are numerous brands that are dedicated to those with food allergies and intolerances. Products include a wide variety of individual flours; substitutes for gluten, milk, casein, soy, egg, corn, and nuts; and ready-to-eat breads, bagels, crackers, cookies, cereals, doughnuts, and chocolate chips. Many sites have recipes and product-search sections. Some sites sell only to retailers and also provide a site search for local stores carrying their products. This is a partial listing only and is not intended as an endorsement. Please note that company information may change after publication.

AllergyGrocer.com
www.allergygrocer.com
91 Western Maryland Parkway
Unit #7
Hagerstown, MD 21740
(800) 891-0083

Applegate Farms
www.applegatefarms.com
750 Rt. 202 South, 3rd floor
Bridgewater, NJ 08807-5530
(866) 587-5858

Arrowhead Mills
www.arrowheadmills.com
The Hain Celestial Group
4600 Sleepytime Drive
Boulder, CO 80301
(800) 434-4246

Aunt Candice Foods
www.auntcandicefoods.com
P.O. Box 93
Oak Grove, MI 48863

Authentic Foods
www.authenticfoods.com
1850 W. 169th Street, Suite B
Gardena, CA 90247
(800) 806-4737

Autism Network for Dietary Intervention (ANDI)
ANDI Bars and links to other product source sites
www.autismndi.com

Best's Kosher
www.bests-kosher.com
3944 S. Morgan St.
Chicago, IL 60609
(773) 650-5900

Ener-G Foods
www.ener-g.com
5960 First Avenue South
P.O. Box 84487
Seattle, WA 98124-5787
(800) 331-5222
See the product search section.

Enjoy Life Foods, LLC
www.enjoylifefoods.com
3810 River Road
Schiller Park, IL 60176-2307
(888) 50-ENJOY

Food Allergy Kitchen
www.foodallergykitchen.com
Diane Hartman
7500 Country Village Drive
Cleves, OH 45002
See Diane's recipes and recipe book on CD.

Garden Spot Distributors
www.gardenspotdist.com
191 Commerce Drive
New Holland, PA 17557
(800) 829-5100

Gillian's Foods
www.gilliansfoods.com
Gillian's Foods
82 Sanderson Ave.
Lynn, Massachusetts 01902

Gluten/Casein Free Grocery Shopping Guide 2008/2009 Edition
www.ceceliasmarketplace.com
Kal-Haven Publishing
PO Box 20383
Kalamazoo, MI 49019

The Gluten-Free Mall
www.glutenfreemall.com
4927 Sonoma Highway, Suite C1
Santa Rosa, CA 95409
(Orders shipped from warehouse in Pennsylvania)
(800) 962-3026

Gluten Free Oats
www.glutenfreeoats.com
578 Lane 9 • Powell, WY 82435
(307) 754-2058 • Fax (516) 723-0924

Gluten Free Oat Products (Lara's) Cream Hill Estates
www.creamhillestates.com
9633 rue Clément
LaSalle, Québec
Canada H8R 4B4
514-363-2066
Toll Free: 1-866-727-3628

GlutenFree.Com
www.glutenfree.com
United-States
glutenfree.com
P.O. Box 840
Glastonbury, CT 06033
Canada (Head Office)
glutenfree.com
2055 Dagenais West
Laval, Qc, H7L 5V1

Glutino
www.glutino.com
2055, Boul. Dagenais Ouest
Laval, Qc, H7L 5V1, Canada
[tel] 1.800.363.3438
[fax] 1.450.629.4781

Kinnikinnick
www.kinnikinnick.com
10940-120 Street
Edmonton, Alberta, Canada T5H 3P7
(877) 503-4466
The best donuts and pancake mixes. Excellent premade bread.

Lundberg Family Farms
www.lundberg.com
5370 Church Street
Richvale, CA 95974
(530) 882-4551
Rice products.

NamasteFoods.com
P.O. Box 3133
Coeur d'Alene, ID 83816
(208) 772-63251
or (866) 258-94931
www.namastefoods.com

Nu World Amaranth
www.nuworldamaranth.com
P.O. Box 2202
Naperville, IL 60567
(630) 369-6819

Pamela's Products
www.pamelasproducts.com
200 Clara Avenue, Ukiah, CA 95482
Phone 707-462-6605

Pacific Natural Foods
www.pacificfoods.com[ED: Site under construction—verify before publication.]
19480 SW 97ᵗʰ Avenue
Tualatin, OR 97062
(503) 692-9666
Nonmilk beverages.

Sweet Sin Bakery
www.glutenfreedesserts.com
Baltimore, MD
Tel:410-366-5777
Fax: 410-366-5788
Cell: 301-305-1491

Twin Valley Mills, LLC
www.twinvalleymills.com
RR1, Box 45
Ruskin, NE 68974
(402) 279-3965
Sorghum flour.

Vance's Foods
www.vancesfoods.com
P.O. Box 627
Gilmer, TX 75644
(800) 497-4834
Dairy-free milk.

Wellshire Farms Inc.
www.wellshirefarms.com
509 Woodstown Road
Swedesboro, NJ 08085
(856) 769-5123

RESTAURANTS

It is not possible to list restaurants and bakeries providing GFCF and hypoallergenic fare. We are listing two of our favorites who so graciously provided us with recipes. There are numerous restaurants providing organic fare and special gluten-free menus. A Web search should be helpful. Also see the *Clan Thompson Celiac Pocket Guide to Restaurants* under Other Resources.

Gluten-Free Restaurant Awareness Program
Search service for GF Restaurants
www.glutenfreerestaurants.org

Grandma Whimsy's Cupboard (Bakery)
640 Highland Way
Hagerstown, MD 21740
(301) 465-9123

Great Sage Restaurant
www.great-sage.com
5809 Clarksville Square Drive
Clarksville, Maryland 21029
(443) 535-9400
An organic vegetarian restaurant offering GFCF options on its adult and children's menus.

Talk About Curing Autism TACA
www.talkaboutcuringautism.org
Select GFCF Diet—Restaurants & Bakeries

OTHER RESOURCES

Autism Education Services: Nadine Gilder
ngilder@worldnet.att.net
1218 Steeplechase Court
Toms River, NJ 08755
(732) 473-9482
Diet counseling.

Clan Thompson Celiac Guides and Software
www.clanthompson.com/index.php3#
■ Celiac Smart List Software (database of more than 5,000 foods)
■ Celiac Pocket Guides to: foods, over-the-counter drugs, prescription drugs, restaurants

Discovery Toys
www.discoverytoysinc.com
Toys, games, books.

Environmental Working Group EWG
www.ewg.org
(children's health, environment, water, food, products, pet health, alerts)
1436 U St. N.W., Suite 100
Washington, DC 20009
(202) 667-6982

Food-Medication Interactions
www.foodmedinteractions.com
The foremost handbooks and software on food/herb/medication reactions
■ Food-*Medication Interactions* (handbook) by Zaneta Pronsky
■ *Herb-Drug Interaction Handbook* by Sharon Herr
P.O. Box 204
Birchrunville, PA 19421-0204
(800) 746-2324

GF Meals
Frozen meals shipped nationwide
www.gfmeals.com
Ventura Blvd., #22
Woodland Hills, CA 91364
(888) 700-5610

Listing of Heath Care Providers with Expertise in ADHD & Autism
Autism Research Institute
Defeat Autism Now!
www.autismwebsite.com/practitioners/us_lc.htm

Organic Consumers Association
www.organicconsumers.org
Information on organics, genetic engineering, food safety, farm issues, safe toys.

Our Green House
www.ourgreenhouse.com
Natural organic eco-friendly products for children, pets, home. Includes toys.
365 South Main Street
Newtown, CT 06470
(203) 364-1484

Rotation Diets: Dr. Sally Rockwell
www.drsallyrockwell.com
Complete guide to rotation diets. Personalized diet plans including computer programs for rotation.
(206) 547-1814

Acknowledgments

PAMELA J. COMPART, MD

This book could not have been written without the input and support of so many people; in many ways, this was a community effort.

My deep gratitude and thanks go out to:

All my friends who nourished me, with both food and emotional support, through my medical training and residency and beyond, and who are likely stunned that my name is on a cookbook;

My incredible colleagues at HeartLight Healing Arts, my integrated/holistic medical practice, who inspire me daily with their clinical astuteness, the bigness of their hearts, and the brightness of their lights;

All the friends, colleagues, and patients who contributed recipes and testimonials; and all the teachers and healers who came before, whose shoulders I stand on.

Special thanks and abiding gratitude go to Jennifer Sima, RN, who labored above and beyond the call of duty, who collected, collated, and taste-tested innumerable recipes, and who provided me with unflagging faith and support during the writing of this book.

This book would not have been possible without the incredible knowledge and creativity of my colleague and coauthor, Dana Laake, whose brilliance and dedication to her work are unparalleled.

Thanks beyond measure and words go to my parents, who gave me unwavering support through all the various changes in my career till I landed at this place, which gives me such joy.

I thank my brothers, who, after they stopped laughing and realized I wasn't kidding about being asked to write a cookbook, supported me 110 percent.

Last, but certainly not least, I give thanks to my patients and their families, who inspire me daily to be better and do better. I get so much more from them than they do from me.

Pamela J. Compart, MD

DANA GODBOUT LAAKE, RDH, MS, LDN

With gratitude and humility, I honor the candle lighters—the mentors and colleagues who have generously endowed so many with their knowledge. It is a privilege to have known and learned from each one, and my commitment is to perpetuate the legacy. As a college freshman, I chose the path less traveled and began a journey that has given me far more sunny days than bumps and disappointments. Early on, I realized that I was in the childhood of the medicine of the future, and was being taught by exceptional visionaries who would long be remembered as the pioneers in the field. More than the journey itself, it is the traveling companions I joined along the way who made the trip extraordinary. With great pleasure, I honor and thank them.

Those who left their legacy and whose work continues past their deaths were the courageous pioneers and visionaries in science, medicine, research, nutrition, and education. They lit the way for so many of us, endured much opposition, and with noble humility, prevailed.

- Emanuel Cheraskin, MD, DMD, physician, dentist, researcher, and expert in the fields of nutritional medicine and dental health—who lit the first candle for me and whose friendship I enjoyed for three decades.

- Linus Pauling, Ph.D.; quantum chemist; expert in physics, quantum mechanics, molecular biology, and nutritional biochemistry; recipient of two Nobel Prizes, for Chemistry and Peace; author of over 1,000 articles and books; and whose scientific contributions were compared to those of Galileo, Newton, and Einstein. To learn from him was the highest privilege.

- Hans Selye, MD, Ph.D., DSC, researcher, educator, author; the first to recognize and describe the stress effect as a disease. He continued his teaching well into the seventh decade of life, and I count myself as fortunate to have been taught so well.

- Carl Pfeiffer, MD, Ph.D., author, educator, researcher, and expert in nutritional biochemistry and the relationship of nutrition to mental illness and behavioral disorders. Named in his honor, the Pfeiffer Treatment Center continues his pioneering work under the direction of William Walsh, Ph.D.

- Mildred Seelig, MD, MPH, MACN, world-renowned magnesium researcher; past president, executive director, and journal editor of the American College of Nutrition; and considered the "grandmother" of magnesium. She sparked my fascination with magnesium that continues today.

> "If you have knowledge, let others light their candles at it.
>
> —M. Fuller

- William (Billy) Crook, MD (AAAP Emeritus), pediatrician, author of numerous books on childhood food allergies and yeast-related illness. He never tired of teaching, even in the eighth and final decade of his life. While in Washington, DC, for advocacy trips, he made time for many of us to gather and draw insights from his deep well of knowledge.

- Bernard Rimland, Ph.D, research psychologist, author, founder of the Autism Research Institute and the Autism Society of America (ARI) and cofounder of Defeat Autism Now! He is credited with changing the prevailing view of autism, in the field of psychiatry, from and emotional illness—widely thought to be caused by "refrigerator mothers"—to the current recognition that autism is a neurodevelopment biological disorder. Because of Dr. Rimland's efforts, the ARI data bank, the world's largest, contains over 35,000 detailed case histories of autistic children and continues to grow—expanding our understanding and ability to treat.

I am thankful for the mentors, scientists, researchers, and educators who continue to devote their lives to the "new" medicine and biomedical interventions. In these pioneers the future has already arrived.

- Doris Rapp, MD, board-certified environmental medical specialist, pediatric allergist, and author of numerous books, including *Is This Your Child* and *Our Toxic World, A Wake Up Call*. She continues to educate, write, and advocate.

- Jon Pangborn, Ph.D., Ch.E, educator, author, innovator, and expert in nutritional biochemistry and laboratory testing. As cofounder of Defeat Autism Now!, he has advanced the field of biomedical interventions in autism. What he taught me about nutritional biochemistry became the foundation for all that followed.

- Sidney McDonald Baker, MD, board certified in pediatrics and obstetrics, educator, and expert in the environmental and biochemical aspects of chronic health problems. He is associate editor of *Integrative Medicine*, cofounder of Defeat Autism Now!, and author of many books, including the most current, *Detoxification and Healing*. His teaching and sincerity are equally inspiring.

- Leo Galland, MD, internationally respected expert in nutritional medicine, listed in *America's Top Doctors*, author, and director of the Foundation for Integrated Medicine. He is a role model for so many.

- Jeffrey Bland, Ph.D., researcher, author, educator, and internationally recognized expert in nutritional biochemistry. He served as senior research scientist at the Linus Pauling Institute, authored over 150 papers and five books, and produces an audiosubscription series called *Functional Medicine Update*. He lectures on subjects years before they become mainstream information—bringing the future to the present. He is the Socrates of nutrition, a mentor, and has had the most consistent impact on my practice for over twenty-seven years.

- George Mitchell, MD, who had the courage twenty-seven years ago to venture into the field of preventive medicine and nutrition. As colleagues and friends, we collaborated in patient care and providing educational courses. I am forever grateful for the opportunity to be his student and for his introducing me to most of the visionaries and pioneers I am honoring. His search for knowledge is endless.

There are special colleagues I am pleased to acknowledge and thank.

- Lisa Lewis, Ph.D. and Karyn Seroussi, innovators, authors, and cofounders of the Autism Network of Dietary Intervention, Inc (ANDI). In 1998, Lisa set the standard with the first GFCF book, *Special Diets for Special Kids*, followed in 2000 by Karyn's book, *Unraveling the Mystery of Autism and Pervasive Developmental Disorder: A Mother's Story of Research and Recovery*. Their recent book *The Encyclopedia of Dietary Interventions for the Treatment of Autism and Related Disorders* is another first.

- Kelly Dorfman, MS, LDN and Patricia S. Lemer, Med, NCC cofounders of Developmental Delay Resources, and tireless advocates for multidisciplinary approaches to autism spectrum disorders and all the children with special needs.

- Julie Matthews, nutritionist extraordinaire and author of *Nourishing Hope* and *Cooking To Heal* which are treatment roadmaps for healthy eating and special diets.

- Victoria Wood, RD, MS, LDN, licensed nutritionist. She remains a consistent valued resource and friend.

- Richard Layton, MD, pediatrician with expertise in allergy, preventive medicine, autism, and behavioral disorders. His excellence in patient care is remarkable.

- Irv Rosenberg, PD; Mickey Weinstein, PD; and Ron Keech, PD, who will always be for me "The Apothecary" and friends for life.

- Pamela J. Compart, MD, developmental pediatrician and coauthor. Her dedication to patients and tenacious thirst for knowledge are exceeded only by her personal and professional integrity. Possessing a natural curiosity, she has been willing to explore what is new and challenging, with the wisdom to question and confirm. I am grateful for her invitation to share the journey of this book. We are cohesive in our gratitude to our patients, from whom we learn the most, and in our shared vision for a book that can make a significant difference in the lives of those who need it most—the children.

Countless thoughtful friends, family, and patients have helped make this book possible by providing recipes, kitchen testing, and editing. Pam Compart and I stand in awe of the children, who have truly been our teachers, some of whom provided their own testimonials and recipes. Earlier, we acknowledge all those who have contributed, which is not nearly the significance each one deserves.

- My dear friend and assistant, Teresa Griswold, as part of the team on this book, diligently and thoughtfully typed and critiqued the recipes.

- Encouragment and help came from all the "girls": the Garrett Park Craft Club, Bunco B's and the STNY club.

- Always, I depend on Pam Foster, for fifty-two years of devotion and support in every thing I have ever attempted whether sensible or not.

All of us are the culmination of the hopes and dreams of every generation of our ancestors. What they pass on, what they teach—eventually becomes us. With respect and admiration, I am especially grateful for my parents, Bill and Dotty Beers, for believing their daughters could do anything, for the priceless gift of self-esteem, and for providing what every child deserves—a functional, loving childhood based in integrity and filled with humor.

- And to my younger, but wiser, sister, Susan Clark, for her love, honesty, true friendship, and outrageously funny stories.

- And to her son, Tim, who after years of refusing to eat "all the green stuff" in my refrigerator, eventually sold natural products and wheatgrass juice.

In our pacthwork quilt of a family, we say that we are not victims of divorce, we are the beneficiaries of the enrichments that life's changes can bring. So we embrace all and count as blessings the Godbouts, Laakes, Clarks, Reddings, Trainers, Browns, and Wilsons. Pete and I are fortunate to have in our lives eight children who have taught us well, enriched our lives, surrounded us with humor, and are the blessings that really count.

- Six of them, who did not grow under my heart, but grew in it:

Sons Steve and Pete Laake, Jr. who took the "step" out of "stepsons" and have given great joy and pride in who they are and how they live their lives. As adolescents, adjusting to the new family was easy, but the new foods were a challenge—overcome with wit and a willingness to try any new food at least once—and also carry extra money to buy something else at the local mall.

Christina and Michael Godbout—more than Rich and Greg's siblings—they have always been our children too.

Daughters-in-law—Colleen Godbout and Carron Laake—daughters within our hearts and for whom there always was a place in this family that only they could fill, and to sweet Marisa Goffe whose place awaits.

- And the two who grew *under* my heart and *in it*—Rich and Greg Godbout, who in fulfilling their own dreams, have made their parents proud—all of us. Inspiring and dedicated, their wit and infectious exuberance for life is a constant in our lives. Thanks for enduring a childhood filled with my culinary experiments in healthy cooking—buckwheat pancakes, green salad dressings, mystery sauces, and vitamin C in the saltshaker.

- To our grandchildren, whose "souls dwell in the house of tomorrow," Peter Winston Laake III, Ella Redding Godbout, and Kathryn Grace Laake (Kit) who really are "grand" children and absolute proof that life is meant to go on.

- And always, I am grateful for the "wind beneath my wings," who came into my life twenty-six years ago bearing the gifts of his two remarkable sons and who patiently provides guidance and wisdom infused with great love and wit—my husband, my love, my problem solver and best friend, who still takes my breath away, Pete Laake.

Dana Godbout Laake

About the Authors

PAMELA J. COMPART, MD

Pamela J. Compart, M.D. is a developmental pediatrician in Columbia, Maryland. She did her pediatric training at Children's National Medical Center in Washington, DC and fellowship training in Behavioral and Developmental Pediatrics at the University of Maryland School of Medicine. She combines traditional and complementary medicine approaches to the treatment of ADHD, autism, and other behavioral and developmental disorders. Dietary changes and use of nutritional supplements complement traditional treatments such as appropriate educational placement and speech therapy, occupational therapy, and other therapies. She is also the director of HeartLight Healing Arts, a multi-disciplinary integrated holistic health care practice, providing services for children, adults, and families.

DANA LAAKE, MS, LDN

Dana Godbout Laake is a licensed nutritionist in Kensington, Maryland. Within her practice, Dana Laake Nutrition, she provides preventive and therapeutic medical nutrition services. An honors graduate from Temple University (health sciences, dental hygiene), she received her master's degree in nutrition from the University of Maryland. She was recipient of the Temple University 50th Anniversary Outstanding Alumnus award. Dana was coauthor of the legislation that established licensure boards for dietetics and nutrition in both Maryland and Washington, DC. In addition to writing, media presentations, and accreditation as a provider of professional continuing education courses, Ms. Laake has been a Maryland legislative assistant on health issues and has served four gubernatorial appointments on two health care regulatory boards (dentistry and dietetics). She has hosted a live radio show, Health Talk 2000. Her practice includes nutritional evaluation and treatment of the full spectrum of health issues affecting adults and children with special needs. She resides in Kensington with her husband, Peter Laake, and they have four sons and three grandchildren.

Index